AMERICAN JOURNAL of PUBLIC HEALTH
NOVEMBER 2025
Issue 11

AJPH

A PUBLICATION OF THE
AMERICAN PUBLIC HEALTH ASSOCIATION

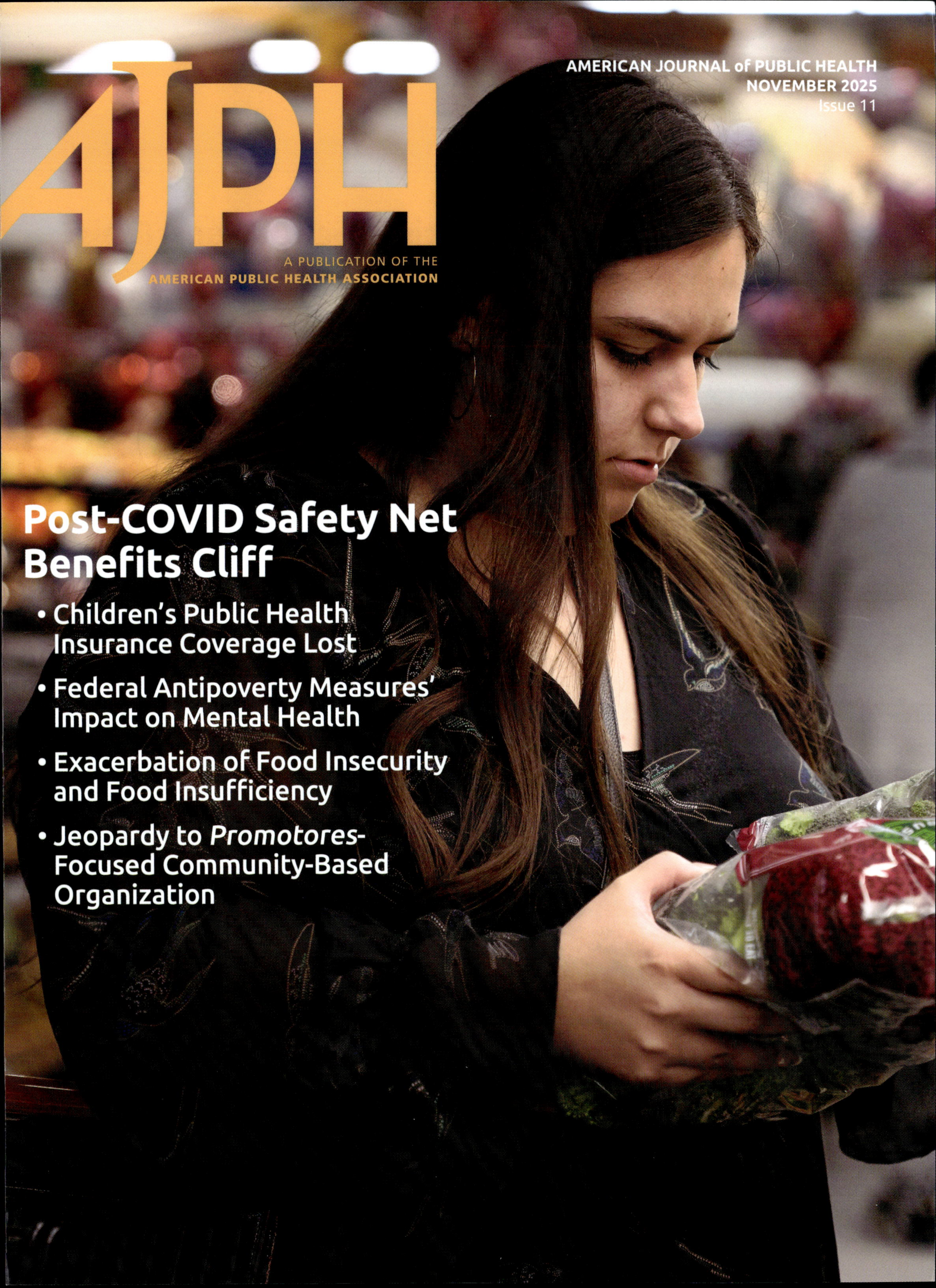

Post-COVID Safety Net Benefits Cliff

- Children's Public Health Insurance Coverage Lost
- Federal Antipoverty Measures' Impact on Mental Health
- Exacerbation of Food Insecurity and Food Insufficiency
- Jeopardy to *Promotores*-Focused Community-Based Organization

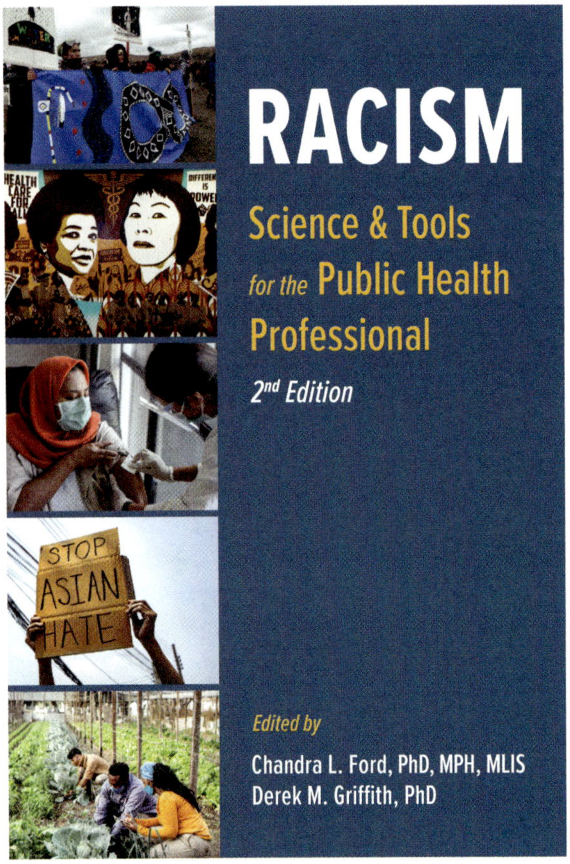

ISBN 978-0-87553-352-0, 600 PP.,
2025, SOFTCOVER

Racism: Science and Tools for the Public Health Professional, 2nd edition

Chandra L. Ford, PhD, MPH, MLIS, and Derek M. Griffith, PhD

Racism: Science and Tools for the Public Health Professional, 2nd edition enables public health professionals to address the health impacts of racism. This vital title also responds to the watershed events of the past five years: the COVID-19 pandemic and its intersection with overt forms of racism across all socioecological levels, the 2020 murder of George Floyd by Minneapolis police and the unprecedented domestic and global movements toward racial justice that transpired, and other major global events.

APHABOOKSTORE.ORG

APHA PRESS

AN IMPRINT OF AMERICAN PUBLIC HEALTH ASSOCIATION

APHA
AMERICAN PUBLIC HEALTH ASSOCIATION
For science. For action. For health.

AJPH®, published monthly, is the official Journal of the American Public Health Association®, 800 I St NW, Washington, DC 20001-3710; (202) 777- APHA; TDD (202) 777-2500. APHA is a nongovernmental professional society founded in 1872, representing all disciplines and specialties in public health.

The *American Journal of Public Health*® (*AJPH*) (print ISSN: 0090-0036; electronic ISSN: 1541- 0048), first published in 1911, is the official journal of the American Public Health Association® (APHA). The oldest and largest organization of public health professionals in the world, APHA represents approximately 30 000 members from more than 50 occupations of public health.

Submissions: Visit www.editorialmanager.com/ajph or ajph.edmgr.com for online manuscript preparation and submission guidelines. Contributions of original unpublished research, social science analyses, scholarly essays, critical commentaries, departments, and letters to the editor are welcome. Questions? Write ajph.submissions@apha.org or call APHA at (202) 777-2469.

Print plus online subscriptions: Institutional price (print copy with online access for a single institution and all authorized users, regardless of geographic location) varies by size of organization and ranges from $993–$1445 for US organizations, and $1073–$1526 for international organizations (air delivery); multiple campuses not permitted without special arrangement. Details of the tiered pricing system at https://subscriptionoffice.com/pages/apha-landing-page. To order, write apha.subscriptions@apha.org.

Online-only subscriptions: Institutional price for one institution and its authorized users (regardless of geographic location) is $878–$1307. To order, write apha.subscriptions@apha.org. For academic consortia or multisite corporate subscriptions, contact apha.subscriptions@apha.org.

Print-only subscriptions: Institutional price is US $701, $782 international.

Back print issues: A limited number of print issues are for sale. Single copies are US $65, $75 international (air delivery). Shipping included; prepay only. To order, write apha.subscriptions@apha.org.

Reprints: For prices and ordering information on 50 or more reprints, check the Reprints section at www.ajph.org. To order smaller quantities of reprints (rush delivery), use the "Purchase Article" link on the article site itself.

Electronic access: Online articles more than 10 years old are available free for personal use at www.ajph.org. Recent articles are available through pay-per-view: single PDF article for $24, single issue access for 24 hours for $33, or entire site access for 24 hours for $38.

Postal information: Periodicals postage paid at Washington, DC, and additional mailing offices. Postmaster: Send address changes to American Journal of Public Health, 800 I St NW, Washington, DC 20001-3710.

Address changes: Send to AJPH, Membership Department (members) or AJPH Subscriptions (subscribers), APHA, 800 I St NW, Washington, DC 20001-3710. Or write to membership.mail@apha.org (members) or apha.subscriptions@apha.org (subscribers).

Advertising: For pricing and other information, see www.ajph.org. Please write to brian.selzer@apha.org or call (202) 777-2470 for other advertising opportunities. Ask about special exhibit packages and sponsorships. Acceptance of advertising by the *Journal* does not imply endorsement of products.

Indexes: Publications that index or abstract articles from *AJPH* include the following: Ageline, Assia (Applied Social Science Index and Abstracts), Biological Abstracts, Chemical Abstracts, CINAHL, Criminal Justice Abstracts, EMBASE, EMCare, Environmental Abstracts, e-psyche, ERIC, ETOH (Alcohol and Alcohol Problems Science Database), Excerpta Medica, Food Science and Technology, General Science Index, Grateful Med, Hospital Literature Index, Human Resources Abstracts, International Pharmaceutical Abstracts (IPA), Medline, Physical Education Index, Pollution Abstracts, Psychological Abstracts, PsychINFO, Safety Science Abstracts, Sage Family Studies Abstracts, Sage Human Resources Abstracts, Science Citation Index, SCOPUS, SIIC Data Bases, Social Work Research and Abstracts, and Statistical Reference Index (SRI)/LexisNexis.

Medscape Publishers' Circle

AJPH

A PUBLICATION OF THE
AMERICAN PUBLIC HEALTH ASSOCIATION

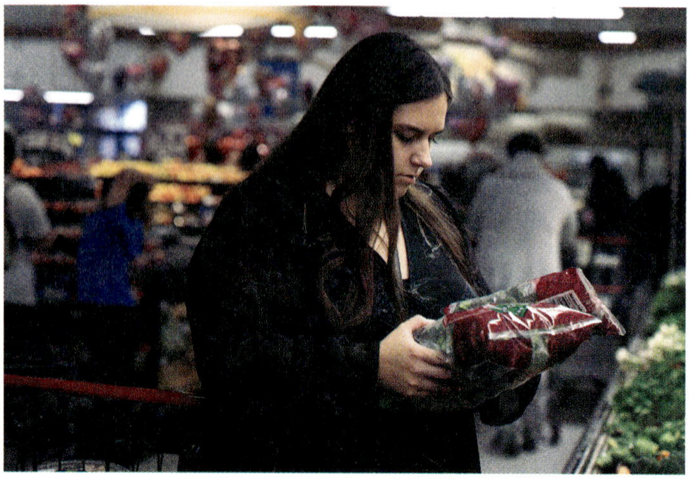

COVER: Jaqueline Benitez shops for groceries at a supermarket in Bellflower, California, on Monday, February 13, 2023. "It's such a lifesaver," said Benitez, who depends on California's SNAP benefits to help pay for food. "Food is such a huge expense. It's a little nerve-wracking to think about not having that."

Cover concept and selection by Aleisha Kropf. Photo by Allison Dinner/Associated Press. Printed with permission.

APHA
AMERICAN PUBLIC HEALTH ASSOCIATION
For science. For action. For health.

Promoting public health research, policy, practice, and education is the *AJPH* mission. As we widen our scope to embrace global issues, we also sharpen our focus to support the needs of public health practitioners. We invite contributions of original unpublished research, opinion and commentary, and letters to the editor.

The *Journal* is printed on acid-free recycled paper.

OPEN ACCESS ONLINE ONLY PODCAST DATA SUPPLEMENT AVAILABLE

EDITOR'S CHOICE

1765 Investments in the Social Safety Net Should Outlast Crises
D. H. Roby

OPINIONS, IDEAS, & PRACTICE

EDITORIALS

1767 Standing Up for Core Principles in Departments of Social and Behavioral Sciences in Public Health: Department Chairs Speak Out
S. B. Austin, J. E. Cohen, S. Cooper, K. M. Emmons, G. C. Gee, K. M. Green, M. Hawk, D. Hudson, T. Kershaw, D. Operario, K. M. Ribisl, C. E. Rodriguez-Diaz, J. M. Sacheck, B. Shaw, K. J. Sikkema, and M. W. Vander Weg

1773 The Supreme Court's 2024–2025 Term: Eroding Public Health, Health Equity, and Access to Justice
D. G. Aaron and W. E. Parmet

1779 A Call for Formal Reporting Standards for Legal Research in Public Health Studies
C. D. Schmit, S. Burris, S. Abdool Karim, B. A. Barsky, S. Grant, A. Schnake-Mahl, L. Tonti, M. D. Douglas, K. M. Nelson, A. J. Goodin, K. Underhill, M. J. P. Poirier, J. Y. Bae, E. Piekarz-Porter, R. Weber-Fares, S. Z. Ingber, and J. F. Chriqui

1783 Why Building Power Is Key to Protecting Academic Public Health and Advancing Health Equity
C. L. McMurtry, M. L. Givens, Z. D. Bailey, N. Graetz, P. J. Fleming, R. J. Petteway, J. Pacheco, S. E. Gollust, J. C. Heller, H. E. Lee, K. M. P. Porter, S. Johnson, J. D. Michener, A. M. W. LeBrón, A. K. Bailey, J. Bloyd, M. Creary, and I. J. Ornelas

1789 The Plight of Marginalized Populations in 2025: The Assault on Health Equity Through a Systems Lens
S. H. Woolf, M. H. Chin, V. M. Murry, and G. C. Gee

1795 Gender Affirmation Research Is Not Gender Ideology Extremism, It Is Science
A. J. Restar, K. E. Gamarel, and D. Operario

1800 Sense of Assurance, Safety, and Security (SASS) in Youths: A Public Health Perspective
L. D. Kubzansky, S. H. Davis, R. Rastogi, G. A. Woolverton, E. Zhang, and C. H. Liu

1805 Firearm Violence Prevention in Peril: A Call to Defend Our Public Safety Infrastructure
D. C. Semenza, T. S. Richmond, S. Rajan, M. E. Betz, C. Branas, S. A. L. Buggs, S. Hargarten, J. Richardson, F. P. Rivara, A. Rowhani-Rahbar, T. L. Sharpe, D. W. Webster, and J. M. Pizarro

1809 Protecting Health Equity Research Among Latinos Who Use Drugs Amid Heightened Immigration Enforcement
M. Pinedo and C. Escobar

1812 Political Decisions, Personal Consequences: Abortion Bans Threaten the Health of All Pregnant People
D. J. Horvath

NOTES FROM THE FIELD

1814 Managing Mental Health Crisis Calls Received by a US Poison Center: A Statewide Collaboration Between the Georgia Poison Center, 911, and 988
M. R. Dernbach, S. Hon, G. Lopez, N. J. Kaslow, J. E. Carpenter, K. Tanner, A. Rucker-Wright, D. Peel, A. Corley, R. D. Solis, T. P. Moran, B. W. Morgan, P. Filkins, G. Whitaker, E. Conaway, B. Cibulas, S. Arkin, D. Arnold, and R. J. Geller

COVID-19 BENEFITS CLIFF

1818 Falling Further Over the US Safety Net Benefits Cliff After COVID-19
V. M. Mays and M. S. Livings

1821 Pandemic-Era Increases in SNAP Benefits Reduced Food Insufficiency
M. Bitler and D. W. Schanzenbach

RESEARCH & ANALYSIS

COVID-19 BENEFITS CLIFF

1824 Pandemic-Related Funding Termination and Structural Drivers of Inequities: A Case Study of a *Promotores/as*-Focused Community-Based Organization
A. M. W. LeBrón, M. Michelen, P. J. Cantero, G. I. Montiel, L. Ruiz, K. Razaghi, L. Pantoja, J. Jimenez, M. Ramirez, A. Bracho, and J. Billimek

1836 Lived Experiences of Families Navigating Safety Net Expansions and Retractions During the Pandemic: A Qualitative Study
N. Fernández-Viña, L. C. H. Fernald, R. Hamad, K. E. Jackson, and W. Gosliner

1848 Children's Insurance Stability and Coverage Inequities During the COVID-19 Continuous Coverage Provisions
E. L. Eliason, A. Vasan, and D. B. Nelson

1858 Expansion of the Earned Income Tax Credit for Young Adults and Mental Health of US Home Renters, 2021–2023
A. K. Ali and W. Lyu

OPEN-THEMED RESEARCH

1868 Dialectical Processes of Health Framework as an Alternative to Social Determinants of Health Framework
S. R. Friedman, S. M. Walters, A. E. Jordan, D. C. Perlman, G. K. Nikolopoulos, P. Mateu-Gelabert, D. Rossi, and J. Eisenberg-Guyot

1877 How Anti-Immigrant Policies Impact Research Among Latinx and Undocumented People Who Use Drugs
Z. K. Coronado, S. L. Koenders, K. R. Knight, J. Lechuga, A. M. López, and C. Martinez

1887 Blood Transfusions for Pregnancy Loss in Texas Before and After Abortion Bans, 2017–2023
A. Nagle, G. Samari, L. Thaxton, and A. Gemmill

1895 Abortion Restrictions and Infant Mortality in the United States, 2018–2023
M. R. Anderson, G. Burtch, and B. N. Greenwood

1903 Social-Ecological Correlates of Involvement in Firearm-Related Violence in a Nationally Representative Survey of Adults
K. R. Mehari, J. N. Coleman, L. T. Stevens, A. D. Farrell, and P. N. Smith

1913 Silicosis Surveillance in California, 2019–2024: Tracking an Epidemic
J. Flattery, C. Woolsey, J. C. Fazio, S. A. Gandhi, A. Heinzerling, R. J. Harrison, and K. J. Cummings

1922 Multiple Social Demographics and Disparities in Smoking Cessation During Pregnancy in the United States, 2016–2022: An Intersectional Analytic Framework
Y. Cheng, C. C. W. Lim, R. M. Carrillo-Larco, and X. Xu

1933 Changes in E-Cigarette and Cigarette Sales in California and Neighboring States Following a Law Prohibiting Flavored Tobacco Product Sales
F. R. M. Ali, A. M. Leventhal, M. C. Diaz, E. W. Crane, and K. Marynak

1938 Differences in Breastfeeding Rates Among African Americans, Black Immigrants, and Hispanic Black Individuals Compared to Other Race/Ethnicity Groups for Infants Born Between 2011 and 2022, United States
A. A. Roess and R. C. Robert

BACKMATTER

OTHER DEPARTMENTS

1943 Statement of Ownership

1944 Subscription Form

Investments in the Social Safety Net Should Outlast Crises

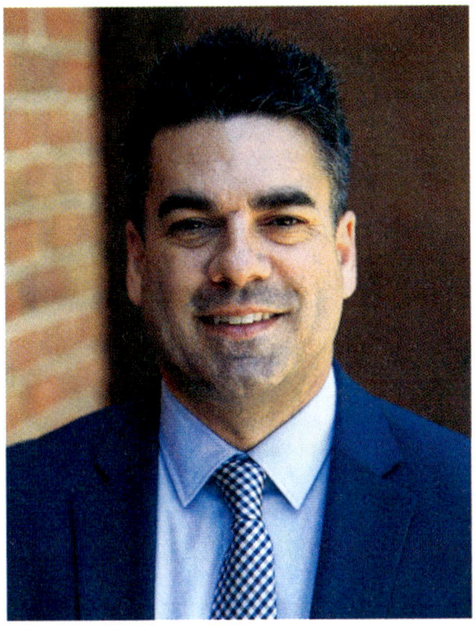

Dylan H. Roby, PhD
Department of Health, Society, and Behavior, UC Irvine Joe C. Wen School of Population & Public Health

The US public health and social safety net are underfunded, creating gaps in services for those in need. During economic crises, natural disasters, or public health emergencies, the federal, state, and county structures and agencies we rely on to support public health needs are often able to get additional resources through emergency declarations by leveraging new federal or state spending designed to address immediate crises. By supplementing Medicaid matching funds or allocating new temporary spending at the federal level, an influx of resources can often help local communities address the pandemic or flood they are facing. Our local safety net is often supported by a combination of federal grant funds (e.g., grants to community clinics or local public health agencies) and federal–state partnerships like Medicaid and the Children's Health Insurance Program that incentivize states and local programs to ramp up or expand programs using federal matching funds.

Now, our federalist model to address crises through local and state agencies is being eroded. New legislation (like HR1, the "Big, Beautiful Bill") explicitly changes Medicaid and Supplemental Nutrition Assistance Program (SNAP) policy to reduce federal support and place a larger burden on states, while attitudes around the role of government in the Trump administration promise to dissolve the processes and structures we rely on to address state and local crises through prompt action administratively and legislatively. Cancelling federal grants to fund public health services and shrinking federal support for programs administered by the states is dangerous. If the Federal Emergency Management Agency, Centers for Disease Control and Prevention, and Centers for Medicare and Medicaid Services are unable to provide short-term funds or grant waivers or be nimble in the face of catastrophe, we will be flat-footed and ineffective when responding to new challenges.

HR1 places barriers on Medicaid and SNAP that will exacerbate disparities and leave us unable to respond to future pandemics, economic downturns, or other crises. Placing work requirements on Medicaid, reducing federal matching funds flowing into state Medicaid programs, and placing higher burdens on states to fund the shortfalls in Medicaid, SNAP, and other programs will make it that much harder to respond. We should anticipate more people falling through the cracks, with higher rates of uninsurance, poverty, and avoidable death. States with means might be able to fill some gaps, while creating others, because of their own budget situation. However, the impact will be worse in lower-income states with a higher reliance on federal support.

While the "obvious" response for many states is to cut programs, states that want to protect their residents and ensure stability will need to invest more state and local funds into protective and responsive systems for public health and social services. For example, California has a millionaire tax to fund county mental health services, and other states use taxes on specific goods to fund social services and education. States will need to establish larger rainy-day funds and budget surpluses to offset federal losses and address uncertainty.

In this issue's special section, four research teams found that health and social policy changes driven by the urgency of a pandemic served to stabilize family incomes, insurance coverage, food availability, and nonprofit support organizations. These learnings should be emphasized in future policy decisions and deserve to be supported as long-term interventions and tools to

AJPH November 2025, Vol. 115, No. 11

improve economic and health conditions broadly, rather than only in the face of crisis. The articles explored existing policy mechanisms to improve the flow of resources to populations in need, which is far more efficient than creating new programs. All these programs are now gone because of the "unwinding" of the public health emergency; they represented a missed opportunity to address entrenched problems of poverty, uninsurance, and food insecurity. AJPH

DOI: https://doi.org/10.2105/AJPH.2025.308271

ORCID iD:
Dylan H. Roby https://orcid.org/0000-0001-5005-9287

Standing Up for Core Principles in Departments of Social and Behavioral Sciences in Public Health: Department Chairs Speak Out

S. Bryn Austin, ScD, Joanna E. Cohen, PhD, MHSc, Spring Cooper, PhD, Karen M. Emmons, PhD, Gilbert C. Gee, PhD, Kerry M. Green, PhD, Mary Hawk, DrPH, LSW, Darrell Hudson, PhD, MPH, Trace Kershaw, PhD, Don Operario, PhD, Kurt M. Ribisl, PhD, Carlos E. Rodriguez-Diaz, PhD, MPH, Jennifer M. Sacheck, PhD, Benjamin Shaw, PhD, MPH, Kathleen J. Sikkema, PhD, and Mark W. Vander Weg, PhD

ABOUT THE AUTHORS

S. Bryn Austin and Karen M. Emmons are with the Department of Social and Behavioral Sciences, Harvard T. H. Chan School of Public Health, Boston, MA. Joanna E. Cohen is with the Department of Health, Behavior and Society, Johns Hopkins Bloomberg School of Public Health, Baltimore, MD. Spring Cooper is with the Department of Community Health and Social Sciences, CUNY School of Public Health and Health Policy, New York, NY. Gilbert C. Gee is with the Department of Community Health Sciences, UCLA Fielding School of Public Health, Los Angeles, CA. Kerry M. Green is with the Department of Behavioral and Community Health, University of Maryland School of Public Health, College Park, MD. Mary Hawk is with the Department of Behavioral and Community Health Sciences, University of Pittsburgh School of Public Health, Pittsburgh, PA. Darrell Hudson is with the Department of Health Behavior and Health Equity, University of Michigan School of Public Health, Ann Arbor. Trace Kershaw is with the Department of Social and Behavioral Sciences, Yale School of Public Health, New Haven, CT. Don Operario is with the Department of Behavioral, Social, and Health Education Sciences, Emory University Rollins School of Public Health, Atlanta, GA. Kurt Ribisl is with the Department of Health Behavior, University of North Carolina Gillings School of Global Public Health, Chapel Hill. Carlos E. Rodriguez-Diaz is with the Department of Community Health Sciences, Boston University School of Public Health, Boston, MA. Jennifer M. Sacheck is with the Department of Behavioral and Social Sciences, Brown University School of Public Health, Providence, RI. Benjamin Shaw is with the Division of Community Health Sciences, University of Illinois Chicago School of Public Health, Chicago. Kathleen J. Sikkema is with the Department of Sociomedical Sciences, Columbia University Mailman School of Public Health, New York, NY. Mark W. Vander Weg is with the Department of Community and Behavioral Health, University of Iowa College of Public Health, Iowa City.

We are living in a pivotal moment that is reshaping the foundation of public health. Departments of social and behavioral sciences face unprecedented challenges because of recent US federal actions threatening both our discipline and the broader field. Although the entire public health enterprise faces these pressures, our programs are especially vulnerable for their conceptual and methodological approaches to address health equity—defined by the Centers for Disease Control and Prevention (CDC) as "the state in which everyone has a fair and just opportunity to attain their highest level of health."[1] This work centers marginalized populations, employs multilevel critical frameworks to analyze health disparities, and partners with communities directly affected by social inequities. This work also requires challenging and transforming unjust systems—principles increasingly at odds with current federal priorities.

As department chairs, we witness how recent federal actions undermine our principles and disrupt our mission to advance research, education, and service promoting the health of all populations—especially those with greatest needs. We also see the toll on faculty, staff, students, alumni, communities, and government partners on the front lines of public health. In this moment, we must advocate for our field, its people, and the communities we serve, and develop strategies to sustain our contributions to science, teaching, and public service.

A DEFINING TIME IN OUR FIELD

Since January 2025, federal actions affecting the Department of Health and Human Services—including agencies such as the National Institutes of Health (NIH), the Food and Drug Administration, the CDC, the Centers for Medicare & Medicaid Services, the Health Resources and Services Administration, the Substance Abuse and Mental Health Services Administration, the Agency for Healthcare Research and Quality, and others—have reshaped

AJPH November 2025, Vol. 115, No. 11

the priorities of the nation's primary public health and research institutions.[2] These agencies have historically partnered with universities to advance science and foster collaborations that improve health. Yet, in the wake of abrupt political reorganizations, thousands of grants and contracts awarded to health researchers have been terminated.[3,4]

According to Grant Witness—an independent project to "track the termination of grants of scientific research agencies under the Trump administration in 2025"—an estimated 5053 NIH grants were terminated as of August 15, 2025.[5] A separate analysis using public data sources estimated losses exceeding $2 billion in funding for mental health and substance use grants alone as of April 11, 2025.[6] Although some awards (1239) have been reinstated, these figures remain fluid as additional federal actions may prompt future waves of grant terminations.

Terminations have targeted topics such as HIV, sexual and gender minority health, COVID-19, vaccine hesitancy, immigrant and refugee health, climate change, and global health. These topics disproportionately affect historically marginalized populations and have long been priorities for social and behavioral science research.[7–9] Projects using terminology such as "cultural competency," "discrimination," "gender," "inclusion," "racism," "intersectionality," "LGBT," and "social justice" are also under scrutiny.[10–12] Investigators in our departments affected by terminations have been told their research "no longer effectuates agency priorities" and is considered "antithetical to the scientific inquiry" and delivers "low returns on investment."[13]

What is notable about these topical areas now under attack is that they are grounded in science—a process driven by inquiry, skepticism, and evidence. Our field proceeds from the premise that ideas must be rigorously investigated, a central principle of the scientific method guiding the peer review process. Community voices add accountability by shaping research priorities to meet population health needs. Replacing scientific judgment with political preference erodes research integrity and risks public health decisions being driven by ideology rather than evidence.

Termination letters are often issued without notice, overriding peer review and forcing immediate work stoppages. These abrupt actions jeopardize research participants, disrupt community partnerships, and cause widespread job losses—from senior professionals to recent graduates. The result is not only displacement of skilled workers but also the loss of invaluable historical knowledge and community trust. Those who drive these executive decisions seem to have forgotten the lesson clearly demonstrated during the COVID-19 pandemic—the importance of maintaining a robust public health workforce.

Simultaneously, universities are under mounting political attack.[14] Curricular content once safeguarded under the banner of academic freedom is now scrutinized for perceived misalignment with prevailing political ideologies.[15] Programs in social and behavioral sciences are at heightened risk, given our focus on topics including structural racism, sexual and gender minority health, sexual and reproductive justice, legacies of discriminatory social systems, and intersectional stigmas. Campus advocacy is also surveilled, and international students may face severe consequences without due process.[16]

Scholars and institutions face pressures to capitulate to external forces.[17] Freezes in federal funding threaten the basic operations of higher education and scientific research. Grant applications are being funded at a slower rate, while proposed reductions in indirect cost rates jeopardize the infrastructure sustaining research nationwide. Faculty and staff who rely on grant funding bear the heaviest burdens. Senior leaders, meanwhile, are under pressure to comply with federal directives to protect their institutions from further harm. In response to financial uncertainty, many institutions have imposed hiring freezes, raising the risk that scientific and service contributions will stagnate or regress. Pathways for the new generation of scholars—especially grant-funded students and postdoctoral fellows—are being eroded, threatening to diminish the scope and impact of future work in our field.

Beyond the broad risks to academic institutions and scientific research, current policy decisions pose tangible threats to the practice of public health. These harms will manifest indirectly, through the erosion of evidence-based practices in key areas such as maternal health, infectious diseases, food and motor vehicle safety, and treatment of cancer and other chronic diseases, among others,[18] and directly, through the elimination of critical programs. Initiatives to prevent drowning, enhance workplace safety, reduce infant mortality, and support tobacco cessation have already been cut. At the time of writing, a $56 million program that partners with emergency providers to reduce drug overdose and improve substance use outcomes is slated for elimination.[19] Similarly, the Ryan White HIV/AIDS program, a cornerstone of care for people with HIV, faces hundreds of millions of dollars in funding reductions.[20] These and other impending cuts will result in avoidable loss of life, raising serious questions about how such outcomes align with the administration's stated goal to "Make America Healthy Again."

The situation is unsustainable and unacceptable. We must speak out.

REAFFIRMING CORE PRINCIPLES

As department chairs in the social and behavioral sciences, we reaffirm our commitment to core principles that have long guided our work but are now under active threat. Although our departments differ in meaningful ways (e.g., local and regional priorities, institutional resources, topical strengths, etc.), we stand united in upholding these shared principles. We are confident that many colleagues who are not listed as coauthors share this commitment. These principles are essential not only to the work of our faculty, staff, students, and community partners, but also to safeguarding the integrity of our mission to advance health and equity for all.

Health Equity as a Collective Goal

To improve health for all, we hold health equity as our highest collective goal. Achieving this requires confronting the historical roots of inequities that shape contemporary outcomes.[21] This demands rigorous research that explicitly names and characterizes patterns of health inequity, paired with the moral clarity to declare these patterns unjust and changeable, and the courage to take action toward social change. Pursuing health equity also means centering voices historically marginalized or ignored. Social and behavioral research on health equity is essential for guiding social transformation grounded in inclusion, justice, and evidence.

Community Engagement and Authentic Partnership

To improve health for all, our work must be conducted with and for community partners. Central to this commitment is recognizing community partners as experts in their own right who deserve equal roles in shaping research and action, and acknowledging the limits of siloed perspectives.[22] Authentic partnership requires professional humility, power sharing, and recognition of the potential harms inflicted under the guise of academic or government efficiency, coupled with a responsibility to repairing injustices. Participatory praxis—the process of applying theory and knowledge in real-world contexts—must be recognized as a foundational component of social and behavioral sciences, with community organizing as a core pillar.[23,24] Meaningful engagement demands sustained efforts to foster community trust. This commitment also entails supporting scholars, practitioners, and community members engaged in advancing health for all.

Critical Theories and Methodological Pluralism

To improve health for all, our work must critically examine the multilevel determinants of health, address the structural roots of health inequities, and direct interventions toward those at highest risk. This requires applying theories and conceptual frameworks that interrogate the roles of social structures, commercial forces, power dynamics, systemic racism, gender- and sex-based hierarchies, class inequality, and cultural contexts in shaping downstream health behaviors.[25] Pedagogically, this approach encourages scholars to explore the historical context of contemporary inequities—such as racism, sexism, homophobia, xenophobia, and others—that have marginalized populations and suppressed dissent.[26] Methodologically, social and behavioral research in public health must embrace diverse research approaches—including qualitative, quantitative, mixed-methods, randomized and quasi-randomized trials, and community participatory designs—recognizing that no single epistemological lens can fully capture the complexities of health.[27] To this end, we must reject reductive, overly simplistic models of health and instead advocate for nuanced, multilayered approaches that reflect the complexity necessary to promote equitable population health.

Communication and Knowledge Translation

To improve health for all, our field must invest in the communities that contribute to the creation and production of research. This requires upholding ethical approaches that position research evidence as a tool for social change, particularly in the face of political and social climates that may undermine these efforts. Our departments have a responsibility to ensure that research findings are returned to the communities from which they originated and that community members who contributed to the work receive appropriate recognition and credit. This demands sustained partnerships and institutional support for knowledge translation.[28] Communication between researchers and community members must extend beyond the publication of findings; historic shortcomings to maintaining engagement have contributed to deep-seated distrust and skepticism toward the research enterprise. Ongoing commitments to knowledge dissemination are needed to combat the misinformation and disinformation that threaten public health.

Diverse and Inclusive Department Cultures

To improve health for all, we must embrace diversity in perspectives, positionalities, and approaches—all of which are essential to advancing public health. True diversity, however, does not occur passively; it requires deliberate and sustained action. Our departments must build pathways to ensure access to our programs for scholars of all backgrounds, free from discrimination. We are equally committed to fostering inclusive department cultures where every member feels valued, safe, and respected, thereby creating environments that nurture and support diverse perspectives.

Commitment to Academic Freedom

To improve health for all, our departments must ensure that researchers, students, and practitioners are supported in exploring novel ideas, challenging prevailing assumptions, and pursuing lines of inquiry without fear of censorship or reprisal. Academic freedom is especially essential when posing difficult questions about the fundamental determinants of health and critically evaluating policies and power structures. In the current climate, some researchers have been asked to pivot their work to avoid scrutiny and preserve funding. We express caution that such shifts risk compromising the scientific momentum needed to advance evidence-based health improvements for populations at greatest need.

A CALL TO ACTION

In this defining moment, our principles must be translated into actions that sustain the integrity and impact of the social and behavioral sciences in public health. As department chairs, we have a responsibility to lead by example, fostering environments where the aforementioned principles are upheld and evidence-based inquiry can thrive. Working collaboratively with faculty, students, staff, and institutional leaders, we are positioned to facilitate inclusive dialogue and guide strategies appropriate to our unique settings. The recommendations offered here are neither exhaustive nor prescriptive. Rather, they serve as prompts for dialogue and consideration that might translate into appropriate local actions, informed by the specific impacts of current policies on each institution.

Protect Academic Freedom and Scientific Integrity

Protecting academic freedom and scientific integrity is foundational to the credibility of public health scholarship. Some recommended actions include the following:

- Support policies and practices that protect researchers from undue external influence, particularly in areas of health equity and structural determinants.
- Develop internal guidelines that ensure scholars can pursue research questions and methodologies without political interference.
- Establish departmental processes for responding to concerns about censorship or harassment.

Support Colleagues Facing Threat and Disruption

Protecting our colleagues—especially early-career scholars—requires proactive measures to sustain mentorship, funding, and career advancement in the face of political and financial disruption. Some recommended actions include the following:

- Build departmental structures for enhanced mentorship to early-career scholars.
- Explore opportunities for pilot and bridge funding mechanisms for colleagues affected by funding or policy changes, including mechanisms to support grant-funded students and trainees.
- Develop contingency plans to maintain key research, teaching, and service activities during financial disruptions.
- Advocate for institutional promotion and tenure processes to acknowledge shifts in the funding environment and recognize a broad range of scholarly contributions.

Sustain and Strengthen Community Partnerships

Our departments must adopt clear and intentional strategies to maintain community trust, especially in times of social-political disruption and funding shortfalls. Some recommended actions include the following:

- Continue engagement with community partners during funding gaps.
- Include community representatives in decision-making related to research priorities and program design.
- Recognize and support community-led initiatives that align with departmental expertise and goals.

Support Resilience

Building resilience within academic public health departments is critical to sustaining our people and our mission during periods of uncertainty and threat. Essential strategies include the following:

- Integrate equity-focused and trauma-informed approaches into faculty development and student advising—such as holding dedicated time at faculty meetings and department town halls where members can reflect openly and safely about current events, creating opportunities for colleagues to work together to address shared challenges, and ensuring availability of counseling, wellness, and other supports.[29]
- Foster departmental environments where all members feel respected and able to contribute fully.
- Celebrate colleagues' actions and accomplishments that reinforce professional principles.

Promote Advocacy and Effective Communication

To advance our field's mission and amplify its impact, we must support and equip faculty and students to engage in effective public communication and policy influence. Strategies may include the following:

- Encourage and support faculty and students in communicating research findings to diverse audiences.
- Facilitate participation in professional networks and policy discussions to share evidence-based perspectives.
- Work with other academic and community leaders as well as policymakers in the administrative and legislative branches of government on coordinated policy statements and protocols to promote ethical public health research, education, and practice.

CONCLUSION

We recognize that the concerns, principles, and actions articulated in this essay are not unique to departments of social and behavioral sciences in public health. Peer academic departments throughout public health—including epidemiology, health services, biostatistics, environmental sciences, global health, and others—are also being affected. We also acknowledge that all peer departments have their own capacities, resources, and levels of vulnerability to the impacts of federal actions and reorganizations. Across the country, university responses to recent political actions have varied, reflecting distinct institutional experiences and risk-management approaches. Despite these differences, we encourage academic departments with shared concerns to engage in a process of reflection and praxis aimed at preserving their integrity and our collective mission.

This is not a moment for caution—it is a moment for strategic action. Our ability to advance health equity, train the next generation of public health leaders, and respond to the health challenges of our time depends on our willingness to act collectively. We urge our colleagues and allies to join forces in safeguarding the people, principles, and partnerships that define the social and behavioral sciences in public health. The stakes for our science, our communities, and the public's health could not be higher. AJPH

CORRESPONDENCE

Correspondence should be sent to Don Operario, Department of Behavioral, Social, and Health Education Sciences, Emory University Rollins School of Public Health, 1518 Clifton Road NE, Atlanta, GA 30322 (e-mail: don.operario@emory.edu). Reprints can be ordered at https://www.ajph.org by clicking the "Reprints" link.

PUBLICATION INFORMATION

Full Citation: Austin SB, Cohen JE, Cooper S, et al. Standing up for core principles in departments of social and behavioral sciences in public health: department chairs speak out. *Am J Public Health*. 2025;115(11):1767–1772.

Acceptance Date: August 21, 2025.

DOI: https://doi.org/10.2105/AJPH.2025.308283

ORCID iDs:
Spring Cooper https://orcid.org/0000-0002-9925-9033

Karen M. Emmons https://orcid.org/0000-0002-0685-6446

Kerry M. Green https://orcid.org/0000-0002-7146-5783

Mary Hawk https://orcid.org/0000-0001-9753-4356

Don Operario https://orcid.org/0000-0003-2467-5048

Kurt M. Ribisl https://orcid.org/0000-0003-3318-8524

Carlos E. Rodriguez-Diaz https://orcid.org/0000-0001-6333-0654

Benjamin Shaw https://orcid.org/0000-0002-4756-495X

Kathleen J. Sikkema https://orcid.org/0000-0003-0371-5119

Mark W. Vander Weg https://orcid.org/0000-0003-3631-0812

CONTRIBUTORS

All authors contributed to the conceptualization and writing of this work.

ACKNOWLEDGMENTS

We are grateful to colleagues in peer departments of social and behavioral sciences and across public health disciplines who stand up for integrity and academic freedom, especially our colleagues whose institutional affiliations prevent them from being directly affiliated with the perspectives expressed here.

Note. The views and opinions expressed in this article are those of the authors and do not necessarily reflect the views of their institutions or their affiliates.

CONFLICTS OF INTEREST

The authors have no conflicts of interest to disclose.

REFERENCES

1. Centers for Disease Control and Prevention. About health equity. February 5, 2024. Available at: https://www.cdc.gov/health-disparities-hiv-std-tb-hepatitis/about/index.html. Accessed August 20, 2025.
2. US Dept of Health and Human Services. Fact sheet: HHS' transformation to make America healthy again. April 2, 2025. Available at: https://www.hhs.gov/press-room/hhs-restructuring-doge-fact-sheet.html. Accessed August 20, 2025.
3. US Dept of Health and Human Services. HHS grants terminated: FY 2020–FY 2024. Tracking accountability in government grants system. Available at: https://taggs.hhs.gov/Content/Data/HHS_Grants_Terminated.pdf. Accessed April 28, 2025.
4. Hatcher AM, Metheny N, Dunkle KL, Fielding-Miller R. A refusal to abandon HIV science. *AIDS.* 2025;39(6):768–770. https://doi.org/10.1097/QAD.0000000000004188
5. Grant Witness Website. Available at: https://grant-witness.us. Accessed August 20, 2025.
6. Beccia AL, Liu L, Delaney S, Zubizarreta D, Ross N, Austin SB. Mapping the costs of mental health- and substance use-related grant cancellations. *medRxiv.* August 2, 2025. https://doi.org/10.1101/2025.08.01.25332818
7. Dhai A. The National Institutes of Health funding withdrawal: decades of progress dismantled in a few weeks. *S Afr Med J.* 2025;115(3):3–4.
8. Kozlov M, Mallapaty S. Exclusive: NIH to terminate hundreds of active research grants. *Nature.* 2025;639(8054):281–282. https://doi.org/10.1038/d41586-025-00703-1
9. Kozlov M, Ryan C. How Trump 2.0 is slashing NIH-backed research—in charts. *Nature.* April 10, 2025. Available at: https://www.nature.com/articles/d41586-025-01099-8. Accessed August 20, 2025.
10. Inside Higher Ed. Federal grant cuts in researchers' own words. April 7, 2025. Available at: https://www.insidehighered.com/opinion/views/2025/04/07/federal-grant-cuts-researchers-own-words-opinion. Accessed April 28, 2025.
11. American Psychological Association. Statement on the cancellation of grants by the National Science Foundation. APA Services Updates. April 24, 2025. Available at: https://updates.apaservices.org/statement-on-the-cancellation-of-grants-by-the-national-science-foundation. Accessed April 28, 2025.
12. US Senate Committee on Commerce, Science, and Transportation. Cruz-led investigation uncovers $2 billion in woke DEI grants at NSF, releases full database. February 11, 2025. Available at: https://www.commerce.senate.gov/2025/2/cruz-led-investigation-uncovers-2-billion-in-woke-dei-grants-at-nsf-releases-full-database. Accessed April 28, 2025.
13. Wu KJ. The NIH's grant terminations are "utter and complete chaos." *The Atlantic.* March 14, 2025. Available at: https://www.theatlantic.com/health/archive/2025/03/nih-grant-terminations/682039. Accessed April 28, 2025.
14. Dirks NB. Academia needs to stick up for itself. *The Atlantic.* March 12, 2025. Available at: https://www.theatlantic.com/ideas/archive/2025/03/trump-columbia-universities/682012. Accessed April 28, 2025.
15. Knott K, Moody J. What to know about Trump's funding threats to colleges. Inside Higher Ed. April 18, 2025. Available at: https://www.insidehighered.com/news/government/politics-elections/2025/04/18/what-know-about-trumps-funding-threats-colleges. Accessed April 28, 2025.
16. Danner C. Why is Trump targeting so many international students? *New York Magazine.* April 19, 2025. Available at: https://nymag.com/intelligencer/article/trump-targeting-international-student-visa-sevis-termination-universities.html. Accessed April 28, 2025.
17. Sentner I, Quilantan B. Universities are caving to Trump with a stunning speed and scope. *Politico.* March 20, 2025. Available at: https://www.politico.com/news/2025/03/20/universities-cave-conservatives-trump-00241765. Accessed April 28, 2025.
18. Centers for Disease Control and Prevention. Ten great public health achievements—United States, 1900–1999. *MMWR Morb Mortal Wkly Rep.* 1999;48(12):241–243.
19. Ameresekere R. Proposed budget cuts to Narcan programs dangerously misunderstand public health aims. *Health Affairs.* July 11, 2025, Available at: https://www.healthaffairs.org/content/forefront/proposed-budget-cuts-narcan-programs-dangerously-misunderstand-public-health-aims. Accessed August 20, 2025.
20. Kates J. Scaling back the nation's HIV response? What the Trump Administration's HHS budget may do. KFF. April 17, 2025. Available at: https://www.kff.org/quick-take/scaling-back-the-nations-hiv-response-what-the-trump-administrations-hhs-budget-may-do. Accessed May 4, 2025.
21. Marmot M, Commission on Social Determinants of Health. Achieving health equity: from root causes to fair outcomes. *Lancet.* 2007;370(9593):1153–1163. https://doi.org/10.1016/S0140-6736(07)61385-3
22. Wallerstein N, Minkler M, Carter-Edwards L, Avila M, Sanchez V. Improving health through community engagement, community organization, and community building. In: Glanz K, Rimer BK, Viswanath K, eds. *Health Behavior: Theory, Research, and Practice.* 5th ed. San Francisco, CA: Jossey-Bass; 2015:277–300.
23. Ford CL, Airhihenbuwa CO. The public health critical race methodology: praxis for antiracism research. *Soc Sci Med.* 2010;71(8):1390–1398. https://doi.org/10.1016/j.socscimed.2010.07.030
24. Minkler M. Linking science and policy through community-based participatory research to study and address health disparities. *Am J Public Health.* 2010;100(suppl 1):S81–S87. https://doi.org/10.2105/AJPH.2009.165720
25. Krieger N. Epidemiology and the web of causation: has anyone seen the spider? *Soc Sci Med.* 1994;39(7):887–903. https://doi.org/10.1016/0277-9536(94)90202-x
26. Fleming PJ. The importance of teaching history of inequities in public health programs. *Pedagogy Health Promot.* 2020;6(4):253–256. https://doi.org/10.1177/2373379920915228
27. Livingood WC, Allegrante JP, Airhihenbuwa CO, et al. Applied social and behavioral science to address complex health problems. *Am J Prev Med.* 2011;41(5):525–531. https://doi.org/10.1016/j.amepre.2011.07.021
28. Kwan BM, Brownson RC, Glasgow RE, Morrato EH, Luke DA. Designing for dissemination and sustainability to promote equitable impacts on health. *Annu Rev Public Health.* 2022;43(1):331–353. https://doi.org/10.1146/annurev-publhealth-052220-112457
29. Tsui EK, Cooper S, Elsayed A, Billings S, Stewart S, Andrews D. When it "feels like we're in this together": toward a trauma-informed public health pedagogy drawing on lived experiences. *Pedagogy Health Promot.* 2023;9(4):275–287. https://doi.org/10.1177/23733799231177045

The Supreme Court's 2024–2025 Term: Eroding Public Health, Health Equity, and Access to Justice

Daniel G. Aaron, MD, JD, and Wendy E. Parmet, JD

ABOUT THE AUTHORS

Daniel G. Aaron is an associate professor of law at the S. J. Quinney College of Law, Salt Lake City, UT. Wendy E. Parmet is the Matthews Distinguished University Professor of Law and faculty codirector, Center for Health Policy and Law, Northeastern University School of Law, Boston, MA.

Decisions by the US Supreme Court can have a powerful impact on public health,[1] as evidenced by the rise of maternal mortality that followed the court's 2022 decision in *Dobbs v Jackson Women's Health Org.* (597 US 215), overturning the constitutional right to abortion,[2,3] and the rise in firearms mortality modeled to result from the Supreme Court's 2022 decision in *New York State Rifle & Pistol Ass'n. v Bruen* (597 US 1), narrowing a state's ability to regulate handguns.[3] The decisions and orders issued during the court's 2025 term were no exception. Several have shifted the law in ways that are likely to have a significant effect on public health.

We explore three different developments that were cemented during the court's 2025 term, and we forecast their impact on public health: executive power over health agencies, protection (or lack thereof) of socially marginalized groups, and access to justice. Importantly, many of these developments emerged from the Supreme Court's emergency docket, often called the "shadow docket." Shadow-docket cases are usually decided without oral argument or meaningful explanation.[4]

AMPLIFYING EXECUTIVE POWER OVER HEALTH AGENCIES

Robust executive authority can be beneficial to public health. It can allow governments to respond quickly to emergencies, such as the COVID-19 pandemic. And in theory, a chief executive officer, such as a president or governor, who cares about health can order agencies to promulgate health-promoting regulations. However, executive authority, especially when it is exercised without the advice and counsel of scientific expertise, can undermine evidence-based policymaking and threaten the rights of individuals and marginalized communities.

Recent articles on the Supreme Court have emphasized the erosion of the deference that judges traditionally afforded to state and federal health agencies.[5–7] With respect to federal agencies, the Supreme Court has overruled a long-standing decision requiring courts to defer to agency rulemaking in many circumstances, curtailed agencies' ability to enforce the law, and restricted agencies' ability to regulate questions of major economic or political significance, arguing that such decisions must be left to Congress.[6,8] Numerous federal health, equity, and environmental policies were felled under these changes—including COVID-19 vaccine requirements for large employers, climate change policies, an interstate air pollution regulation, and the Centers for Disease Control and Prevention's eviction moratorium.[6,7,9,10] According to Erwin Chemerinsky (University of California, Berkeley, School of Law dean), Joe Biden's losses at the Supreme Court were "the toughest series of defeats" a president has faced since the 1930s.[11]

Yet, since Donald Trump's second presidential inauguration, the court has appeared to alter course, halting lower court decisions that would have blocked many of the president's efforts to take control of federal agencies. For example, in 2025's *Trump v Wilcox* (605 US ___ [*Wilcox*]) the court, from the shadow docket, allowed the president to fire members of the National Labor Relations Board and the Merit Systems Protection Bureau, even though Congress established these agencies to be independent of the president. Without naming it, the court's decision in *Wilcox* appears to embrace the "unitary executive theory," which holds that the Constitution grants the president exclusive control over all federal agencies.[12] The court's adoption of this view in *Wilcox* gives the president control of the National Labor Relations Board, which guards workers' right to unionize. This may affect health because unionized

AJPH November 2025, Vol. 115, No. 11

employees are more likely to have health insurance and a regular health care provider.[9] The decision may also affect several other independent agencies that relate to health, including the Federal Trade Commission, which reviews anticompetitive and deceptive practices by pharmaceutical companies, pharmacy benefit managers, and private equity firms in health care.

The court has also greenlit greater presidential control over scientific advisory boards. In *Kennedy v Braidwood Management* (606 US ___ [2025]), the court upheld the US Preventive Services Task Force, whose recommendations determine which preventive services insurance companies must cover without cost sharing. The court emphasized that the US Preventive Services Task Force is constitutional only because the secretary of Health and Human Services has full control over its members and their decisions. As legal scholar of Yale Law School Abbe Gluck explains, the decision is a "potentially pyrrhic victory" for health because, while it upholds the US Preventive Services Task Force, it diminishes the independence and authority of the task force's experts (https://bit.ly/41uOlto). Secretary of Health and Human Services Robert F. Kennedy Jr. has signaled an interest in firing all of the US Preventive Services Task Force's current members and replacing them with ideological allies, who may, for example, raise religious objections to medications like the contraceptive pill or preexposure prophylaxis for HIV.

Signs of executive control over agencies are mounting. In June 2025, Kennedy fired all 17 members of the Advisory Committee on Immunization Practices—the body that issues recommendations about vaccines that determine coverage by insurers. Since then, Kennedy replaced the fired Advisory Committee on Immunization Practices members with eight individuals, some of whom are vaccine skeptics[13]; excluded expert organizations like the American Medical Association from taking part in vaccine decision-making[14]; and appears to be expanding political influence over the US Food and Drug Administration's premarket review of vaccines.[15] Kennedy's actions may make it harder for people in the United States to access vaccines, while also undermining public trust. Although the health impact of these actions have yet to be measured, one thing is clear: the secretary's actions relating to vaccines have been made easier by the Supreme Court's decisions.

The Supreme Court has also paved the way for dismantling other federal health-related agencies. In a series of reorganizations, the administration planned to "practically wipe out" the National Institute for Occupational Safety and Health, cut 83 000 staff at the Department of Veterans Affairs, and eliminate about half of workers at other agencies, including the Department of Energy and the National Oceanic and Atmospheric Association; many other reorganizations remain confidential.[16] A lower court blocked the reorganizations, noting that, if the reorganizations proceed, "agencies will not be able to do what Congress has directed them to do" (https://bit.ly/4mXpYIS). But the Supreme Court intervened in *Trump v American Federation of Government Employees* (606 US ___ [2025]), issuing a two-paragraph order from the shadow docket stating that the government was likely to prevail. Six days later, in a one-paragraph shadow-docket ruling in *McMahon v New York*, the court effectively allowed Trump to shutter the Department of Education, which plays pivotal roles in accrediting universities, administering student loans, and supporting special education.

Such decisions give the president and his political appointees unprecedented authority over federal health agencies, allowing him to command or disassemble them altogether—even when these actions are at odds with public health and an agency's statutory mission.

ESCHEWING PROTECTIONS FOR MARGINALIZED GROUPS

For much of the 20th century, the Supreme Court viewed its role as including the protection of marginalized groups.[17] Such protections can help to ensure that marginalized communities have equal or near equal access to health care, beneficial social services, and political representation, all of which can help to mitigate health inequities.[18] Moreover, invalidating discriminatory laws can protect against structural stigma (i.e., conditions, norms, policies, and practices that constrain stigmatized groups), which is thought to explain a significant fraction of health disparities.[19]

Last term underscored that the Supreme Court no longer accepts that its mission includes protecting socially marginalized groups. Consider 2025's *United States v Skrmetti* (605 US ___ [*Skrmetti*]), involving a Tennessee law, SB1, that prohibited health care interventions for the purpose of helping youths "identify with, or live as, a purported identity inconsistent with the minor's sex." Plaintiffs alleged antitransgender and sex discrimination; for example, someone assigned female at birth could obtain hormones for hirsutism, but someone assigned male at birth could not obtain such hormones to stop hair growth for transition. Even though all major US medical organizations agree that gender-affirming care for transgender youths can be evidence-based and health promoting, even lifesaving,[20] the court upheld the law. According to the majority, SB1 did not discriminate based on sex or transgender status because it banned hormones for gender dysphoria, a medical use, rather than based on identity group. By so doing, the court effectively erased the statute's plain text and opened the door for state laws that block gender-affirming care, even for adults. One court has already relied on *Skrmetti* to deny challenges to cancellations of grants supporting the health of sexual minorities (*American Public Health Assn v National Institutes of Health*, No. 25-1611 [1st Cir. 2025]).

The court has also issued a series of decisions that imperil the health of immigrants. There are 47 million immigrants (14% of the population) living in the United States; in the health care system, 29% of physicians and 24% of direct care staff are foreign-born.[21] Punitive immigration laws can instill fear, anxiety, and trauma and have been shown to reduce utilization of health care services.[22]

Although the court stated in *A.A.R.P. v Trump* (604 US ___ [2025]) that immigrants have a right to due process before they are deported, other decisions—primarily from the shadow docket—have supported the administration's efforts to rapidly deport millions of noncitizens, often with little or no process. For example, in *Noem v Doe* (605 US ___ [2025]) the Supreme Court allowed the Trump administration to strip about 500 000 immigrants of "temporary protected status"—turning immigrants who were present lawfully into unauthorized and deportable residents. Likewise, in *Department of Homeland Security v D.V.D.* (606 US ___ [2025)], the court allowed the Trump administration to deport immigrants to countries with which they have no connection—including war-torn ones considered unsafe, such as South Sudan. Such decisions can be expected to imperil the health of the deportees and add to the fear and trauma in their US communities.

Further, on June 27, 2025, in *Trump v CASA* (606 US ___ [*CASA*]), the court lifted a nationwide injunction from a lower court blocking an executive order ending birthright citizenship. This right—enshrined in the Fourteenth Amendment of the Constitution—ensures that individuals who are born in the United States are full citizens. Every lower court that had reviewed the executive order found it unconstitutional. Although the Supreme Court in *CASA* did not rule on the merits and only blocked one legal avenue—a lower court has already certified a class action and blocked the order using another avenue—*CASA* raises the risk that the executive order will go into effect in some states, leaving many children who are born in the United States stateless and unable to access Medicaid, the Children's Health Insurance Program, and other critical benefits. Hospitals will still be legally required to treat these patients in their emergency departments under the Emergency Medical Treatment and Labor Act (42 USC. § 1395dd [2018]) but will be less able to secure federal or state reimbursement for services if citizenship is stripped.

CLOSING COURTHOUSE DOORS AND REDUCING ACCESS TO JUSTICE

In addition to giving short shrift to legal claims by socially marginalized groups, the Supreme Court has made it more difficult for them to have their claims heard.

In 2025, *Medina v Planned Parenthood South Atlantic* (606 US ___ [*Medina*]), a case challenging a South Carolina law that blocked Planned Parenthood's participation in the state Medicaid program, the Supreme Court ruled that providers and patients generally cannot seek legal redress for violation of the Medicaid Act (Social Security Amendments of 1965, Pub L No. 89–97, 79 Stat. 286). According to the court, because the statute did not use the word "right," the provision was unenforceable by the public. *Medina* will also make it hard for patients and providers to enforce other federal provisions governing health care. The court's decision also means that states can use Medicaid funding as a cudgel to cut off providers of politicized health care without being held accountable for violating the law. (A recent congressional provision purports to "defund" Planned Parenthood but is tied up in court. *Planned Parenthood v Kennedy*, District of Massachusetts, No. 1:25-cv-11913-IT.)

By blocking nationwide injunctions, *CASA* also restricts access to justice. Although the court kept the door ajar for other procedural mechanisms challenging the executive order on birthright citizenship, its condemnation of nationwide injunctions may make it far more difficult for litigants to get broad relief from illegal or unconstitutional executive actions that deny access to health care or violate the rights of marginalized groups.

Many other decisions in 2025 have closed the door on remedies through seemingly narrow procedural rulings. For example, in *J.G.G. v Trump* (No. 25-cv-00766 [DDC 2025]) the court held that many immigrants who want to challenge their detention must proceed

BOX 1— Selected US Supreme Court Cases, 2022–2025

Case (Date)	Case No.	Subject
Dobbs v Jackson Women's Health Center (2022)	19-1392	The constitutional right to terminate a pregnancy
NYSRPA v Bruen (2022)	20-843	The validity of a New York handgun restriction and the scope of the right to bear arms
Trump v Wilcox (2025)	24A966	The power of the president to fire leaders of multiheaded agencies despite Congress's language restricting termination
Kennedy v Braidwood Management (2025)	24-316	The constitutionality of the US Preventive Services Task Force and the power of political officials to fire or overrule task force members
Trump v American Federation of Government Employees (2025)	24A1174	The validity of an executive order planning a broad reorganization of federal agencies
McMahon v New York (2025)	24A1203	The power of the president to dismantle the Department of Education
United States v Skrmetti (2025)	23-477	The validity of a Tennessee ban on transgender health care
A.A.R.P. v Trump (2025)	24A1007	The process required for removal of immigrants under the Alien Enemies Act
Noem v Doe (2025)	24A1079	The validity of the administration's termination of "temporary protected status" for about 500 000 immigrants
Department of Homeland Security v D.V.D. (2025)	24A1153	The validity of the administration's removals to third countries
Trump v CASA (2025)	24A884	The validity of an executive order dispensing with birthright citizenship and the power of federal courts to issue nationwide injunctions
Medina v Planned Parenthood (2025)	23-1275	The ability of patients and providers to sue states for violations of federal statutes, here the Medicaid Act
Trump v J.G.G. (2025)	24A931	The ability of immigrants to challenge removals pursuant to the Alien Enemies Act
Department of Education v California (2025)	24A910	The proper venue for challenging federal education grant terminations
National Institutes of Health v American Public Health Assn (2025)	25A103	The proper venue for challenging federal grant terminations by the National Institutes of Health
Lackey v Stinnie (2025)	23-621	The ability of plaintiffs' attorneys to be paid for preliminary victories that resolve a dispute

through a labyrinthine process called "habeas corpus." This decision will make it more difficult to challenge actions that enhance the stigmatic and direct harms on immigrants we discussed earlier.

Similarly, in *Department of Education v California* (604 US ___ [2025]), the court ruled that challenges to grant terminations cannot be brought in ordinary federal district courts but must instead be filed in the Court of Federal Claims, which focuses on contract disputes against the United States. This ruling makes it more difficult to challenge grant cancellations, which have affected many researchers funded by the National Institutes of Health (NIH). Although lower courts have blocked many NIH grant cancellations, the Trump administration asked the Supreme Court on July 24, 2025, to apply *Department of Education v California* and overrule one lower court's order. On August 21, in *National Institutes of Health v American Public Health Assn* (606 US ___ [2025]), the Supreme Court ruled in a split 4 to 1 to 4 decision from the shadow docket that although the district court could rule on the legality of the policies for terminating grants, challenges to individual grant terminations had to be brought in the Court of Federal Claims. Moreover, because federal law prohibits claims from "substantially the same operative facts" from proceeding simultaneously in both courts, those who want to challenge NIH's policies regarding grants and gain reinstatement of their own grant may have to pick which suit to file first.

Finally, the court sliced the financial rewards for private plaintiffs who win cases against the government. Under 42 US § 1988 (Proceedings in vindication of civil rights), private litigants who prevail can obtain "a reasonable attorney's fee" from the defendant—a source of revenue that has allowed public interest law practices to survive and protect access to justice for minoritized groups, including for health-related matters. Yet in *Lackey v Stinnie* (604 ___ [2025]), the Supreme Court held that fees are only available when a plaintiff wins after a final judgment in the case. Now, litigants who win preliminary remedies cannot receive compensation if the government withdraws an illegal law before the final decision to avoid paying fees. This case erodes access to justice and imperils the ability of marginalized groups to secure representation and have their day in court.[23] In contrast, legal operations financed by business and political interests are likely to remain well funded.

THE US SUPREME COURT AND PUBLIC HEALTH

It is difficult to overstate the enormous impact that the Supreme Court's decisions have had and are likely to have on health.[5,9,10,24] The court's decisions (1) directly affect the workings and composition of health agencies; (2) weaken the rights of patients and vulnerable populations, including transgender people and immigrants; and (3) make it more difficult for individuals and communities to attain justice.

As discussed, many of these developments emerged from the shadow docket. The shadow docket allows the court to change the law rapidly without justifying its decisions to the US public—the main source of the court's legitimacy. The impact of such actions may upend population health and will need to be investigated. Shadow-docket decisions may also be infused with politics: although district courts ruled against the Trump administration in 82 of 87 decisions between May 1 and June 23, 2025, the Supreme Court ruled for the administration in 15 of 16 decisions,[25] raising serious questions about whether the Supreme Court may be protecting the administration from legal oversight.

In this moment, the public health community can no longer afford the luxury of staying outside the arenas of politics and law. They must research empirically the impact of judicial decisions on health, treating the court's decrees as a social determinant of health. They must also educate lawmakers on the impact of court decisions on people and patients, partner with policy and legal experts to inform the public about the important role that courts play in determining the health of individuals and communities, and attempt to combat the misinformation that muddles popular understandings of public health. Should we remain silent, the threats to public health will only grow. AJPH

CORRESPONDENCE

Correspondence should be sent to Daniel G. Aaron, 383 South University St, Salt Lake City, UT 84112 (e-mail: Daniel.Aaron@law.utah.edu). Reprints can be ordered at https://www.ajph.org by clicking the "Reprints" link.

PUBLICATION INFORMATION

Full Citation: Aaron DG, Parmet WE. The Supreme Court's 2024–2025 term: eroding public health, health equity, and access to justice. *Am J Public Health.* 2025;115(11):1773–1778.

Acceptance Date: August 19, 2025.

https://doi.org/10.2105/AJPH.2025.308281

ORCID iD:
Daniel G. Aaron https://orcid.org/0000-0003-4490-7504

CONTRIBUTORS

The authors contributed equally to this work.

ACKNOWLEDGMENTS

D. G. Aaron receives funding from Arnold Ventures, a philanthropic foundation. W. E. Parmet receives funding from ChangeLab Solutions, the Robert Wood Johnson Foundation, and the W. K. Kellogg Foundation.

CONFLICTS OF INTEREST

The authors have no conflicts of interest to disclose.

REFERENCES

1. Gostin LO, Wetter S. The Supreme Court is harming public health and the environment. *JAMA.* 2023;329(18):1549–1550. https://doi.org/10.1001/jama.2023.3564
2. Zhu DT, Zhao L, Alzoubi T, et al. Public health and clinical implications of *Dobbs v Jackson* for patients and healthcare providers: a scoping review. *PLoS One.* 2024;19(3):e0288947. https://doi.org/10.1371/journal.pone.0288947
3. Gaffney A, Himmelstein DU, Dickman S, et al. Projected health outcomes associated with 3 US Supreme Court decisions in 2022 on COVID-19 workplace protections, handgun-carry restrictions, and abortion rights. *JAMA Netw Open.* 2023;6(6):e2315578. https://doi.org/10.1001/jamanetworkopen.2023.15578
4. Vladeck SI. *The Shadow Docket: How the Supreme Court Uses Stealth Rulings to Amass Power and Undermine the Republic.* New York, NY: Basic Books; 2024.
5. Aaron DG, Emery AE. US Supreme Court limits on the power of US health agencies. *JAMA.* 2024;331(17):1441–1442. https://doi.org/10.1001/jama.2024.3723
6. Farmer R, Aaron DG. Loper Bright's deregulatory synergies. *Seton Hall L Rev.* 2025;55(5):1697–1719.
7. Parmet WE, Khalik F. Judicial review of public health powers since the start of the COVID-19 pandemic: trends and implications. *Am J Public Health.* 2023;113(3):280–287. https://doi.org/10.2105/AJPH.2022.307181
8. Parmet WE. The rise, fall, and resurrection of public health law. *Am J Law Med.* 2024;50(3–4):279–293. https://doi.org/10.1017/amj.2025.11
9. Parmet WE. Protecting public health in the courts. *Am J Public Health.* 2025;115(5):687–688. https://doi.org/10.2105/AJPH.2025.308087
10. Wiley LF. The 2023 US Supreme Court term: implications for public health. *Am J Public Health.* 2023;113(3):269–271. https://doi.org/10.2105/AJPH.2022.307210
11. Kruzel J. US Supreme Court dealt Biden historic series of defeats. Reuters. January 20, 2025. Available at: https://www.reuters.com/world/us/us-supreme-court-dealt-biden-historic-series-defeats-2025-01-18. Accessed July 23, 2025.
12. Chabot CK. Interring the unitary executive. *Notre Dame Law Review.* 2022;98(1):129–209. https://doi.org/10.2139/ssrn.3921776
13. Daval CJR, Kesselheim AS. The advisory committee on immunization practices—legal roles, challenges, and guardrails. *JAMA.* 2025;334(8):669–671. https://doi.org/10.1001/jama.2025.11400
14. American Medical Association. Latest ACIP move is dangerous to the nation's health. August 1, 2025. Available at: https://www.ama-assn.org/public-health/prevention-wellness/latest-acip-move-dangerous-nation-s-health. Accessed August 7, 2025.
15. Zettler PJ, Cha S, Despres S, Lurie P. FDA review of Novavax's COVID-19 vaccine—regulatory integrity and deviations from standard practice. *JAMA.* 2025;334(6):479–480. https://doi.org/10.1001/jama.2025.9898
16. *Donald J. Trump v American Federation of Government Employees*, 606 US __ (2025). No. 24A1174 (2025). Available at: https://www.supremecourt.gov/opinions/24pdf/24a1174_h3ci.pdf. Accessed August, 8 2025.
17. Chemerinsky E. *The Case Against the Supreme Court.* New York, NY: Penguin Books; 2014.
18. Dawes DE, Williams DR. *The Political Determinants of Health.* Baltimore, MD: Johns Hopkins University Press; 2020.
19. Hatzenbuehler ML, Phelan JC, Link BG. Stigma as a fundamental cause of population health inequalities. *Am J Public Health.* 2013;103(5):813–821. https://doi.org/10.2105/AJPH.2012.301069

20. Balkan E, Babbs G, Meyers DJ, et al. Gender-affirming surgery for transgender and gender diverse Medicare beneficiaries. *JAMA Netw Open.* 2025;8(5):e258072. https://doi.org/10.1001/jamanetworkopen.2025.8072
21. Santos PMG, Jagsi R, Oronce CIA. Who will care for America? Immigration policy and the coming health workforce crisis. *N Engl J Med.* 2025;393(2):105–107. https://doi.org/10.1056/NEJMp2504949
22. Vernice NA, Pereira NM, Wang A, Demetres M, Adams LV. The adverse health effects of punitive immigrant policies in the United States: a systematic review. *PLoS ONE.* 2020;15(12):e0244054. https://doi.org/10.1371/journal.pone.0244054
23. School SL. The Supreme Court's decision in *Lackey v Stinnie* and what it means for plaintiffs' access to courts. March 3, 2025. Available at: https://law.stanford.edu/2025/03/03/the-supreme-courts-decision-in-lackey-v-stinnie-and-what-it-means-for-plaintiffs-access-to-courts. Accessed July 10, 2025.
24. Parmet WE. *Constitutional Contagion: COVID, the Courts, and Public Health.* Cambridge, UK: Cambridge University Press; 2023.
25. Bonica A. The Supreme Court is at war with its own judiciary. June 25, 2025. Available at: https://data4democracy.substack.com/p/the-supreme-court-is-at-war-with. Accessed August 18, 2025.

A Call for Formal Reporting Standards for Legal Research in Public Health Studies

Cason D. Schmit, JD, Scott Burris, JD, Safura Abdool Karim, LLM, PhD, Benjamin A. Barsky, JD, PhD, Sean Grant, DPhil, Alina Schnake-Mahl, ScD, MPH, Lauren Tonti, JD, MPH, Megan D. Douglas, JD, Kimberly M. Nelson, PhD, MPH, Amie J. Goodin, PhD, MPP, Kristen Underhill, JD, DPhil, Mathieu J. P. Poirier, PhD, MPH, CPH, Jin Yung Bae, JD, MPH, Elizabeth Piekarz-Porter, JD, Regen Weber-Fares, JD, MPH, Susan Zells Ingber, MSPP, AB, and Jamie F. Chriqui, PhD, MHS

ABOUT THE AUTHORS

Cason D. Schmit and Regen Weber-Fares are with the Department of Health Policy and Management, Texas A&M University School of Public Health, College Station, TX. Scott Burris is with the Center for Public Health Law Research, Temple University Beasley School of Law, Philadelphia, PA. Safura Abdool Karim is with the Berman Institute of Bioethics, Johns Hopkins University, Baltimore, MD. Benjamin A. Barsky is with the University of California College of the Law, San Francisco. Sean Grant is with the RAND Corporation, Santa Monica, CA. Alina Schnake-Mahl is with the Department of Health Management and Policy, Urban Health Collaborative, Dornsife School of Public Health, Drexel University, Philadelphia, PA. Lauren Tonti is with the Department of Economics, University of Missouri, Columbia. Megan D. Douglas is with the Department of Community Health and Preventive Medicine, Morehouse School of Medicine, Atlanta, GA. Kimberly M. Nelson is with the Department of Community Health Sciences, Boston University School of Public Health, Boston, MA. Amie J. Goodin is with the Department of Pharmaceutical Outcomes and Policy, Center for Drug Evaluation and Safety, University of Florida, Gainesville. Kristen Underhill is with the Cornell Law School, Ithaca, NY. Mathieu J. P. Poirier is with the School of Global Health, York University, Toronto, Canada. Jin Yung Bae is with the NYU School of Global Public Health, New York, NY. Elizabeth Piekarz-Porter and Jamie F. Chriqui are with the University of Illinois Chicago School of Public Health. Susan Zells Ingber is with Sellers Dorsey, Philadelphia, PA.

Law—the range of policy instruments including statutes, regulations, ordinances, orders, formal guidance, court decisions, or other written standards within legal or organizational frameworks—is a common tool of public health intervention. Law also sets the powers, duties, and limits of government agencies and is woven into the social determinants of health.[1] Researchers from many disciplines use scientific methods to evaluate the impact of law on population health.

There has been significant improvement in policy evaluation methods, followed by greater openness to causal claims, but in one respect, the study of the health effects of laws and legal practices—now often referred to as "legal epidemiology"[2]—appears to be problematic: transparent reporting of the specific methods used to create the legal variables representing the legal exposure. Transparency is a fundamental scientific value and crucial for peer review, replication, and credibility for research consumers. In this editorial, we review the state of the art in scientific legal measurement and the emergence of the transparency problem, and then we suggest a pathway to better reporting practices.

LEGAL RESEARCH TRANSPARENCY IN POLICY EVALUATION

The longitudinal legal data sets typically required in causal inference studies encompass multiple features of laws across many jurisdictions and years. As recently summarized by Barsky et al., creating structured data for legal epidemiology studies entails determining the scope of the research, gathering the text of the laws to be studied ("legal research"), transforming the relevant textual features of the law into structured data for qualitative or quantitative analysis ("coding"), and implementing quality control and documentation procedures.[3] Errors in finding laws within the scope of the study, capturing effective dates or other temporal elements, identifying study-relevant differences in the law, and consistently coding those features risk mismeasurement and misclassification of the legal data. This process may, and perhaps normally should, be carried out by or with lawyers. That said, legal research for scientific purposes has methodological elements—particularly in quality control and documentation—that go beyond those typically used in standard legal research for nonscientific purposes.

There is literature on scientific legal research methods[4–6] and some consensus on the basic elements of good practice,[7] but the extent of their adoption was unmeasured until 2024, when Pepin et al. reviewed 177 studies published between 2009 and 2019 evaluating the health impact of law.[8] The Pepin et al. review exposed substantial deficiencies in the reporting of legal measurement methods. Eight percent of the reviewed studies provided no information at all about the source of their legal data. Forty percent reported obtaining data from a website, which is concerning from a transparency perspective because few websites purport to provide transparently created data for scientific research. Furthermore, papers rarely reported methods details considered important in the existing methods literature, such as the qualifications of the legal research team and details of the legal search. Details of the search strategy and legal databases used are essential to understand the validity of the legal data: just as in a systematic literature review, searching different legal databases will yield drastically different results depending on the search terms and strings used.

The findings of the Pepin et al. review are alarming but not surprising to researchers who focus on the health effects of laws and legal practices.[5,9–12] The results are and have been taken as a call to action to develop formal reporting standards for legal research in public health studies. Aside from being a fundamental scientific value, transparency is essential to allow reviewers and editors to assess the validity of studies during the publication process, as well as to the readers who will draw on the studies in new research and policymaking. While deficiencies in transparency do not necessarily indicate that the methods used or the conclusions reached in a study were faulty, a more stringent review enabled by better reporting of methods can forestall the publication of flawed studies.[13]

LEGAL MEASUREMENT REPORTING STANDARDS TO BENEFIT SCIENCE

Given a general consensus on rigorous methods,[4–7] coupled with the prevalence of poor methods reporting,[8] legal measurement for scientific research is an apt candidate for a formal reporting standard. Reporting standards can help peer reviewers and journal editors identify lapses in reporting and ask authors to repair them.[3] Furthermore, a reporting checklist can increase consistency in legal research practices across disciplines. It also may help researchers who do their own legal research appreciate—and perhaps even master—the nuances of legal measurement. For the many researchers who use legal information or data from third parties (e.g., websites cataloging state laws), reporting standards may help them be better informed, more critical consumers of the legal work of others and report on potential limitations of those legal data sources. Proper reporting is indispensable for researchers who wish to replicate a study and is a primary mechanism for spreading methodological innovations and improvements as researchers are better situated to learn from and build on transparently reported previous work.

The adoption of standards for other research types—for example, CONSORT for randomized trials, and PRISMA for systematic reviews—has benefited all research stakeholders. While not an instant cure,[14] reporting standards can be a tool for motivated researchers, reviewers, and editors to improve the conduct of research and its translation into action. This is, if anything, possibly even more useful in research assessing the impact of law on population health, because it is carried out by scientists from a wide range of disciplines. The Pepin et al. review included studies led by authors trained in economics, epidemiology, health policy, law, medicine, nursing, pharmacy, political science, psychology, public administration, social work, and veterinary medicine, among other fields, working in a diverse array of research institutions.

DEVELOPING REPORTING STANDARDS OF RESEARCH ON LAW

An interdisciplinary and international group of researchers engaged with scientific legal measurement—including experts in law, epidemiology, health services research, health policy, political science, and economics—convened at the Center for Public Health Law Research at Temple University in May 2024. Following the general approach to guideline development in the EQUATOR Network, the group discussed and reached agreement on three key points: that the current state of reporting in research studies was suboptimal, that there was a body of methodological literature and research experience on which a standard could be based, and that a formal reporting standard would improve transparency. The group, calling itself the Legal Measurement Methods Consortium, has registered a standard in development, "Standards for Legal Epidemiology Reporting (STLER)" with the EQUATOR Network,[15] and consortium members are conducting further research on the nature and extent of transparency problems in legal epidemiology. The next step, now in progress, is a Delphi study to develop consensus on the elements to be included in a reporting guideline. A consensus meeting of stakeholders—including researchers, editors, and research consumers—will review the Delphi findings and adopt a reporting standard. After the meeting, the working group will execute a strategy for publication, endorsement, and adoption.

A successful reporting standard requires buy-in and participation not just from researchers but also from reviewers, editors, and people who use research evidence in advocacy and policymaking. Hence, this editorial serves not only as the call for the development of a standard but also as an invitation to the broader public health research community to participate in its development. We invite interested people to contact the corresponding author or access the reporting standard website[15] to indicate their interest in participating in or supporting the development of these reporting standards to move the field toward more rigorous and transparent methodology for research assessing the impact of law on population health.

CONCLUSION

When a report of scientific findings lacks transparency regarding the details of its research process, science is compromised, even if the process was sound. This is just as true when a law is the exposure as when any other intervention or behavior is being evaluated. The concerns we have raised should alarm all stakeholders of research assessing the impact of law on population health, from the researchers that conduct it, the journals that publish it, the funders that support it, the advocacy groups that use it, to the policymakers that rely upon it. To maintain our credibility in the supply chain of evidence-informed policy, the diverse multidisciplinary community of researchers studying the health effects of law must work together to course correct now. The development of a robust reporting standard is the first step. We encourage members of the research community to help us develop these standards—and then to spread them across our many fields and journals and to put them into routine practice. AJPH

CORRESPONDENCE

Correspondence should be sent to Cason D. Schmit, 121 SPHA, 212 Adriance Lab Rd, College Station, TX 77843 (e-mail: schmit@tamu.edu). Reprints can be ordered at https://ajph.org by clicking the "Reprints" link.

PUBLICATION INFORMATION

Full Citation: Schmit CD, Burris S, Abdool Karim S, et al. A call for formal reporting standards for legal research in public health studies. *Am J Public Health*. 2025;115(11):1779–1782.

Acceptance Date: July 4, 2025.

DOI: https://doi.org/10.2105/AJPH.2025.308246

ORCID iDs:

Cason D. Schmit https://orcid.org/0000-0002-7929-7198

Safura Abdool Karim https://orcid.org/0000-0002-4843-9907

Alina Schnake-Mahl https://orcid.org/0000-0002-7775-3022

Lauren Tonti https://orcid.org/0000-0002-6083-4993

Megan D. Douglas https://orcid.org/0000-0003-3666-5664

Kimberly M. Nelson https://orcid.org/0000-0001-8893-5764

Amie J. Goodin https://orcid.org/0000-0002-0020-8720

Kristen Underhill https://orcid.org/0009-0000-0349-2846

Mathieu J. P. Poirier https://orcid.org/0000-0003-3842-0011

Jin Yung Bae https://orcid.org/0000-0002-8389-0971

Elizabeth Piekarz-Porter https://orcid.org/0000-0001-8161-3738

Regen Weber-Fares https://orcid.org/0009-0003-6871-6865

Susan Zells Ingber https://orcid.org/0000-0002-5290-8884

Jamie F. Chriqui https://orcid.org/0000-0003-2538-0276

CONTRIBUTORS

All authors contributed to conceptualization and final approval of the version to be published. All authors contributed to writing the original draft, led by C. D. Schmit. C. D. Schmit, S. Burris, J. F. Chriqui, S. Abdool Karim, B. A. Barsky, and S. Grant contributed to review and editing of the article.

ACKNOWLEDGMENTS

We are grateful for the insights of the Legal Measurement Methods Consortium and the Temple Center for Public Health Law Research for their support in organizing this collaboration.

CONFLICTS OF INTEREST

We have no conflicts of interest to disclose.

REFERENCES

1. Burris S, Wagenaar AC, Swanson J, Ibrahim JK, Wood J, Mello MM. Making the case for laws that improve health: a framework for public health law research. *Milbank Q*. 2010;88(2):169–210. https://doi.org/10.1111/j.1468-0009.2010.00595.x
2. Burris S, Cloud LK, Penn M. The growing field of legal epidemiology. *J Public Health Manag Pract*. 2020;26(suppl 2):S4–S9. https://doi.org/10.1097/PHH.0000000000001133
3. Barsky BA, Schnake-Mahl A, Schmit CD, Burris S. Improving the transparency of legal measurement in health policy evaluation—a guide for researchers, reviewers, and editors. *JAMA Health Forum*. 2025;6(3):e250067. https://doi.org/10.1001/jamahealthforum.2025.0067
4. Anderson E, Thomas S, Treffers RD, Wagenaar AC. Measuring statutory law and regulations for empirical research. In: Wagenaar A, Burris S, eds. *Public Health Law Research: Theory and Methods*. San Francisco, CA: John Wiley & Sons; 2023: 209–232.
5. LaFond C, Toomey TL, Rothstein C, Manning W, Wagenaar AC. Policy evaluation research. Measuring the independent variables. *Eval Rev*. 2000;24(1):92–101. https://doi.org/10.1177/0193841X0002400104
6. Chriqui JF, Piekarz-Porter E, Schermbeck RM, Das A. Assessing policy impacts on chronic disease risk reduction: the science and art of policy rating systems. *Annu Rev Public Health*. 2025;46(1): 331–348. https://doi.org/10.1146/annurev-publhealth-071723-113826
7. Presley D, Reinstein T, Webb-Barr D, Burris S. Creating legal data for public health monitoring and evaluation: Delphi standards for policy surveillance. *J Law Med Ethics*. 2015;43(suppl 1): 27–31. https://doi.org/10.1111/jlme.12210
8. Pepin DA, St Clair Sims R, Khushalani J, et al. A narrative review of literature examining studies researching the impact of law on health and economic outcomes. *J Public Health Manag Pract*. 2024;30(1):12–35. https://doi.org/10.1097/PHH.0000000000001833
9. Pacula RL, Hunt P, Boustead A. Words can be deceiving: a review of variation among legally effective medical marijuana laws in the United States. *J Drug Policy Anal*. 2014;7(1):1–19. https://doi.org/10.1515/jdpa-2014-0001

10. Horwitz JR, Davis C, McClelland L, Fordon R, Meara E. The importance of data source in prescription drug monitoring program research. *Health Serv Res.* 2021;56(2):268–274. https://doi.org/10.1111/1475-6773.13548
11. Burris S. Legal epidemiology: growth, and growing pains. *J Public Health Manag Pract.* 2024;30(1):1–2. https://doi.org/10.1097/PHH.0000000000001836
12. Burris S. Theory and methods in comparative drug and alcohol policy research: response to a review of the literature. *Int J Drug Policy.* 2017;41:126–131. https://doi.org/10.1016/j.drugpo.2016.11.011
13. Lee Y, Choi SW, Lee J. Retracted: Longitudinal study on deterrent effect of drug-induced homicide law on opioid-related mortality across 92 counties and the District of Columbia in the US. *J Drug Issues.* 2022;52(2):131–143. https://doi.org/10.1177/00220426211037614
14. Page MJ, Moher D. Evaluations of the uptake and impact of the Preferred Reporting Items for Systematic reviews and Meta-Analyses (PRISMA) Statement and extensions: a scoping review. *Syst Rev.* 2017;6(1):263. https://doi.org/10.1186/s13643-017-0663-8
15. Equator Network. Reporting guidelines under development for other study designs: STLER: Standards for Legal Epidemiology Reporting. 2025. Available at: https://www.equator-network.org/library/reporting-guidelines-under-development/reporting-guidelines-under-development-for-other-study-designs/#STLER. Accessed May 12, 2025.

Why Building Power Is Key to Protecting Academic Public Health and Advancing Health Equity

Caitlin L. McMurtry, PhD, SM, Marjory L. Givens, PhD, MSPH, Zinzi D. Bailey, ScD, MSPH, Nick Graetz, PhD, MPH, Paul J. Fleming, PhD, MPH, Ryan J. Petteway, DrPH, MPH, Julianna Pacheco, PhD, MA, Sarah E. Gollust, PhD, Jonathan C. Heller, PhD, Hedwig E. Lee, PhD, MA, Keshia M. Pollack Porter, PhD, MPH, Sheri Johnson, PhD, MA, Jamila D. Michener, PhD, MA, Alana M. W. LeBrón, PhD, MS, Amy Kate Bailey, PhD, MA, James Bloyd, DrPH, MA, Melissa Creary, PhD, MPH, and India J. Ornelas, PhD, MPH

ABOUT THE AUTHORS

Caitlin L. McMurtry is with the Brown School, Washington University, St Louis, MO. Marjory L. Givens, Jonathan C. Heller, and Sheri Johnson are with the Population Health Institute, University of Wisconsin-Madison. Zinzi D. Bailey and Sarah E. Gollust are with the School of Public Health, University of Minnesota Twin Cities, Minneapolis. Nick Graetz is with the Department of Sociology, University of Minnesota Twin Cities. Paul J. Fleming and Melissa Creary are with the School of Public Health, University of Michigan, Ann Arbor. Ryan J. Petteway is with the OHSU-PSU School of Public Health, Portland, OR. Julianna Pacheco is with the Department of Political Science, University of Iowa, Iowa City. Hedwig E. Lee is with the Department of Sociology, Duke University, Durham, NC. Keshia M. Pollack Porter is with the Bloomberg School of Public Health, Johns Hopkins University, Baltimore, MD. Jamila D. Michener is with the Department of Government, Cornell University, Ithaca, NY. Alana M. W. LeBrón is with the Joe C. Wen School of Population and Public Health and the Department of Chicano/Latino Studies, University of California, Irvine. Amy Kate Bailey is with the Department of Sociology, University of Illinois Chicago. James Bloyd is with the Collaborative for Health Equity Cook County, Chicago, IL. India J. Ornelas is with the School of Public Health, University of Washington and Fred Hutchinson Cancer Center, Seattle.

Academic public health is at a crossroads. For decades, research in our field has focused on identifying and describing health inequities, differences in health that are unnecessary, avoidable, unfair, and unjust. We have documented recent declines in life expectancy, increases in maternal and infant mortality, and a range of other disease outcomes—all with marked differences by race, ethnicity, geography, education, and class. The field has been called on to reduce these inequities, yet little progress has been made, and in many cases, the gaps have widened.[1,2] Now, federal health agencies, universities, health systems and the communities we serve are in peril. We must ask ourselves: are we willing to address the power structures that jeopardize public health and produce health inequities?

Academic public health must acknowledge that power imbalances are at the root of health inequities.[3] These imbalances persist through laws, policies, institutional practices, and norms leveraged by powerful actors.[4–6] Community organizing is a process of building power across people to address shared interests and priorities through direct and collective action.[7] Community organizing frameworks teach us that power is built and maintained via dominant power (e.g., unilateral power, power over) and relational power (e.g., power that engages, power with, transformative processes, and visioning). Advancing health equity requires addressing these types of power in two ways: (1) building power by cultivating the capacity of people who are disproportionately burdened by health inequities and who therefore have the most at stake and (2) breaking power by weakening and destabilizing the societal, economic, and political forces (or structural determinants) that perpetuate health inequity.[8] Academic public health must enhance its capacity as a strategic partner and join communities in local and national power-building movements.[3]

In this essay, we present the collective analysis of the Health and Power Organizing Project (HPOP), a group of public health academics committed to using community organizing and power-building principles to advance health equity and change the incentive structures within academia. HPOP was initiated in 2023 by faculty and staff at the University of Wisconsin Population Health Institute with funding support from the W. K. Kellogg Foundation. Informed by a community organizing approach, HPOP emerged by tapping into existing networks to identify and invite initial members based on a demonstrated commitment to advancing health equity, an understanding of the relationship between power and public health, and a desire to transform systems connected to public health academia.

Consistent with the goal of building relational power, a diverse group in terms of disciplinary fields, levels of seniority, and identities met to take the initial steps toward establishing this base-building formation. This process prioritized relationship building across members and cocreation of a shared analysis, goals, strategies, and governance of HPOP. Recognizing the importance of integrating academic and community knowledge into our analysis, we also interviewed community-based practitioners and community organizers. Our analysis reflects the critical conversations we had in retreats and virtual meetings over the first two years as a first step in achieving our longer-term goals. We define the nature of the problem and offer opportunities to intervene on the factors we view as the root of the challenge; specific strategies must emerge from the relationships created through organizing. We are not the first, and will not be the last, to reveal the layered power asymmetries driving health inequities; our shared analysis builds on the work of past scholars who have created space for a radical reimagination of our field.[9,10]

ANALYSIS OF THE POWER ECOSYSTEM

In this section, we define the nature of the problem by identifying challenges and offering opportunities for intervention. The political environment is rapidly evolving, but to transform the power ecosystem, academic public health faces challenges at three levels: systemic, institutional, and individual. These levels are based on the social ecological model and reflect our interest in showing how factors at each level impact one another. We describe these levels below and provide select examples in Box 1.

Systemic Level

At the systemic level, leaders of powerful institutions (e.g., corporations, universities, government) develop, spread, and apply worldviews and policies that erode equity. We see this in the censorship and termination of federal research grants related to climate change; lesbian, gay, bisexual, transgender, and queer health; racial and ethnic health disparities; and others.[11] It is also visible in the widespread backlash against teaching about historical injustices, including the legacy of slavery and racial exploitation in the United States. These efforts will have profound implications for scientific research and how we teach public health in the future if students arrive in our classes with little knowledge of the historical context of health inequities. As a preference for "colorblind" racial ideology and hostility toward the concept of equity, itself, becomes normalized, so, too, grows the need for advocates of health equity. Unless we work together to challenge this intellectual backsliding, institutions will continue to exploit and marginalize those with less power. We must respond by building power among those most affected and breaking the power of leaders opposed to equity. Accomplishing this means weakening the ways in which institutions benefit from these practices.[12,13]

Within higher education, academic institutions and professional organizations uphold norms about bias and neutrality that are rooted in inequity and limit the potential to imagine transformative research and action.[14,15] Knowledge produced by academic researchers is considered valid while community-based knowledge is disregarded or minimized. These dynamics cement power solely within established, "legitimate" actors and organizations—many of whom have constructed our current, ineffectual practices. It also erodes relationships with communities who might otherwise participate in cocreating solutions to health inequities and hinders the ability of academics to improve population health.

When it comes to changing the incentives required to transform these practices, progress is often slow or nonexistent because accrediting bodies require consensus across diverse academic institutions and political contexts.[16] Accreditation standards serve as benchmarks for conveying our principles and ethics to students. The federal government is seeking to erode those standards and eliminate accreditation bodies.[17] Allowing these changes would jeopardize the field by worsening the education of new leaders in health equity.

In addition, funders, academics, and civil society have shaped the rules so that communities most affected by health inequities are neither informing public health research and practice, nor are they organized to do so. Even when entities like the National Institutes of Health claim an interest in health equity and correcting power imbalances in research, they rarely fund communities to do this work, and more recently, they have eliminated programs that fund community-driven health equity research.[18] When we rely on funders to determine the direction of the field, changes in leadership (and their attendant priorities) can be

AJPH November 2025, Vol. 115, No. 11

BOX 1— Analysis of the Power Ecosystem and Select Examples of How Power Is Wielded to Influence Health Equity

Level	Analysis
Systemic	Leaders of powerful institutions develop, spread, and apply worldviews and policies that erode equity. • The National Institutes of Health and Environmental Protection Agency have censored and terminated health equity grants in the areas of lesbian, gay, bisexual, transgender, and queer individuals' health; HIV; vaccines; race/ethnicity; and environmental justice. • The Office of Health Equity was eliminated and there have been cuts at the Office of Minority Health and the National Institute on Minority Health and Health Disparities. • Programs designed to ameliorate racial injustices, including affirmative action, have been prohibited, which will lead to less racial/ethnic student diversity.
	Academic institutions and professional organizations uphold norms rooted in inequity that limit transformative research and action. Advocacy or community-based participatory research (CBPR) is often viewed as antithetical to impartiality or lacking rigor.
	Accrediting bodies require consensus across diverse contexts, slowing progress to transform academic practices. • Institutions prohibited by state law from teaching topics related to equity have tried to erode public health competencies. • Executive Orders direct authorities to "hold accountable" accrediting bodies that advance "unlawful 'diversity, equity, and inclusion' requirements" by monitoring, suspending, denying, or terminating accreditation recognition.
	Funders, academics, and civil society have shaped rules so that communities are neither informing research, nor organized to do so. • They set the academic research agenda through their strategic priorities, often with little or no input from communities most affected. • Funders rarely address the power dynamics necessary to position communities to advance health equity.
	Policymakers, when they engage with scientific evidence, often do so in limited or symbolic ways to inform (or confirm) their decisions. • Much scientific research is never translated into policy; many policies are enacted despite overwhelming evidence to the contrary. • Many policymakers distrust science and scientists, are hostile toward equity, and hold conspiratorial beliefs.
Institutional	Most funders do not grant awards for structural change and often view action research as "advocacy," which they do not support. Grant review criteria prioritize a narrow notion of rigor over community needs and incremental progress over structural change.
	Accrediting bodies in higher education do not prioritize organizing (power-building) and policy change in public health training. None of public health's foundational competencies address how to affect policy processes, politics, or power structures.
	Academic institutions often lack trusting relationships with communities because of harms that are rarely acknowledged or reconciled. • Trusting relationships often hinge on personal relationships, leaving them vulnerable to departures and funding changes. • Institutions rely on soft-money positions, requiring researchers to fund their salary or benefits through external support. • Instruction is often geared toward accreditation criteria rather than toward broader critical thinking.
	Academic institutions and disciplines hold norms that limit diversity in the types of research conducted by faculty and students. Grant and publication opportunities prioritize analyses of secondary data sources over CBPR, encourage methods that lack critical analyses of praxis norms, and are shaped by White supremacy, like using race in ways that imply genetic differences.
Individual	Academics are often trained, hired, or incentivized to focus on discrete studies rather than activities leading to structural change. Individuals do not always see themselves as part of social change efforts.
	As researchers, we have not organized ourselves to push for health equity or defend public health and are not prepared to do so. • Only about 25% of US faculty members are unionized, leading to vulnerability when trying to change work conditions and incentives. • Without collective power, it can feel precarious to take public positions on "controversial" topics.
	As instructors, we often lack practically relevant, solution-oriented tools to teach students how to build and break power. In staying out of politics, faculty limit their ability to meaningfully guide students seeking to engage in advocacy.

Note. Please see Appendix A (available as a supplement to the online version of this article at https://ajph.org) for a full list of Box 1 references.

profoundly destabilizing and have widespread implications for scientific knowledge now and in the future.

Finally, policy outcomes are often disconnected from scientific evidence in important ways. When policymakers do consult scientific evidence, they often engage with it in limited or symbolic ways to inform (or confirm) their decisions.[19,20] Academics often study the preferred policies of lawmakers, rather than their constituents, leading to "policy-based evidence-making," rather than evidence-based policymaking. Some lawmakers are actively hostile to science and use their power to restrict action by government, academic institutions, and individual researchers rather than to advance progress.[21]

Institutional Level

At the institutional level, most funders within academic public health do not grant awards for structural change, often viewing community-based research as "advocacy," which they do not support. This is due, in part, to fears of maintaining their federal tax-exempt status. Instead, grant review criteria prioritize "rigor" over community needs. Rather than facilitating opportunities for marginalized communities to equitably collaborate with academic partners, funders elevate their own philanthropic priorities—an approach that is fundamentally antithetical to the principle of "nothing about us without us."[22]

In higher education, accrediting bodies do not prioritize organizing and policy change in public health training. Such knowledge is crucial if we hope to prevent backsliding in public health and prepare future practitioners to enact the types of transformative change necessary for health equity.

Academic institutions often lack trusting relationships with surrounding communities because of ongoing and historic harms that are rarely acknowledged, much less reconciled.[23] Universities increasingly operate as extraction-oriented bureaucracies, where students are customers. Institutions of higher learning sell education as a commercial product and expand their campuses in ways that displace long-standing local businesses and residents. As universities stockpile billions in their endowments and grow ever-larger real estate portfolios, they often fail to incentivize faculty for repairing or building equitable relationships, nor do they adequately recognize the interests of community partners in setting academic research priorities.[24] When universities do build trusting relationships with community partners, rarely are these relationships institutional. Instead, they often hinge on personal relationships between specific faculty and community organizations, leaving these relationships vulnerable to departures and funding changes.

Academic institutions often reward peer-reviewed publications and grant funding over activities that lead to structural change.[25] They also fail to meaningfully invest in faculty appointments and research centers and instead rely on external support, which constrains scholarship to funders' priorities. That funding is now under threat, jeopardizing the workforces of schools of public health, medicine, and others nationwide. Academia is under siege by the federal government, state legislatures, and interest groups with ideological agendas like the elimination of tenure and diversity, equity, and inclusion practices. Despite this, many colleges and universities still do not perceive their role as political actors or use their power to transform systems.[21] This inhibits their ability to protect their students, staff, faculty, and institutional sustainability and prevents them from demonstrating the value of education and research.

In addition, academic institutions and academic disciplines hold norms that limit diversity in the types of research conducted by faculty and students.[24] They prioritize publication volume over community-engaged research and the use of methodologies shaped by White supremacy.[26–28] Changing these practices can be difficult because scholars with privileged social statuses hold power within academic institutions and control admissions, faculty hiring and retention, and curricular decisions.[26] This underscores the importance of initiatives to embrace viewpoint diversity in scholarship and diversify institutional leadership. It also explains why political resistance to change these efforts is often fierce.

Individual Level

At the individual level, academics working in public health are often trained, hired, and incentivized to focus their energy on research rather than activities that lead to structural transformation. Regardless of whether we envision our roles as academics narrowly or expansively, most of us are ill-equipped to address the central role of politics and power in health equity.[29] As researchers, we have not organized ourselves sufficiently to push for health equity or defend public health and have little preparation to do so. Many of us feel isolated and powerless because we are trained in methods suited for slow, incremental change.[26] We lack relationships with like-minded scholars or those who could use our research as a tool for change (e.g., journalists, policymakers). Still further, most researchers do not study the power-related root causes that create health inequities, (e.g., profit or political incentives) nor how to change them.[24,30]

As instructors, we often lack practically relevant, solution-oriented tools to teach students how to build and break power. Many of our syllabi focus on tweaks to what currently exists rather than encouraging consideration of what could be. This can exclude knowledge and ways of knowing that are best at challenging existing power relations.[28,31] If we do not see or treat students as generators of solutions, we will condemn them to studying—and perpetuating—the status quo.

WHAT WE CAN DO TO BUILD AND BREAK POWER

These factors necessitate a radical change if we are to shift academic public health toward advancing the goal of achieving health equity. We are angered and disheartened by the lack of progress our fields have made over the last 20 years and dismayed by the dismantling of health equity efforts happening in real time. In response, we are determined to reimagine academic public health and drive social change. We believe public health scholars need to share and build power with communities facing inequities now more than ever.

We aim to strengthen our capacity to break and build power so that we can innovate what we research and teach, hold ourselves accountable to the communities we are entrusted to serve, and increase our impact. We encourage colleagues to reflect on how their own actions might inadvertently perpetuate power imbalances—for example, by considering how we teach students about the structural determinants of health and their relationship to power. We must improve our capacity to organize and build power by forging relationships with colleagues and community organizing groups and advocating accreditation competencies focused on understanding power and its effects on systemic change. We can promote institutional change by examining how our own institutions perpetuate power imbalances and harm, while demanding action to repair relationships with surrounding communities. We can share models for transforming academic institutions to incentivize activities that address inequities, such as adopting promotion and tenure criteria that prioritize impact. Finally, we can create long-term strategic partnerships with organizing groups at the local and national level so that we can become trusted allies and engage in the political work necessary for change. This includes meaningfully connecting with local communities to learn about their needs, assisting with power-building efforts already underway, and encouraging them to hold us accountable. We can also build partnerships with scholars at other universities to resist federal, state, and local policy changes that jeopardize health equity.

As an example of applying a community organizing approach, we are working to grow our relational power within HPOP by building trusted relationships (power) and eliciting the experiences and insights of a wide base of people to inform future collective action. Careful to build power before program (e.g., direct action), our power-building process has involved

1. identifying health equity leaders through one-on-one meetings with academics to understand each person's self-interests, unique and shared pressures, and visions for the future;
2. building relationships with people across different organizations (e.g., groups working to build power to protect academic freedom and health equity initiatives);
3. building community organizing skills;
4. organizing house meetings with our base to collect personal stories that inform our shared analysis and motivate base-building; and
5. holding regular assemblies with HPOP stewards to continue to build relationships, identify shared pressures, and ratify decisions as we expand our organizing approach.

We are also building awareness through presentations and gatherings at public health conferences. Each of these efforts sharpens our shared analysis and helps build a strong network founded in authentic relationships to inform future collective action for health equity. Toward this end, we encourage readers with similar interests to reach out to the authors of this article to learn more about being in relationship with HPOP and to begin building power in their own networks and institutions. We hope that sharing our analysis will lead to broader conversations within our field about the need to build and break power to protect public health and achieve health equity. AJPH

CORRESPONDENCE

Correspondence should be sent to India Ornelas, Box 351621, University of Washington, 3980 15th Ave NE, Seattle, WA 98195 (e-mail: iornelas@uw.edu). Reprints can be ordered at https://www.ajph.org by clicking the "Reprints" link.

PUBLICATION INFORMATION

Full Citation: McMurtry CL, Givens ML, Bailey ZD, et al. Why building power is key to protecting academic public health and advancing health equity. *Am J Public Health*. 2025;115(11): 1783–1788.

Acceptance Date: May 30, 2025.

DOI: https://doi.org/10.2105/AJPH.2025.308210

ORCID iDs:
Caitlin L. McMurtry https://orcid.org/0000-0003-2617-7085

Marjory L. Givens https://orcid.org/0009-0000-7967-0389

Zinzi D. Bailey https://orcid.org/0000-0002-5708-3754

Nick Graetz https://orcid.org/0000-0002-4362-2059

Paul J. Fleming https://orcid.org/0000-0001-9150-1254

Ryan J. Petteway https://orcid.org/0000-0001-9312-5192

Julianna Pacheco https://orcid.org/0000-0002-1166-6612

Sarah E. Gollust https://orcid.org/0000-0001-6109-5953

Jonathan C. Heller https://orcid.org/0000-0001-5509-089X

Keshia M. Pollack Porter https://orcid.org/0000-0001-5363-5462

James Bloyd https://orcid.org/0000-0003-1273-9016

India J. Ornelas https://orcid.org/0000-0003-2957-6452

CONTRIBUTORS

This essay has 18 authors, all of whom have worked closely with the Health and Power Organizing Project since its inception. It presents our shared analysis of threats to population health and health equity, the result of collective intellectual efforts since 2023. All authors made substantial contributions to this article. M. L. Givens facilitated the project, and I. J. Ornelas led the development of the article, with writing assistance from C. L. McMurtry. All authors contributed to the shared analysis and contributed to the drafting or revisions of the essay.

ACKNOWLEDGMENTS

This work was supported in part by grant funding from the W. K. Kellogg Foundation (award 6011577-2022).

We would like to thank Rae Brooks, Katie Zinler, Kim Gilhuly, and Soraya Willems for thought partnership in this work.

CONFLICTS OF INTEREST

The authors have no conflicts of interest to disclose.

REFERENCES

1. Whitehead M. The concepts and principles of equity and health. *Int J Health Serv.* 1992;22(3):429–445. https://doi.org/10.2190/986L-LHQ6-2VTE-YRRN
2. World Report on Social Determinants of Health Equity. Geneva, Switzerland: World Health Organization; 2025.
3. Heller JC, Fleming PJ, Petteway RJ, Givens M, Pollack Porter KM. Power up: a call for public health to recognize, analyze, and shift the balance in power relations to advance health and racial equity. *Am J Public Health.* 2023;113(10):1079–1082. https://doi.org/10.2105/AJPH.2023.307380
4. Karatekin C, Gresham B, Barnes AJ, Corcoran F, Kritzik R, Mason SM. Re-politicizing the WHO's social determinants of health framework. *Health Promot Int.* 2024;39(5):daae122. https://doi.org/10.1093/heapro/daae122.
5. Heller JC, Givens ML, Johnson SP, Kindig DA. Keeping it political and powerful: defining the structural determinants of health. *Milbank Q.* 2024;102(2):351–366. https://doi.org/10.1111/1468-0009.12695
6. Reynolds MM, Galea S. Advancing the study of power: opportunities and priorities for understanding population health inequities. *Am J Public Health.* 2025;115(6):883–889. https://doi.org/10.2105/AJPH.2025.308015
7. Alinsky SD. *Rules for Radicals: A Pragmatic Prier for Realistic Radicals.* New York, NY: Random House; 1971.
8. Michener J. Health justice through the lens of power. *J Law Med Ethics.* 2022;50(4):656–662. https://doi.org/10.1017/jme.2023.5
9. Krieger N. ENOUGH: COVID-19, structural racism, police brutality, plutocracy, climate change—and time for health justice, democratic governance, and an equitable, sustainable future. *Am J Public Health.* 2020;110(11):1620–1623. https://doi.org/10.2105/AJPH.2020.305886
10. Jones CP. Toward the science and practice of anti-racism: launching a national campaign against racism. *Ethn Dis.* 2018;28(suppl 1):231–234. https://doi.org/10.18865/ed.28.S1.231
11. Kozlov M, Ryan C. How Trump 2.0 is slashing NIH-backed research—in charts. *Nature.* 2025;640(8060):863–865. https://doi.org/10.1038/d41586-025-01099-8
12. Coon SR, Parker L. Racial evasion policy: university leadership responses to incidents of racism in the age of neoliberalism. *J Crit Educ Policy Stud.* 2021;19(2):344–369. Available at: http://www.jceps.com/wp-content/uploads/2021/09/19-2-13-luarsep.pdf. Accessed September 9, 2025.
13. Michener J. Entrenching inequity, eroding democracy: state preemption of local housing policy. *J Health Polit Policy Law.* 2023;48(2):157–185. https://doi.org/10.1215/03616878-10234156
14. Espino MM, Ariza J. "We're not going to overcome institutional bias by doing nothing": Latinx/a/o student affairs professionals as advocates for equity. *Educ Sci.* 2022;12(10):716. https://doi.org/10.3390/educsci12100716
15. Ray V. A theory of racialized organizations. *Am Sociol Rev.* 2019;84(1):26–53. https://doi.org/10.1177/0003122418822335
16. Bender MC. Trump signs executive order targeting college accreditors. *New York Times.* April 23, 2025. Available at: https://www.nytimes.com/2025/04/23/us/politics/trump-executive-order-university-accreditors.html. Accessed May 7, 2025.
17. The White House. Reforming accreditation to strengthen higher education. April 23, 2025. Available at: https://www.whitehouse.gov/presidential-actions/2025/04/reforming-accreditation-to-strengthen-higher-education. Accessed August 27, 2025.
18. National Institutes of Health. Community Partnerships to Advance Science for Society (ComPASS). April 8, 2025. Available at: https://commonfund.nih.gov/compass. Accessed May 7, 2025.
19. Bogenschneider K, Corbett T. *Exploring the Disconnect Between Research and Policy.* London, UK: Routledge; 2010.
20. Gollust SE, Seymour JW, Pany MJ, Goss A, Meisel ZF, Grande D. Mutual distrust: perspectives from researchers and policy makers on the research to policy gap in 2013 and recommendations for the future. *Inquiry.* 2017;54:46958017705465. https://doi.org/10.1177/0046958017705465
21. Michener J, LeBrón AMW. Racism, health, and politics: advancing interdisciplinary knowledge. *J Health Polit Policy Law.* 2022;47(2):111–130. https://doi.org/10.1215/03616878-9517149
22. Charlton JI. *Nothing About Us Without Us: Disability Oppression and Empowerment.* Oakland, CA: University of California Press; 2000.
23. Scharff DP, Mathews KJ, Jackson P, Hoffsuemmer J, Martin E, Edwards D. More than Tuskegee: understanding mistrust about research participation. *J Health Care Poor Underserved.* 2010;21(3):879–897. https://doi.org/10.1353/hpu.0.0323
24. Fleming PJ, Stone LC, Creary MS, et al. Antiracism and community-based participatory research: synergies, challenges, and opportunities. *Am J Public Health.* 2023;113(1):70–78. https://doi.org/10.2105/AJPH.2022.307114
25. Cassil A. Disrupting the status quo: redesigning academic incentives to prioritize social impact in health services research. Meeting Report. AcademyHealth. September 2021. Available at: https://academyhealth.org/sites/default/files/publication/%5Bfield_date%3Acustom%3AY%5D-%5Bfield_date%3Acustom%3Am%5D/distrupting_the_status_quo_september2021.pdf. Accessed February 15, 2025.
26. Bailey ZD, Krieger N, Agénor M, Graves J, Linos N, Bassett MT. Structural racism and health inequities in the USA: evidence and interventions. *Lancet.* 2017;389(10077):1453–1463. https://doi.org/10.1016/S0140-6736(17)30569-X
27. Givens ML, Gennuso KP, Pollock EA, Johnson SL. Deconstructing inequities – transparent values in measurement and analytic choices. *N Engl J Med.* 2021;384(19):1861–1865. https://doi.org/10.1056/NEJMms2035717
28. Petteway RJ. On epidemiology as racial-capitalist (re) colonization and epistemic violence. *Crit Public Health.* 2023;33(1):5–12. https://doi.org/10.1080/09581596.2022.2107486
29. Jessani NS, Ling B, Babcock C, Valmeekanathan A, Holtgrave DR. Advocacy, activism, and lobbying: how variations in interpretation affects ability for academia to engage with public policy. *PLOS Glob Public Health.* 2022;2(3):e0000034. https://doi.org/10.1371/journal.pgph.0000034
30. Pacheco J, Gollust SE, Callaghan T, Motta M. A call for measuring partisanship in US public health research. *Am J Public Health.* 2024;114(8):772–776. https://doi.org/10.2105/AJPH.2024.307691
31. Manalo-Pedro E, Walsemann KM, Gee GC. Whose knowledge heals? Transforming teaching in the struggle for health equity. *Health Educ Behav.* 2023;50(4):482–492. https://doi.org/10.1177/10901981231177095

The Plight of Marginalized Populations in 2025: The Assault on Health Equity Through a Systems Lens

Steven H. Woolf, MD, MPH, Marshall H. Chin, MD, MPH, Velma M. Murry, PhD, and Gilbert C. Gee, PhD

ABOUT THE AUTHORS

Steven H. Woolf is with the Department of Family Medicine and Population Health, Virginia Commonwealth University School of Medicine, Richmond, VA. Marshall H. Chin is with the Department of Medicine, University of Chicago, Chicago, IL. Velma M. Murry is with the Department of Human and Organizational Development, Vanderbilt University, Nashville, TN. Gilbert C. Gee is with the Department of Community Health Sciences, Fielding School of Public Health, University of California Los Angeles.

Note. The ideas expressed in this editorial are those of the authors and do not necessarily represent the views or policies of their employers or other organizations with which they are associated.

The health equity literature frequently alludes to systemic, structural, and institutional racism, but often fails to connect the dots between these systems and health outcomes. How exactly are health inequities produced by structures and institutions within our society? Scholars have examined the role of diverse systems, including not only health care but also education, housing, economic development and employment, safety net programs, law and justice, foreign policy, immigration, and the media. Past policies like redlining and restrictive covenants are often cited as historical examples in which policymakers took overt action to alter structures and institutions to segregate and exclude marginalized groups.

The events of 2025 remind us that history repeats itself. We describe a concerted effort by today's policymakers to restore restrictions on marginalized populations on a massive scale by targeting systems, structures, and institutions in virtually every area of public policy. Specifically, this article details how federal and state policies enacted in 2025 served to decrease access to opportunity structures for economic vitality, education, housing, justice, and health care. At breathtaking speed, the administration weaponized the state; pushed legal boundaries to dismantle diversity, equity, and inclusion (DEI) initiatives; and threatened dissenters with legal and financial retaliation. It decimated the nation's scientific infrastructure, seeking not only to censor data and impede scholarship but also to erase the historical narrative of how racism produced today's inequities. This strategy served to weaken efforts to call out and understand inequitable policies and solve the nation's struggle with racism.

The population health consequences of the events of 2025 are profound, not only because of the attacks on the nation's public health infrastructure but also because they directly affected the social drivers of health (e.g., education, income, employment, housing, access to health care). Looking forward, the long-term impact is likely to deepen inequities, because the rollback of civil rights protections reviewed in this article poses a disproportionate risk to all Americans who are marginalized on the basis of their race/ethnicity, gender, sexual orientation, socioeconomic status, disability, or religion—including low-income White Americans. Deepening inequity also poses a threat to the nation, sowing division, weakening the economy, and sapping the nation's vitality and security. In the end, marginalized people—be they White or people of color—will bear the brunt of the damage.

A SYSTEMS PERSPECTIVE ON 2025

The 2024 campaign season saw an abrupt shift in the national conversation about racism and social justice. Politicians used DEI (a term ostensibly referring to hiring and school admission policies to widen opportunities for historically marginalized populations) as a pretext for assailing civil rights protections broadly and for further enriching the elite by redirecting resources away from marginalized groups. Politicians played off the emotions of an aggrieved populace, whose zero-sum mentality stoked fears of displacement by an increasingly diverse population. The anti-DEI movement became a vehicle for revolting against all efforts to widen opportunity for historically marginalized groups and a rallying cry for those with White supremacist sentiments. Clever political strategists seized the moment, pulling off a stunning

AJPH November 2025, Vol. 115, No. 11

reversal in language that rebranded DEI as racist and discriminatory. They used poll-tested words (e.g., "woke," "radical") to stir resentment and applied divide-and-conquer strategies to turn marginalized communities against each other.

The anti-DEI movement was codified in a flurry of executive orders[1] that not only eliminated DEI offices and staff but also targeted civil rights reforms that had widened opportunities for historically marginalized populations. The executive orders seemed intended to marginalize all groups, with the exception of cisgendered White males, favoring the wealthy. Programs at any federal agency that catered to people of color were cunningly rebranded as "reverse discrimination" in violation of civil rights, as were programs for those who identified as lesbian, gay, bisexual, transgender, queer or questioning, and other diverse sexual orientations and gender identities (LGBTQ+). The president ended enforcement of the "disparate impact" principle, which for 50 years had barred policies that, intentionally or not, exert a disproportionate effect on a demographic group.[1] The prosecution of DEI was expanded to DEI-A, deprioritizing accessibility measures for disabled Americans.[1] In addition to exercising his legal powers, the president used intimidation and extortion to pressure institutions to meet his demands.

With little subtlety, people of color were singled out for insults and policy changes across government, from layoffs and program terminations to the removal of historical materials from government buildings and cemeteries. The common themes behind these efforts were to decrease access to opportunity for marginalized populations, revise the historical narrative about racism, and pressure institutions to adopt anti-DEI policies. The administration implemented this agenda in every sector of public policy: education, housing, employment, social welfare programs, the law, voting rights, immigration, environmental policy, science, health care, and more.

Education

The administration dismantled programs meant to broaden educational opportunities for students of color, threatening legal action or loss of federal funding if schools, colleges, and universities failed to comply.[1] Saying that it was combating anti-Semitism, the administration targeted elite academic institutions like Harvard University, withholding billions of dollars in federal grants unless they revised policies related to DEI and international students.[2] The federal government and many states also began altering curricula to remove content labeled as DEI.[3] The Department of Education began investigating accreditation bodies for requiring schools to meet DEI-related accreditation requirements.

Housing

The administration reduced housing assistance for low-income households, a population overrepresented by Black and Hispanic residents.[4] It instituted plans to slash rental assistance, eliminate Section 8 vouchers that help low-income residents secure housing, and cancel funding for community programs on homelessness and disaster recovery.[4] It took steps to weaken the 1968 Fair Housing Act, which prohibited discrimination in the rental, sales, and financing of housing.[4] It cut funding to the Fair Housing Program, closed hundreds of fair housing cases, terminated the US Interagency Council on Homelessness, and rolled back support for chronically unhoused people.[4]

Economic Development and Employment

The administration altered the equal employment opportunity provisions of the 1964 Civil Rights Act, which protect workers against job discrimination.[1] Federal staff lost civil service protections and were instructed to report coworkers engaging in DEI. As DEI offices closed throughout the government, large and small employers across the country followed suit.[5] Policies to aid the poor and middle class were also targeted, as when the president rescinded a Biden-era increase in the minimum wage.[1] The administration declared English the official language, likely reincarnating racist bans on non-English languages in workplaces.[1]

Safety Net Programs

The administration and Congress sought large reductions in discretionary spending, focusing on cutting disbursements for Medicaid and safety net programs such as the Supplemental Nutrition Assistance Program, disproportionately affecting families with children, elderly individuals, and those with disabilities.[6] Policymakers also sought cuts in Temporary Assistance for Needy Families, the Social Services Block Grant, the Administration for Community Living, and the Low-Income Home Energy Assistance Program, among others. The administration's plans to shift safety net responsibilities to states raised concern among states that lacked the resources to absorb the demand.[7]

Criminal Justice

In a disturbing pivot, the Civil Rights Division of the Department of Justice shifted its focus to prosecuting violations of the president's DEI orders.[8] The administration retreated from prosecuting corruption and white-collar criminals.[9] It rolled back efforts to prosecute police misconduct, dismissing lawsuits and consent decrees (court-ordered agreements with police departments),[10] and took steps to prioritize arrests over criminal justice. The administration strengthened police immunity, pressured cities to increase arrests, and reinstituted the death penalty.[9] Programs to alleviate mass incarceration were defunded, including those supporting violence intervention, youth justice, alternatives to incarceration, reentry, and victim services.[9] The Bureau of Justice Statistics removed gender and gender identity from surveys, eliminating the ability to track hate crimes and violence against transgender persons.

Voting Rights

Efforts to weaken protections of the Voting Rights Act of 1965 were pursued by the administration and many states. The Department of Justice dropped lawsuits over gerrymandering to dilute the voting strength of Black and Latino voters.[11] Although the federal code already bars noncitizens from voting in federal elections, the White House and Congress took steps to require documentary proof of citizenship (e.g., passports), which White citizens can more readily access than citizens of color.[1,12] They also threatened to withhold federal funding from states that counted absentee and mail-in ballots received after Election Day, a tactic known to suppress minority votes.[13]

Immigration

The administration embraced xenophobia, treating people from other countries as inherently dangerous. It focused heavily (but not exclusively) on migrants from Latin America.[14] For example, the administration turned away asylum seekers crossing the United States–Mexico border but made an exception for White Afrikaners from South Africa. The administration ended the international refugee program, revoked visas for international students, eliminated temporary protected status for immigrants, and challenged birthright citizenship.[1,15] People of color were surveilled, apprehended, arrested, and sometimes transferred without due process from prisons to remote detention centers or other countries.[14] Notably, the administration invoked the Alien Enemies Act of 1798 to deport Venezuelan immigrants to El Salvador.[15]

Environmental Policy

Programs addressing the environment, climate change, and severe weather—which disproportionately affect vulnerable low-income and minoritized communities—were eliminated.[1] The administration relaxed environmental regulations on industries, canceled investments in clean energy, terminated programs to deal with severe weather, and reduced funding for disaster recovery assistance. It ended programs to address extreme heat, which disproportionately affects people of color living in urban heat islands. Environmental justice programs that reduce harmful exposure of low-income and minority communities to nearby highways and industrial sites were eliminated.[16]

Health Care

The administration sought to cut funding for public insurance programs that serve low-income families, including Medicaid and subsidies to low-income applicants under the Affordable Care Act. It sought to cut funding for the Prevention and Public Health Fund, suicide prevention programs for LGBTQ+ youths, tribal and minority health programs (including deep cuts to the Indian Health Service), HIV/AIDS clinics, mental health services, and training of health care workers to serve in underrepresented communities.[17] Conservative states tightened restrictions on reproductive health services, disproportionately affecting low-income and minoritized women who could not travel elsewhere. Black infant mortality in these states increased by 11%.[18]

Research and Data

In addition to massive cuts in staffing and funding of federal research agencies and the termination of hundreds of grants to universities and other research centers, the administration expressly prohibited research with any ties to DEI, sexual orientation and gender identity, and climate science.[1] Agencies removed or modified thousands of webpages and data sets on these topics, a strategy that served to make inequities invisible. Fearing repercussions, university faculty conducting research on health equity issues—many of them scholars of color—felt pressured to remove their names as authors, reword manuscripts and grant proposals to avoid terms that agencies would flag, or abandon projects altogether.[19] Journal editors were contacted by a US attorney investigating whether their practices, including the publication of papers on health equity, conflicted with the president's agenda.

Arts and Culture

The administration removed the first Black director of the National Library of Congress, ordered the Smithsonian Institution to remove "improper" exhibits depicting the history of racism, and called for restoring controversial monuments (e.g., Confederate memorials).[1] The National Museum of African American History and Culture lost its director and was at risk for closure.[20] Funding for community-based arts programs, many of which featured ethnic art or were located in low-income communities, was slashed.[21]

Media

The president targeted the free press, an important vehicle for social justice, and attacked media outlets responsible for unfavorable media coverage.[22] The administration ordered the end of federal funding for National Public Radio and the Public Broadcasting Service,[1] while simultaneously joining forces with conservative social media to fill the information space with divisive content, such as that disseminated by Elon Musk, to advance misleading narratives around racism. For example, the White House and conservative media circulated unrelated photographs to promote a false story of White genocide in South Africa.[23]

CONCLUSION

This situation—the permeation of racism in multiple sectors by systems of discrimination—has occurred before. For example, policies and social norms in the Jim Crow Era saturated virtually all institutions and structures of the United States. However, the institutions of democracy that bolstered the Civil Rights Movement and its emergence from Jim Crow, such as an intact judicial system, are now in jeopardy. In the past, Supreme Court rulings on school desegregation, voting rights, and fair housing met with resistance but were ultimately executed. The 2025 administration is now openly defying court orders and threatening judges whose rulings they find disagreeable. The leaders of Congress, an institution that once passed historic civil rights bills, have abandoned their responsibility to check the power of the executive branch. Past presidents who disliked laws would still enforce them, as when Eisenhower dispatched federal troops to the South, whereas today's Supreme Court has granted full immunity against crimes committed as official acts of the presidency.

At this writing (June 2025), it is difficult to predict how many of the administration's actions, now tied up in litigation, will prevail, but the trajectory is concerning. Experts on tyranny are warning that the president is seizing untrammeled powers, that a constitutional crisis is erupting, that American democracy is giving way to authoritarianism, and that a descent into fascism, once unimaginable, could easily occur.[24] Time will tell whether, years hence, these fears are alarmist or prescient.

For marginalized Americans, what is clear from history is that their needs are likely to be sidelined by the powerful unless an organized social movement demands change. History teaches that change occurs when movements focus on reforming systems and collective engagement with communities. Throughout 2025, the administration picked off institutions, one at a time. Universities, law firms, media companies, and other targets often stood alone in court, missing the opportunity to achieve greater impact by joining forces. Absent the coordinated leverage exerted by past civil rights movements—filling the streets, engaging in boycotts, and voting for change—the current administration's agenda is likely to prevail, and inequities will tragically deepen. For the public health community, which will find itself documenting the widening gaps in life expectancy and other health outcomes, the moral imperative in the face of cruelty is clear.[25] It must uphold its values, to protect the needy, denounce racism and other forms of discrimination, and advocate social justice—regardless of political retribution.

Additional references are available in a supplement to the online version of this article at https://ajph.org. AJPH

CORRESPONDENCE

Correspondence should be sent to Steven H. Woolf, MD, MPH, Department of Family Medicine and Population Health, Virginia Commonwealth University School of Medicine, 830 East Main St, Suite 5035, Richmond, VA 23298-0212 (e-mail: steven.woolf@vcuhealth.org). Reprints can be ordered at https://www.ajph.org by clicking the "Reprints" link.

PUBLICATION INFORMATION

Full Citation: Woolf SH, Chin MH, Murry VM, Gee GC. The plight of marginalized populations in 2025: the assault on health equity through a systems lens. *Am J Public Health*. 2025;115(11):1789–1794.

Acceptance Date: June 16, 2025.

DOI: https://doi.org/10.2105/AJPH.2025.308221

ORCID iDs:

Steven H. Woolf https://orcid.org/0000-0001-9384-033X

Marshall H. Chin https://orcid.org/0000-0003-1924-5641

Velma M. Murry https://orcid.org/0000-0003-2663-2738

Gilbert C. Gee https://orcid.org/0000-0002-1716-9465

CONTRIBUTORS

G. C. Gee originated the editorial. S. H. Woolf served as lead author. M. H. Chin, V. M. Murry, and G. C. Gee collaborated with S. H. Woolf to review and edit article drafts.

CONFLICTS OF INTEREST

S. H. Woolf serves as senior fellow at the Center for American Progress and has received funding from the National Collaborative for Health Equity. M. H. Chin reported receiving grants or contracts separate from this work from the Agency for Healthcare Research and Quality, California Health Care Foundation, Health Resources and Services Administration, Kaiser Foundation Health Plan, Merck Foundation, National Institute of Diabetes and Digestive and Kidney Diseases (NIDDK), Patient-Centered Outcomes Research Institute, and Robert Wood Johnson Foundation; that he is a member of the Bristol-Myers Squibb Company Health Equity Advisory Board, Blue Cross Blue Shield Health Equity Advisory Panel, Essential Hospitals Institute Innovation Committee, Institute for Healthcare Improvement and American Medical Association National Initiative for Health Equity Steering Committee for Measurement, National Committee for Quality Assurance Expert Work Group on role of social determinants of health data in health care quality measurement, Council of Medical Specialty Societies Encoding Equity in Clinical Research and Practice Alliance Advisory Committee, and Advisory Board for the America's Health Insurance Plans 2025 Annual Conference; co-chaired the Health Equity Advisory Team for the Centers for Medicare & Medicaid Services Health Care Payment Learning and Action Network; and was a member of the National Advisory Council of the National Institute on Minority Health and Health Disparities, the Health Disparities and Health Equity Working Group of the NIDDK, Families USA Equity and Value Task Force Advisory Council, National Academy of Medicine Council, Centers for Disease Control and Prevention (CDC) and American College of Physicians Advisory Committee I Raise the Rates: Promotion of Influenza Immunization through Interprofessional Partnership, and The Joint Commission Health Care Equity Certification Technical Advisory Panel; and was a subject matter expert for the Institute for Healthcare Improvement Health Equity Alliance Accelerator. He has received honoraria from Sutter Health and Genentech (Sutter Health supports the Institute for Healthcare Improvement Health Equity Alliance Accelerator in part with funding provided by Genentech) and received support for attending meetings and travel from America's Health Insurance Plans. V. M. Murry has received funding from the National Institutes of Health, CDC, Spencer Foundation, and Patient-Centered Outcomes Research Institute. She is a member of the National Advisory Mental Health Research Council and the National Academy of Medicine, and has served on several National Academies Consensus Study Committees and Workshop Forums. In the past three years, G. C. Gee has received funding from the National Institutes of Health, the California Academic Health Department and California Alliance of Academics and Communities for Health Equity, the California Endowment, the Robert Wood Johnson Foundation, The Mellon Foundation, the Australian Research Council, and the Sierra Foundation. He has also served as the co-chair of the Board of Social and Community Sciences subcommittee of the Scientific Counselors for the Environmental Protection Agency (EPA), and on the executive committee of the Board of Scientific Counselors for the EPA. He has also served as a member of the National Advisory Committee for the Evidence for Action, and was a content expert, consultant, or on the advisory board for the Connect for Cancer Prevention Study, the Time Use Project for Health and Well-Being, California Center for Population Research, a data safety and monitoring board for Massachusetts General Hospital, the *Health Affairs* journal, and the National Longitudinal Survey of Youth 2026.

REFERENCES

1. The White House. Presidential actions. Available at: https://www.whitehouse.gov/presidential-actions/?s=. Accessed May 30, 2025.
2. Bender MC. All the actions the Trump administration has taken against Harvard. *New York Times.* May 22, 2025. Available at: https://www.nytimes.com/2025/05/22/us/politics/harvard-university-trump.html?searchResultPosition=14. Accessed May 30, 2025.
3. Schwartz S. A wave of new legislation aims to ban DEI in public schools. *Education Week.* March 26, 2025. Available at: https://www.edweek.org/leadership/a-wave-of-new-legislation-aims-to-ban-dei-in-public-schools/2025/03. Accessed May 30, 2025.
4. Wheeler S. Updated list of all Trump's actions that impact housing. *Housingwire.* May 22, 2025. Available at: https://www.housingwire.com/articles/updated-list-of-all-trumps-actions-that-impact-housing. Accessed May 30, 2025.
5. Goldberg E, Krolik A, Boyce L. How corporate America is retreating from DEI. *New York Times.* March 13, 2025. Available at: https://www.nytimes.com/interactive/2025/03/13/business/corporate-america-dei-policy-shifts.html. Accessed May 30, 2025.
6. Bogage J. What's in Republicans' giant tax and immigration bill? *Washington Post.* May 14, 2025. Available at: https://www.washingtonpost.com/business/2025/05/13/republican-trump-tax-immigration-plan. Accessed May 30, 2025.
7. Kallins L, Katz E. How proposed changes to federal safety net programs could affect the states. National Conference of State Legislatures. May 2, 2025. Available at: https://www.ncsl.org/state-legislatures-news/details/how-proposed-changes-to-federal-safety-net-programs-could-affect-the-states. Accessed May 30, 2025.
8. Jurecic Q. Justice department releases slate of memos from Attorney General Bondi. *Lawfare.* Available at: https://www.lawfaremedia.org/article/justice-dept.-releases-slate-of-memos-from-attorney-general-bondi. Accessed June 17, 2025.
9. Michaels D, Vanderford R, Fanelli J. Trump administration retreats from white-collar criminal enforcement. *Wall Street Journal.* April 13, 2025. Available at: https://www.wsj.com/finance/regulation/trump-doj-white-collar-law-enforcement-4d27b06d. Accessed May 30, 2025.
10. Johnson C, Lucas R. Trump DOJ dismisses investigations of police in several cities, including Minneapolis. *NPR.* May 21, 2025. Available at: https://www.npr.org/2025/05/21/nx-s1-5406262/trump-administration-dismisses-police-investigations-minneapolis-george-floyd. Accessed June 16, 2025.
11. Wang HL. Under Trump, the Justice Department is stepping away from some voting rights cases. *NPR.* March 31, 2025. Available at: https://www.npr.org/2025/03/24/nx-s1-5332145/voting-rights-act-1965-justice-department. Accessed May 30, 2025.
12. Bomboy S. Understanding voter registration changes proposed by Congress and the president. National Constitution Center. April 10, 2025. Available at: https://constitutioncenter.org/blog/understanding-voter-registration-changes-proposed-by-congress-and-the-president. Accessed May 30, 2025.
13. Hing AK. The right to vote, the right to health: voter suppression as a determinant of racial health disparities. *J Health Dispar Res Pract.* 2020;12(6):48–62. https://doi.org/jhdrp/vol12/iss6/5
14. US Immigration and Customs Enforcement. ICE enforcement and removal operations statistics. Available at: https://www.ice.gov/statistics. Accessed May 30, 2025.
15. Watson T, Zars J. 100 days of immigration under the second Trump administration. Brookings. April 29, 2025. Available at: https://www.brookings.edu/articles/100-days-of-immigration-under-the-second-trump-administration. Accessed May 30, 2025.
16. Volcovici V, Lynch SN, Mason J. Trump administration cuts environmental justice programs at EPA, DOJ. *Reuters.* February 6, 2025. Available at: https://www.reuters.com/world/us/trump-administration-cuts-environmental-justice-programs-epa-doj-sources-say-2025-02-06. Accessed May 30, 2025.
17. Sun LH, Johnson CY, Roubein R, Achenbach J, Lauren W. Internal budget document reveals extent of Trump's proposed health cuts. *Washington Post.* April 16, 2025. Available at: https://www.washingtonpost.com/health/2025/04/16/hhs-budget-cut-trump. Accessed May 30, 2025.
18. Gemmill A, Franks AM, Anjur-Dietrich S, et al. US abortion bans and infant mortality. *JAMA.* 2025;333(15):1315–1323. https://doi.org/10.1001/jama.2024.28517
19. Bibbins-Domingo K, Bonow RO, Bressler NM, et al. Reaffirming the JAMA Network commitment to the health of patients and the public. *JAMA.* 2025;333:1121–1122. https://doi.org/10.1001/jama.2025.2405

20. Bowley G, Pogrebin R, Schuessler J. National African American museum faces uncertainty without its leader. *New York Times.* May 9, 2025. Available at: https://www.nytimes.com/2025/05/06/arts/design/smithsonian-national-african-american-museum-kevin-young.html. Accessed June 1, 2025.
21. Reizman R. Casualties in Trump's war on the arts: the small museums keeping local history alive. *The Guardian.* May 25, 2025. Available at: https://www.theguardian.com/us-news/2025/may/25/small-museums-trump-cuts-arts-funding. Accessed June 1, 2025.
22. James M. FCC commissioner sounds alarms about free speech 'chilling effect' under Trump. *Los Angeles Times.* May 29, 2025. Available at: https://www.latimes.com/entertainment-arts/business/story/2025-05-29/fcc-commissioner-discusses-protecting-free-speech. Accessed June 1, 2025.
23. Mwai P, Murphy M, Horton J, Cheetham J. Fact-checking Trump's Oval Office confrontation with Ramaphosa. *BBC.* May 22, 2025. Available at: https://www.bbc.com/news/articles/ce9vxve994ro. Accessed June 1, 2025.
24. Shore M, Snyder T, Stanley J. We study fascism, and we're leaving the US. *New York Times.* May 14, 2025. Available at: https://www.nytimes.com/2025/05/14/opinion/yale-canada-fascism.html. Accessed May 30, 2025.
25. Chin MH, Muramatsu N, Pollack HA. Cruelty and health inequity. *J Gen Intern Med.* 2023;38(12):2821–2823. https://doi.org/10.1007/s11606-023-08263-8

Gender Affirmation Research Is Not Gender Ideology Extremism, It Is Science

Arjee J. Restar, PhD, MPH, Kristi E. Gamarel, PhD, EdM, and Don Operario, PhD

ABOUT THE AUTHORS

Arjee J. Restar is with the Department of Social and Behavioral Science, Yale University School of Public Health, New Haven, CT. Kristi E. Gamarel is with the Department of Health Behavior and Health Equity, and the Institute for Social Research Population Studies Center, University of Michigan School of Public Health, Ann Arbor. Don Operario is with the Department of Behavioral, Social, and Health Education Sciences, Emory University Rollins School of Public Health, Atlanta, GA, when this article was written.

The recent termination of National Institutes of Health (NIH) grants focused on gender affirmation research is an unprecedented attack on scientific inquiry. Following Executive Order 14168, issued January 20, 2025, federal agencies—including the NIH—were directed to recognize only "two sexes, male and female" as "immutable" and "grounded in fundamental and incontrovertible reality."[1] The order explicitly prohibits funding for programs that "promote gender ideology," leading to the cancellation of studies on transgender, nonbinary, and other gender-diverse (hereafter, "trans") population health across multiple NIH institutes.[2,3]

According to ongoing tracking initiatives monitoring these cancellations, more than 8.5% of NIH-funded research studies on trans health (195 out of 2100) have been terminated, with six having "frozen funding" and 101 currently in a "possibly reinstated" status as of July 20, 2025.[3] These terminated grants include research, training, and infrastructure projects.[3] In many cases, principal investigators of terminated grants reported that their terminations were explicitly attributed to alleged noncompliance with the executive order's ban on "gender ideology extremism."[2,3] Termination notices claimed that such research "no longer effectuates agency priorities," dismissing it as "unscientific," offering "little identifiable return on investment," and failing to "enhance the health of many Americans," while allegedly ignoring "biological realities."[1]

These assertions profoundly mischaracterize rigorous, evidence-based research on gender affirmation as mere ideology. In fact, it is the order itself—driven by ideological motives rather than scientific reasoning—that introduces a dangerous epistemological distortion. This politicization of science undermines both the integrity of gender-related research and the foundational principles that sustain scientific progress across topics and disciplines.

Gender affirmation research is the interdisciplinary scientific investigation of the multilevel processes—medical, psychosocial, legal, policy—by which trans people affirm their gender identity.[4,5] What fundamentally distinguishes gender affirmation research from ideology is its epistemological foundation. Science advances through empirical observation, testable hypotheses, reproducible methods, and systematic peer review[6,7]—all while maintaining a commitment to uncertainty and revision in the face of new evidence.[8] These core principles of scientific inquiry have been established across disciplines and serve as the foundation for evidence-based knowledge production.[9] Gender affirmation research exemplifies these principles using rigorous methodological approaches, including population-based sampling, validated measurement instruments, statistical adjustment for confounding, longitudinal cohort designs, and community-engaged research frameworks.[10–16] These tools ensure that findings are grounded in observable reality—not in ideology or assumption.

GENDER-AFFIRMING RESEARCH FOLLOWS SCIENTIFIC PRINCIPLES

Empirical evidence clearly demonstrates that gender affirmation research adheres to established scientific standards and yields measurable, translational results—hallmarks of credible science. This body of research has consistently shown that gender-affirming care is associated with significant improvements in health outcomes. Systematic reviews and population-based studies repeatedly find that gender-affirming care improves quality of life and reduces psychological distress, suicidality, and all-cause mortality at clinically

AJPH November 2025, Vol. 115, No. 11

meaningful levels.[11,15,17–21] These findings underscore the practical and ethical imperative of supporting this research—not silencing it.

Over the past several decades, gender affirmation research has directly informed the development of evidence-based clinical practice guidelines adopted by major medical organizations, including the World Professional Association for Transgender Health, the American Academy of Pediatrics, and the Endocrine Society.[22,23] Studies in this field have led to the refinement of surgical techniques, resulting in improved patient outcomes and reduced complication rates for gender-affirming procedures.[22,23] Scientific research advancements in gender-affirming care have also contributed to the safety optimization of tailored hormone therapy protocols according to individual health needs (i.e., precision medicine approaches), enabling more personalized and effective treatment.[23]

Gender affirmation research has also shaped comprehensive care models that integrate medical, mental health, and social services, resulting in improved patient satisfaction and mental health outcomes compared with fragmented care.[4,15] Furthermore, these studies have informed institutional, state, and federal policies, contributing to the reduction of health care disparities and the expansion of insurance coverage for gender-affirming care.[5]

These findings have been replicated across diverse geographic contexts and health care settings and through a variety of methodological designs in the United States[12] and globally.[13] Such reproducibility is a cornerstone of credible science and sharply distinguishes it from ideological assertion. Far from being fringe or speculative, gender-affirming care is supported by a growing, interdisciplinary body of evidence.[13] And when methodological challenges do arise—as in the widely discussed 2019 study examining causal inference in the relationship between gender-affirming care and mental health outcomes[24]—the scientific community responds not with denial but with deeper inquiry and empirical refinement.[14]

This approach stands in stark contrast to ideologically driven reviews, such as the Cass Review of gender identity services for children and young people in the United Kingdom[25] and the Department of Health and Human Services Review of Treatment of Pediatric Gender Dysphoria in the United States,[26] both of which have been criticized for their flawed methodologies, including selective interpretation of evidence and predetermined conclusions that discount the experiences and needs of transgender individuals.[27]

Conversely, comprehensive systematic reviews adhering to scientific review standards—such as the recent review by Utah's Department of Health and Human Services—demonstrate how a balanced review of the state of science can acknowledge both strengths and limitations of the current evidence base.[14] Reviews of gender affirmation research must continue to prioritize methodological rigor, critical inquiry, knowledge refinement, and the advancement of population health—principles that stand in marked contrast to ideologically driven approaches that seek to confirm predetermined beliefs rather than engage with the full scope of scientific evidence.

Gender affirmation research exemplifies methodological pluralism—a foundational tenet of scientific advancement that directly opposes ideological rigidity.[7] Where ideology—whether political, religious, or cultural—often demands adherence to a single, immutable belief, science thrives on multiplicity and openness to revision. This pluralistic approach enables triangulation across varied study designs, producing more robust and comprehensive insights than any one method could achieve alone.[7] Research in this area draws on a rich array of disciplines—including endocrinology, psychology, public health, epidemiology, biostatistics, legal studies, and health policy—each offering distinct methodologies and perspectives to deepen our understanding of gender and its intersections with health.[13]

A clear example is the work of Sevelius et al., who developed the gender affirmation conceptual framework, which explicitly integrates multiple theoretical frameworks to understand the unique needs of trans women of color.[28,29] The gender affirmation framework has been expanded to include multiple domains of gender affirmation[4] and move beyond the individual level on analysis.[28–30]

From longitudinal cohort studies to qualitative ethnography, from randomized controlled trials to community-based participatory research, bibliometric analysis shows that gender affirmation research has consistently employed rigorous designs that test explicit hypotheses, address uncertainty, and progressively refine knowledge.[28] This epistemic breadth is not a flaw: it is a scientific strength, grounded in the very ethos of inquiry and critical examination. Far from ideological, it is science at its most robust.

GENDER AFFIRMATION SCIENCE IS GROUNDED IN DATA, NOT IDEOLOGY

Ideology is defined by its reliance on fixed axioms and its resistance to revision—even in the face of contradictory evidence. Executive Order 14168's assertion that biological sex is "immutable" and "grounded in fundamental and incontrovertible reality" exemplifies this rigidity, disregarding decades of scientific research that has illuminated the biological complexity of sex. This includes well-documented research on chromosomal variation, hormone receptor diversity, and differences in sexual development.[31,32] Current estimates indicate that approximately 0.018% to 1.7% of births involve some form of intersex condition or difference in sex development, depending on the definitions and diagnostic criteria used,[33–35] thereby affecting millions of individuals whose biological reality challenges the binary sex framework reinforced by the executive order.

Research has consistently documented the psychological and physical harms of enforcing binary norms through nonconsensual medical interventions on intersex individuals, including elevated risks of mental health problems, sexual dysfunction, and loss of fertility.[35,36] Gender affirmation research does not ignore these complexities: it engages them directly through evidence-based methodologies that distinguish between sex assigned at birth, gender identity, and physiological traits.[37,38] Far from rejecting biology, the field of gender affirmation research integrates biological, medical, psychosocial, and legal dimensions of health using rigorous, multidimensional analyses. Researchers in this space employ carefully developed and validated measures that far exceed the reductive binary framework imposed by ideologically driven mandates.

This work is guided by recommendations from and for epidemiologists to precisely measure gender and avoid the pitfalls of erasing nonbinary and intersex individuals in data collection systems[16] and to move toward expansive frameworks and modalities.[39,40] Consequently, contemporary frameworks for understanding gender recognize it as a multidimensional construct, moving beyond simplistic binary categorizations to acknowledge the full spectrum of human gender diversity.

These frameworks begin with the understanding that both sex and gender are shaped by complex interactions among genetic, epigenetic, anatomical, biological, physiological, cognitive, environmental, historical, and cultural factors,[16,39,40] challenging any singular or static definition and emphasizing the dynamic nature of human development. These triangulated practices reflect scientific integrity, not dogma. Not only is the claim that gender affirmation research "ignores biological realities" false, it is a projection of the very ideological distortion it alleges. By insisting on a rigid binary that contradicts observable data, Executive Order 14168 undermines the scientific values it claims to uphold.

More importantly, the existence of trans populations is not a theoretical abstraction but an empirically grounded reality, documented across cultures and centuries.[41,42] Although the executive order's definition of gender negates and erases the existence of trans people,[1] historical and anthropological evidence and records consistently affirm the presence of gender-diverse individuals in a wide range of societies. Examples include the *hijras* of South Asia, *kathoey* (or third-gender) individuals in Thailand, the *babaylan* of the Philippines, Two-Spirit identities among Indigenous North American peoples, and the *muxe* of the Zapotec people—many of whom have long held respected and culturally significant roles.[16,43] Science must begin from this truth—that trans people have always existed and do exist—if it is to preserve its integrity. To ignore, deny, or refuse to measure gender with such extensive evidence of gender diversity is not an act of neutrality or objectivity but an ideologically motivated act of distortion and erasure of empirical reality.[16,41,42] It is a deliberate ideological stance masquerading as science.

DEFENDING SCIENCE AGAINST IDEOLOGICAL ATTACKS

When political mandates override evidence and undermine lines of research inquiry, the consequences extend far beyond any single field. Such actions erode public trust in science, compromise health outcomes, and silence the voices of communities already relegated to the margins of care. Trans people face direct harms; additionally, their families report elevated psychological distress, and health care providers and researchers face moral injury, professional burnout, and a chilling effect when barred from delivering standard-of-care treatments.[44] Moreover, the erosion of public trust in the science of gender and health contributes to the proliferation of misinformation, disinformation, and pseudoscientific claims about trans people, which have been directly linked to increased discrimination, violence, and legislative attacks on trans rights across multiple states.[44–46]

When ideologically driven narratives about gender-affirming care are elevated above scientific consensus and weaponized through policy to legitimize misinformation and penalize noncompliance, public confidence in medical guidance deteriorates. This discourages trans individuals from seeking essential, evidence-based care, jeopardizing both individual and public health.[45,47,48] These harms do not occur in isolation: they contribute to a broader erosion of trust in medical science and clinical practice as a whole.

The implications of Executive Order 14168 on trans population health outcomes are not simply rhetorical: they are measurable and verifiable. Emerging studies have documented the harmful effects of antitrans legislation, which include increased depression, anxiety, and suicidality in this population.[49–51] With a growing number of state bills seeking to restrict, ban, or criminalize gender-affirming care[52] and the US Supreme Court's six to three majority decision in *United States v Skrmetti*[53] upholding state bans on gender-affirming care for trans youth, the future of access remains uncertain and determined by state governments.

The data are clear: trans youths who need but are denied gender-affirming care report nearly double the rate of suicidal ideation compared with those who receive it.[54] According to the Trevor Project's 2024 National Survey, 39% of LGBTQ+ (lesbian, gay, bisexual, transgender, queer or questioning, and all subsects) youths seriously considered suicide in the past year, including 46% of transgender and nonbinary youths.[55] In this context, continued efforts to deny and restrict gender-affirming care are not medically unjustifiable or ethically indefensible—especially in the absence of any scalable, evidence-based suicide prevention strategies specifically designed to meet the needs of trans youths.[52]

These are not theoretical harms—they are immediate, observable, and documentable public health crises. The politicization and mischaracterization of gender affirmation research as an extremist ideological agenda is likely to have direct and measurable consequences, contributing to increased morbidity and mortality among trans individuals. In this sociopolitical climate, the scientific community must not remain passive. The scientific community holds an urgent ethical and professional obligation to confront disinformation, defend the integrity of gender-related health research, and advance empirically grounded, equity-focused interventions. When such research is defunded or politically targeted, the pipeline needed to produce life-saving evidence is severed, jeopardizing the future of health equity for all communities.

Research on gender affirmation is neither ideological extremism nor a political agenda—it is science, advancing. Scientists must speak clearly, practice dissent, and resist politicization. AJPH

CORRESPONDENCE

Correspondence should be sent to Arjee Javellana Restar, Laboratory of Epidemiology and Public Health, 60 College St, New Haven, CT 06510 (e-mail: arjee.restar@yale.edu). Reprints can be ordered at http://www.ajph.org by clicking the "Reprints" link.

PUBLICATION INFORMATION

Full Citation: Restar AJ, Gamarel KE, Operario D. Gender affirmation research is not gender ideology extremism, it is science. *Am J Public Health*. 2025;115(11):1795–1799.

Acceptance Date: June 13, 2025.

DOI: https://doi.org/10.2105/AJPH.2025.308220

ORCID iD:
Arjee J. Restar https://orcid.org/0000-0003-2992-8198

CONTRIBUTORS

A. J. Restar drafted the article. All authors contributed substantially to the conceptualization, analysis, and interpretation of the work; edited and reviewed the article; and approved of the final published version and agree to be accountable for all aspects of the work.

CONFLICT OF INTEREST

The authors have no conflicts of interest to disclose.

REFERENCES

1. Executive Office of the President. Defending Women From Gender Ideology Extremism and Restoring Biological Truth to the Federal Government. Executive order 14168. *Fed Regist*. 2025; 90(9):8615–8618. Published January 20, 2025.
2. Reardon S. NIH kills existing grants on transgender issues. *Science*. 2025;387(6739):1136. https://doi.org/10.1126/science.adx3896
3. Ross N, Delaney S. Grant watch. Weekly terminated NIH grants report. July 16, 2025. Available at: https://grant-watch.us/docs/2025-07-16_weekly_report_confirmed_term.pdf. Accessed May 29, 2025.
4. Reisner SL, Radix A, Deutsch MB. Integrated and gender-affirming transgender clinical care and research. *J Acquir Immune Defic Syndr*. 2016;72(suppl 3):S235–S242. https://doi.org/10.1097/QAI.0000000000001088
5. Scheim AI, Restar AJ, Zubizarreta D, et al. Legal gender recognition and the health of transgender and gender diverse people: A systematic review and meta-analysis. *Soc Sci Med*. 2025;378: 118147. https://doi.org/10.1016/j.socscimed.2025.118147
6. Popper K. *The Logic of Scientific Discovery*. London, England: Routledge; 1959.
7. Ludwig D, Ruphy S. Scientific pluralism. November 3, 2021. Available at: https://plato.stanford.edu/entries/scientific-pluralism. Accessed July 20, 2025.
8. Committee on Science, Engineering, and Public Policy. *On Being a Scientist: A Guide to Responsible Conduct in Research*. 3rd ed. Washington, DC: National Academies Press; 2009.
9. Kuhn TS. *The Structure of Scientific Revolutions*. 3rd ed. Chicago, IL: University of Chicago Press; 1997.
10. Pattar BS, Gulamhusein N, Rytz CL, et al. Characterization of the literature informing health care of transgender and gender-diverse persons: a bibliometric analysis. *PLoS One*. 2024;19(10): e0309169. https://doi.org/10.1371/journal.pone.0309169
11. Christensen JA, Oh J, Linder K, et al. Systematic review of interventions to reduce suicide risk in transgender and gender diverse youth. *Child Psychiatry Hum Dev*. 2025;56(1):88–100. https://doi.org/10.1007/s10578-023-01541-w
12. Scheim AI, Baker KE, Restar AJ, Sell RL. Health and health care among transgender adults in the United States. *Annu Rev Public Health*. 2022;43: 503–523. https://doi.org/10.1146/annurev-publhealth-052620-100313
13. Scheim AI, Rich AJ, Zubizarreta D, et al. Health status of transgender people globally: a systematic review of research on disease burden and correlates. *PLoS One*. 2024;19(3):e0299373. https://doi.org/10.1371/journal.pone.0299373
14. Utah Department of Health and Human Services. Section 239: Systematic medical evidence review of hormonal transgender treatment report. October 1, 2024. Available at: https://le.utah.gov/xcode/Title26B/Chapter1/C26B-1-S239_2024100120240501.pdf. Accessed July 20, 2025.

15. Wernick JA, Busa S, Matouk K, Nicholson J, Janssen A. A systematic review of the psychological benefits of gender-affirming surgery. *Urol Clin North Am.* 2019;46(4):475–486. https://doi.org/10.1016/j.ucl.2019.07.002
16. Restar AJ, Lett E, Menezes NP, et al. Getting precise about gender and sex measurement: a primer for epidemiologists. *Am J Epidemiol.* 2024;193(12):1861–1867. https://doi.org/10.1093/aje/kwae144
17. Yee K, Lind BK, Downing J. Change in gender on record and transgender adults' mental or behavioral health. *Am J Prev Med.* 2022;62(5):696–704. https://doi.org/10.1016/j.amepre.2021.10.016
18. Reisner SL, Pletta DR, Keuroghlian AS, et al. Gender-affirming hormone therapy and depressive symptoms among transgender adults. *JAMA Netw Open.* 2025;8(3):e250955. https://doi.org/10.1001/jamanetworkopen.2025.0955
19. Puckett JA, Price S, Dunn T, et al. Legal gender affirmation, psychological distress, and physical health issues: indirect effects via enacted stigma. *Sex Res Soc Policy.* 2024;21:1112–1122. https://doi.org/10.1007/s13178-024-00971-y
20. van Leerdam TR, Zajac JD, Cheung AS. The effect of gender-affirming hormones on gender dysphoria, quality of life, and psychological functioning in transgender individuals: a systematic review. *Transgend Health.* 2023;8(1):6–21. https://doi.org/10.1089/trgh.2020.0094
21. Hughes LD, King WM, Gamarel KE, Geronimus AT, Panagiotou OA, Hughto JM. Differences in all-cause mortality among transgender and non-transgender people enrolled in private insurance. *Demography.* 2022;59(3):1023–1043. https://doi.org/10.1215/00703370-9942002
22. Coleman E, Radix AE, Bouman WP, et al. Standards of care for the health of transgender and gender diverse people, version 8. *Int J Transgend Health.* 2022;23(suppl 1):S1–S259. https://doi.org/10.1080/26895269.2022.2100644
23. Hembree WC, Cohen-Kettenis PT, Gooren L, et al. Endocrine treatment of gender-dysphoric/gender-incongruent persons: an endocrine society clinical practice guideline. *J Clin Endocrinol Metab.* 2017;102(11):3869–3903. https://doi.org/10.1210/jc.2017-01658
24. Bränström R, Pachankis JE. Reduction in mental health treatment utilization among transgender individuals after gender-affirming surgeries: a total population study. *Am J Psychiatry.* 2020;177(8):727–734. https://doi.org/10.1176/appi.ajp.2019.19010080
25. Cass H. Independent review of gender identity services for children and young people. 2024. Available at: https://cass.independent-review.uk/home/publications/final-report. Accessed May 29, 2025.
26. US Department of Health and Human Services. HHS releases comprehensive review of medical interventions for children and adolescents with gender dysphoria. May 1, 2025. Available at: https://www.hhs.gov/press-room/gender-dysphoria-report-release.html. Accessed May 29, 2025.
27. Noone C, Southgate A, Ashman A, et al. Critically appraising the Cass Report: methodological flaws and unsupported claims. *BMC Med Res Methodol.* 2025;25(1):118–128. https://doi.org/10.1186/s12874-025-02581-7
28. Sevelius J, Chakravarty D, Neilands TB, HRSA SPNS Transgender Women of Color Study Group, et al. Evidence for the model of gender affirmation: the role of gender affirmation and healthcare empowerment in viral suppression among transgender women of color living with HIV. *AIDS Behav.* 2021;25(suppl 1):64–71. https://doi.org/10.1007/s10461-019-02544-2
29. Sevelius JM. Gender affirmation: a framework for conceptualizing risk behavior among transgender women of color. *Sex Roles.* 2013;68(11–12):675–689. https://doi.org/10.1007/s11199-012-0216-5
30. Gamarel KE, King WM, Mouzoon R, et al. A "tax" on gender affirmation and safety: costs and benefits of intranational migration for transgender young adults in the San Francisco Bay area. *Cult Health Sex.* 2021;23(12):1763–1778. https://doi.org/10.1080/13691058.2020.1809711
31. Holterhus P-M, Kulle A, Busch H, Spielmann M. Classic genetic and hormonal switches during fetal sex development and beyond. *Med Genet.* 2023;35(3):163–171. https://doi.org/10.1515/medgen-2023-2036
32. Witchel SF. Disorders of sex development. *Best Pract Res Clin Obstet Gynaecol.* 2018;48:90–102. https://doi.org/10.1016/j.bpobgyn.2017.11.005
33. Fausto-Sterling A. *Sex/Gender: Biology in a Social World.* New York, NY: Routledge; 2012.
34. Human Rights Watch. "I want to be like nature made me": medically unnecessary surgeries on intersex children in the US. June 25, 2017. Available at: https://www.hrw.org/report/2017/07/25/i-want-be-nature-made-me/medically-unnecessary-surgeries-intersex-children-us. Accessed July 20, 2025.
35. Wiesemann C, Ude-Koeller S, Sinnecker GH, Thyen U. Ethical principles and recommendations for the medical management of differences of sex development (DSD)/intersex in children and adolescents. *Eur J Pediatr.* 2010;169(6):671–679. https://doi.org/10.1007/s00431-009-1086-x
36. Carpenter M. Intersex human rights, sexual orientation, gender identity, sex characteristics and the Yogyakarta Principles plus 10. *Cult Health Sex.* 2021;23(4):516–532. https://doi.org/10.1080/13691058.2020.1781262
37. National Academies of Sciences, Engineering, and Medicine. *Measuring Sex, Gender Identity, and Sexual Orientation.* Washington, DC: National Academies Press; 2022.
38. Alpert AB, Hernandez T, Ruddick R, et al. Disentangling gender, sex, and biology: a mixed methods study of gender identity data collection tools. *Patient Educ Couns.* 2025;130:108473. https://doi.org/10.1016/j.pec.2024.108473
39. Darwin H. Challenging the cisgender/transgender binary: nonbinary people and the transgender label. *Gender Soc.* 2020;34(3):357–380. https://doi.org/10.1177/0891243220912256
40. Ashley F. "Trans" is my gender modality: a modest terminological proposal. In: Erickson-Schroth L, ed. *Trans Bodies, Trans Selves: A Resource by and for Transgender Communities.* 2nd ed. New York, NY: Oxford University Press; 2022:2.
41. Feinberg L. Transgender liberation: a movement whose time has come. In: Stryker S, Whittle S, eds. *The Transgender Studies Reader.* New York, NY: Routledge; 2013:205–220.
42. Feinberg L. *Transgender Warriors: Making History From Joan of Arc to Dennis Rodman.* Boston, MA: Beacon Press; 1997.
43. Public Broadcasting Service. A map of gender-diverse cultures. October 2023. Available at: https://www.pbs.org/independentlens/content/two-spirits_map-html. Accessed May 29, 2025.
44. Hughes LD, Kidd KM, Gamarel KE, Operario D, Dowshen N. "These laws will be devastating": provider perspectives on legislation banning gender-affirming care for transgender adolescents. *J Adolesc Health.* 2021;69(6):976–982. https://doi.org/10.1016/j.jadohealth.2021.08.020
45. Meade NG, Lepore C, Olezeski CL, McNamara M. Understanding and addressing disinformation in gender-affirming health care bans. *Transgend Health.* 2024;9(4):281–287. https://doi.org/10.1089/trgh.2022.0198
46. McNamara M, McLamore Q, Meade N, Olgun M, Robinson H, Alstott A. A thematic analysis of disinformation in gender-affirming healthcare bans in the United States. *Soc Sci Med.* 2024;351:116943. https://doi.org/10.1016/j.socscimed.2024.116943
47. Elischberger HB. Science v. fiction: Gen Z's skepticism of disinformation used to justify anti-trans legislation in the USA. *Sex Res Soc Policy.* 2025;22(1):49–68. https://doi.org/10.1007/s13178-024-01035-x
48. Lepore C, Alstott A, McNamara M. Scientific misinformation is criminalizing the standard of care for transgender youth. *JAMA Pediatr.* 2022;176(10):965–966. https://doi.org/10.1001/jamapediatrics.2022.2959
49. Restar A, Layland EK, Hughes L, et al. Antitrans policy environment and depression and anxiety symptoms in transgender and nonbinary adults. *JAMA Netw Open.* 2024;7(8):e2431306. https://doi.org/10.1001/jamanetworkopen.2024.31306
50. Truszczynski M, Truszczynski N, Estevez RI, Elliott AE. Does policy matter? The impact of state and city anti-discrimination policy on the discrimination experiences of trans and nonbinary people. *Sex Res Soc Policy.* 2022;19(4):1786–1794. https://doi.org/10.1007/s13178-022-00762-3
51. Lee WY, Hobbs JN, Hobaica S, DeChants JP, Price MN, Nath R. State-level anti-transgender laws increase past-year suicide attempts among transgender and non-binary young people in the USA. *Nat Hum Behav.* 2024;8(11):2096–2106. https://doi.org/10.1038/s41562-024-01979-5
52. Restar AJ, Layland EK, Davis B, Thompson H, Streed C. The public health crisis state of transgender health care and policy. *Am J Public Health.* 2024;114(2):161–163. https://doi.org/10.2105/AJPH.2023.307523
53. *United States v Skrmetti, Attorney General and Reporter for Tennessee, et al.* No. 23-477. Argued December 4, 2024—Decided June 18, 2025.
54. Herman JL, Brown TN, Haas AP. Suicide thoughts and attempts among transgender adults: findings from the 2015 U.S. Transgender Survey. September 2019. Available at: https://williamsinstitute.law.ucla.edu/publications/suicidality-transgender-adults. Accessed July 20, 2025.
55. Nath R, Matthews D, DeChants J, et al. US National Survey on the Mental Health of LGBTQ+ Young People. 2024. Available at: https://www.thetrevorproject.org/survey-2024. Accessed July 20, 2025.

Sense of Assurance, Safety, and Security (SASS) in Youths: A Public Health Perspective

Laura D. Kubzansky, PhD, MPH, Seetha H. Davis, BA, Ritika Rastogi, PhD, G. Alice Woolverton, PhD, Emily Zhang, MA, and Cindy H. Liu, PhD

ABOUT THE AUTHORS

Laura D. Kubzansky and Seetha H. Davis are with the Department of Social and Behavioral Sciences, Harvard T. H. Chan School of Public Health, Boston, MA. At the time of this work, Ritika Rastogi, G. Alice Woolverton, and Cindy H. Liu were with the Department of Pediatrics, Brigham and Women's Hospital, Boston, MA. Emily Zhang is with the Lynch School of Education and Human Development, Boston College, Boston, MA.

AJPH November 2025, Vol. 115, No. 11

As noted in the 2021 US Surgeon General Advisory, mental health problems among youths have been rising over the last two decades, and these trends have only accelerated since 2020.[1] Although physical and mental health are often viewed as separate health domains, a growing body of research demonstrates that mental health generally precedes and predicts physical health and healthy aging.[2] Thus, mental health matters not only in its own right but also for its long-term impacts on life span health. The troubling downward and sustained trends in population mental health among US youths have major implications for the future health of US society, for decades to come.

The accelerated rise in mental health problems among US youths has led to ongoing debate about potential contributors and calls for more mental health services. Investigators have pointed to factors such as excessive social media use, racism, and climate change as key contributors.[1,3–5] They posit that the social environment has become more toxic for youths and is increasingly failing to provide conditions that promote healthy development and well-being. If true, even major efforts to increase access to and availability of high-quality mental health services, though critical for alleviating suffering, will be insufficient for reversing the observed trends. A more systematic understanding of how the social environment shapes the observed trends will help to identify and evaluate upstream factors that enhance the capacity of individuals to thrive while yielding important new targets for prevention and intervention within public health.

It has been 80 years since psychologist Abraham Maslow proposed a hierarchy of needs in which he described sense of safety as a fundamental need.[6] Humanist theories more generally have defined sense of safety as feeling psychologically secure, as a result of feeling protected from both physical and psychological harm.[7] Similar ideas have been proposed in other disciplines, variously emphasizing different elements of safety such as feeling secure (i.e., feeling protected, having someone to rely on)[8] and having a sense of assurance in the conditions providing security. Research on attachment underscores the neurobiological and evolutionary underpinnings of feeling safe, whereby infants' early bonds with their primary caregivers provide the foundation for life span health and functioning.[8] Organizational and workplace literature defines the concept of psychological safety as arising when individuals feel comfortable taking interpersonal risks in the workplace.[9,10] Other perspectives focus on context, considering how external factors like neighborhood disorder, school climate, or social exclusion may diminish one's sense of safety and assurance in the security of a particular environment (e.g., one's neighborhood).[11–13] Taken together, this work suggests that having confidence in one's safety and security is shaped by the social environment and is foundational for healthy development and functioning.

With this as context, we suggest that sense of assurance, safety, and security is an overlooked and underappreciated factor that can help explain when and how the socioecological context affects youth mental health and well-being. We posit that large-scale societal shifts in the United States have produced conditions that fail to foster this sense among youths, and this partly underlies the mental health problems they are confronting. Society's capacity to provide a sense of assurance, safety, and security has rarely been a focus in health research and, to our knowledge, this notion of safety, broadly defined, is not routinely assessed and monitored. Without a clear definition or capacity to monitor, any subtle or gradual declines in such feelings of safety and security among youths can easily escape notice. Population science researchers who focus on social or environmental determinants of health may take society's capacity to foster a sense of safety and security for granted or assume that the need is unsatisfied only among the most disadvantaged individuals. However, if many social trends (e.g., higher prevalence of gun violence in schools, greater social disconnectedness) lead to feelings of unsafety and insecurity, then we may have finally reached a tipping point whereby population levels of feeling safe and secure are problematically low, in turn leading to the reduction of emotional well-being and the acceleration in mental health disorders among youths.

Although specific factors related to safety (e.g., bullying in school, neighborhood crime) have received some attention in public health and epidemiology, research on safety more broadly defined has been conducted across a range of disciplines, including sociology, psychiatry, and psychology. For example, insecurity has been defined as a social phenomenon with relevance to health; scholars suggest that a sense of insecurity is shaped by contextual factors (e.g., economic instability) and social experiences (e.g., lack of social trust), and that it affects growth and development by interfering with individuals' capacity to develop and maintain a stable sense of self and well-being.[13] In the Generalized Unsafety Theory of Stress, Brosschot et al. propose that a sense of safety is integrally linked to stress and its relation to health.[14] More specifically, stress responses arise not only in response to threats but also more ubiquitously when information about safety in the environment is absent. This theory directly ties safety to health via its effects on stress perceptions and stress-related responses. Some empirical research also links unsafety with various aspects of health. For example, evidence shows that living in unsafe neighborhoods is associated with worse child health.[15,16] Other work suggests that perceptions of unsafety in specific environments (e.g., schools, neighborhoods) may contribute to worse health in childhood as well as fewer health-promoting behaviors, setting children up for poorer health in adulthood.[17] Building on these prior theories and frameworks regarding security, safety, and unsafety, we first propose and define a concept that represents the feeling of confidence one has in being safe and secure—the sense of assurance, safety, and security—and then describe a framework that can be used to understand when and how this sense of assurance, safety, and security may impact health.

CONCEPTUALIZING SENSE OF ASSURANCE, SAFETY, AND SECURITY

We define sense of assurance, safety, and security (hereafter referred to as SASS) as a cognitive-affective perception that one is protected from harms, which can be both proximal and distal. First, the extent to which individuals perceive and evaluate themselves to be safe should be differentiated from circumstances that might engender a sense of safety. In prior work evaluating safety in relation to health, sense of safety was not routinely directly measured but rather was inferred based on exposures to sources of unsafety, such as neighborhood violence or exposure to trauma. Although such exposures likely reduce one's SASS, measuring only these conditions is insufficient, as it conflates external and objective circumstances with internal subjective experiences, which may differ. Thus, in recognizing that SASS is at least partly shaped by the social and physical environment, a critical first step for population-based research when considering the health effects of SASS is to separate factors that promote or hinder capacity for safety (i.e., external circumstances) from a person-centered, subjective sense of feeling assured, safe, and secure (i.e., internal subjective experiences). This distinction is similar to one drawn in research on stress, which carefully distinguishes stressors—factors that have the potential to induce feelings of stress (e.g., conditions that are demanding or difficult)—from the perception or feeling of stress (e.g., believing that demands exceed one's capacity to cope).[18]

Second, we posit that the absence of unsafety may not translate directly to having SASS. That is, individuals who are not directly threatened, or fail to report sources of unsafety, may not necessarily feel protected from harm. For example, objectively safe environments (e.g., a neighborhood with low crime rates) may lack the resources needed to foster SASS (e.g., social capital, accessible playgrounds). Thus, the absence of physical or emotional threats may be necessary but not sufficient to engender SASS. By extension, factors that lead to SASS could differ from those that lead to a sense of unsafety. Of note, past studies have tended to assess safety by measuring either the presence of factors that make environments unsafe (e.g., neighborhood crime, bullying at school) or perceptions of unsafety in specific environments, rather than identifying whether and how individuals feel safe generally.

Third, we posit that, similar to other cognitive and affective attributes (e.g., sense of belonging, self-esteem),[19,20] there are probably individual differences in the propensity to have higher or lower SASS levels and that individuals experience a global SASS that is generally stable across contexts (e.g., family, school, workplace) and domains (e.g., psychological, social, and physical safety). However, our definition also recognizes that individuals' SASS levels are responsive to their immediate environment (within-person variation) and to their past experiences (between-person variation), and can change over the course of development (age-associated variation). From a developmental perspective, experiencing a sense of unsafety may not be problematic.[21,22] Indeed, adolescents are generally more oriented toward novelty-seeking or risk-taking relative to older adults, which might prompt youths to seek out factors or environments that can evoke a transient sense of unsafety. However, too strong a sense of unsafety can foster unhealthy risk-taking, as individuals may feel they have nothing to lose. As such, although individuals may have a general baseline SASS, this state is not immutably fixed and can change because of naturally occurring experiences, developmental processes, and direct or intentional intervention (e.g., creating a culture of respect in the workplace[23]).

Fourth, we posit that SASS is shaped by societal events, norms, and broader public discourse, embedded within cultures and societal structures—all of which may shift over time. From a research perspective, this could drive substantial differences across cohorts and periods regarding factors needed to engender SASS and who is most likely to experience strong SASS. For example, the COVID-19 pandemic radically altered individuals' SASS when engaging in mundane activities such as going to school or to the grocery store. In addition, recent policy shifts regarding abortion and reproductive rights in the United States may lead girls, women, and others with childbearing capacity to feel more unsafe overall, particularly during their reproductive years.

Importantly, we distinguish our definition of SASS from that of "safetyism." Put forth by Lukianoff and Haidt, the concept refers to an overarching belief within society that feeling safe is sacrosanct and must be preserved at all costs.[24] The authors note that the concept of safety is not well-defined and point out that in current discourse, safety has come to refer primarily to whether individuals feel emotionally safe. A culture of safetyism promotes the notion that any emotional discomfort represents a lack of safety; under this assumption, emotional discomfort is framed as unacceptable and requiring intervention. In contrast to the idea of safetyism, our proposed conceptualization of SASS espouses a distinct definition that goes beyond notions of "safety" exclusively, including, among other features, the following:

1. Both physical and emotional safety are relevant;
2. There are periods and environments in which feeling less safe may be developmentally appropriate; and
3. Emotional discomfort can occur with a range of experiences, including those that are normative and objectively safe.

A NEW CONCEPTUAL MODEL FOR HEALTH

Our model (Figure 1) recognizes that individuals are embedded within social and physical environments, and it illustrates how SASS fits within the larger set of factors that influence youth health; these include not only antecedents of SASS but also its downstream effects by highlighting linkages between SASS and other psychological, social, biological, and behavioral processes that, in turn, affect health and well-being. Many sources of safety and unsafety are a product of structural-level factors or derived from culture and policy at the local or national level. Sources may also derive from meso- or individual-level factors (e.g., living in areas with low social capital, experiencing discrimination), and effects vary depending on developmental context across the life span. The model further highlights that sources of unsafety can differ from sources that promote assurance, safety, and security; sources can be derived from interpersonal and material factors; and sources can occur at more proximate or distal levels (for examples, see Table A, available as a supplement to the online version of this article at http://www.ajph.org).

As further illustrated in Figure 1, upstream determinants of SASS occur within a dynamic environment, and the extent to which any given factor affects an individual's SASS depends on other factors that can be either extrinsic or intrinsic to the individual. For example, individuals in a more nurturing environment may experience a given source of unsafety (e.g., a neighborhood with high crime) as less threatening because their immediate environment is supportive.[14] Consequences of SASS for

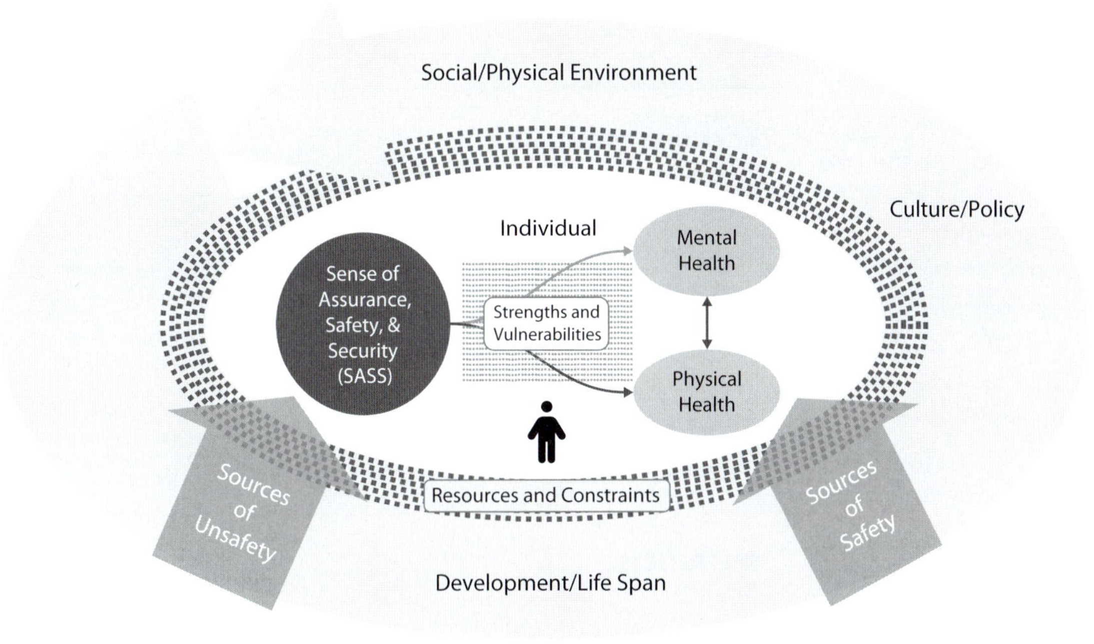

FIGURE 1— Conceptual Model of Sense of Assurance, Safety, and Security (SASS) and Health

Note. An individual's SASS is shaped by the social and physical environment within which sources of safety and unsafety are embedded at the macro, meso, and micro levels. How sources of safety and unsafety are experienced is filtered through other resources and constraints within the individual's environment. The effects of SASS on mental and physical health depend on an individual's other strengths and vulnerabilities. Overall, these relationships may differ depending on the timing of experiences and developmental period.

subsequent health will also depend on an individual's other strengths (e.g., strong cognitive abilities) and vulnerabilities (e.g., predisposition to distress), and their current period of development and life span.

CALL TO ACTION

Declines in youth SASS driven by changes at individual, interpersonal, and structural levels may significantly contribute to the accelerated rate of youth mental health problems. As such, the SASS concept may provide a novel target for intervention and prevention strategies to improve population health. With a clear conceptual definition, SASS can be operationalized, assessed reliably in the population, and tracked over time. Next steps for research involve developing valid measures of SASS, identifying antecedents, and assessing the extent to which SASS may be modified and by what means. We must establish whether SASS causally affects health and, if so, the mechanisms underlying this association. Examining the effects of SASS on health and well-being requires rigorous study designs, including experimental and longitudinal approaches. Further research to determine what promotes (or disrupts) SASS in youths is paramount. Finally, monitoring levels of SASS routinely can help predict mental health trends among youths, providing opportunities to address problems before they become entrenched. Although neighborhood safety or school safety has been assessed in national surveys, there is no national surveillance on global SASS among youths (or adults). Given globalization and the ubiquitousness of social media, worldwide and community events can profoundly affect individuals. Thus, tracking distal and proximal experiences and their effects on SASS is critical.

Building on our conceptual model and evidence to date, SASS may be considered a health asset, a factor that increases the likelihood that youths will thrive. Thus, additional recommendations for work include promoting youth SASS as a public health priority when considering socioecological determinants of health. Investment is urgently needed from government and philanthropic organizations to fund researchers in developing valid measures of SASS and building the evidence base linking SASS to health. In addition, policymakers need to commit to tracking trends and creating conditions that increase the likelihood of SASS. Awareness about the consequences of having or failing to have SASS among youths is necessary to engage funders and policymakers toward this initiative.

We have long known that conditions perceived as highly threatening can impair health and functioning.[14] Less work has addressed what environmental conditions are needed to foster healthy functioning among youths, and if the absence (or removal) of threatening conditions is sufficient to promote thriving at a population level. Building on our SASS framework, we propose that more is needed, and having conditions that foster SASS is an underappreciated determinant of youth health. We hope that bringing this perspective forward will provide new avenues for improving youth mental health and population health more broadly. AJPH

CORRESPONDENCE

Correspondence should be sent to Laura D. Kubzansky, 677 Huntington Ave, Boston, MA 02115 (e-mail: lkubzans@hsph.harvard.edu). Reprints can be ordered at https://www.ajph.org by clicking the "Reprints" link.

PUBLICATION INFORMATION

Full Citation: Kubzansky LD, Davis SH, Rastogi R, Woolverton GA, Zhang E, Liu CH. Sense of assurance, safety, and security (SASS) in youths: a public health perspective. *Am J Public Health*. 2025;115(11): 1800–1804.

Acceptance Date: July 3, 2025.

DOI: https://doi.org/10.2105/AJPH.2025.308241

ORCID iDs:

Laura D. Kubzansky https://orcid.org/0000-0002-4039-2235

Seetha H. Davis https://orcid.org/0000-0002-2332-3430

Ritika Rastogi https://orcid.org/0000-0002-1998-7795

G. Alice Woolverton https://orcid.org/0000-0001-9961-4659

Emily Zhang https://orcid.org/0000-0002-8809-8473

Cindy H. Liu https://orcid.org/0000-0001-6985-5961

CONTRIBUTORS

L. D. Kubzansky and C. H. Liu conceptualized the study, drafted the manuscript, critically revised the manuscript, and approved of the final manuscript as submitted. S. H. Davis, R. Rastogi, G. A. Woolverton, and E. Zhang participated in conceptual development and literature synthesis, critically revised the manuscript, and approved of the final manuscript as submitted.

ACKNOWLEDGMENTS

This work was supported by a grant from Hopelab Foundation.

The authors thank Amber Song and Professor Andrew Oswald for their contributions to this project.

CONFLICTS OF INTEREST

The authors have no conflicts of interest to disclose.

HUMAN PARTICIPANT PROTECTION

This work did not include human participants.

REFERENCES

1. *Protecting Youth Mental Health: The US Surgeon's Advisory*. Rockville, MD: Office of the Surgeon General; 2021.
2. Sumner JA, Koenen KC, Kubzansky LD. The long arm of mental health: new urgency with the COVID-19 pandemic. *Am J Health Promot*. 2021; 35(2):311–312. https://doi.org/10.1177/0890117120983982c
3. Morley J, Cowls J, Taddeo M, Floridi L. Public health in the information age: recognizing the infosphere as a social determinant of health. *J Med Internet Res*. 2020;22(8):e19311. https://doi.org/10.2196/19311
4. Paradies Y, Ben J, Denson N, et al. Racism as a determinant of health: a systematic review and meta-analysis. *PLoS One*. 2015;10(9):e0138511. https://doi.org/10.1371/journal.pone.0138511
5. Ragavan MI, Marcil LE, Garg A. Climate change as a social determinant of health. *Pediatrics*. 2020; 145(5):e2019316. https://doi.org/10.1542/peds.2019-3169
6. Maslow AH. A theory of human motivation. *Psychol Rev*. 1943;50(4):370–396. https://doi.org/10.1037/h0054346
7. Taormina RJ, Gao JH. Maslow and the motivation hierarchy: measuring satisfaction of the needs. *Am J Psychol*. 2013;126(2):155–177. https://doi.org/10.5406/amerjpsyc.126.2.0155
8. Eisenberger NI, Master SL, Inagaki TK, et al. Attachment figures activate a safety signal-related neural region and reduce pain experience. *Proc Natl Acad Sci U S A*. 2011;108(28):11721–11726. https://doi.org/10.1073/pnas.1108239108
9. Edmondson A. Psychological safety and learning behavior in work teams. *Adm Sci Q*. 1999;44(2): 350–383. https://doi.org/10.2307/2666999
10. Edmondson AC, Lei Z. Psychological safety: the history, renaissance, and future of an interpersonal construct. *Annu Rev Organ Psychol Organ Behav*. 2014;1(1):23–43. https://doi.org/10.1146/annurev-orgpsych-031413-091305
11. Weiner J, Francois C, Stone-Johnson C, Childs J. Keep safe, keep learning: principals' role in creating psychological safety and organizational learning during the COVID-19 pandemic. *Front Educ*. 2021;5:618483. https://doi.org/10.3389/feduc.2020.618483
12. Higgins M, Ishimaru A, Holcombe R, Fowler A. Examining organizational learning in schools: the role of psychological safety, experimentation, and leadership that reinforces learning. *J Educ Change*. 2012;13(1):67–94. https://doi.org/10.1007/s10833-011-9167-9
13. Valente R, Valera Pertegas S. Ontological insecurity and subjective feelings of unsafety: analysing socially constructed fears in Italy. *Soc Sci Res*. 2018;71:160–170. https://doi.org/10.1016/j.ssresearch.2017.11.007
14. Brosschot JF, Verkuil B, Thayer JF. Generalized Unsafety Theory of Stress: unsafe environments and conditions, and the default stress response. *Int J Environ Res Public Health*. 2018;15(3):464. https://doi.org/10.3390/ijerph15030464
15. Theall KP, Shirtcliff EA, Dismukes AR, Wallace M, Drury SS. Association between neighborhood violence and biological stress in children. *JAMA Pediatr*. 2017;171(1):53–60. https://doi.org/10.1001/jamapediatrics.2016.2321
16. Beck AF, Huang B, Ryan PH, Sandel MT, Chen C, Kahn RS. Areas with high rates of police-reported violent crime have higher rates of childhood asthma morbidity. *J Pediatr*. 2016;173:175–182.e1. https://doi.org/10.1016/j.jpeds.2016.02.018
17. Pistella J, Ioverno S, Rodgers MA, Russell ST. The contribution of school safety to weight-related health behaviors for transgender youth. *J Adolesc*. 2020;78:33–42. https://doi.org/10.1016/j.adolescence.2019.12.001
18. Epel ES, Crosswell AD, Mayer SE, et al. More than a feeling: a unified view of stress measurement for population science. *Front Neuroendocrinol*. 2018;49:146–169. https://doi.org/10.1016/j.yfrne.2018.03.001
19. Braun L, Gollner R, Rieger S, Trautwein U, Spengler M. How state and trait versions of self-esteem and depressive symptoms affect their interplay: a longitudinal experimental investigation. *J Pers Soc Psychol*. 2021;120(1):206–225. https://doi.org/10.1037/pspp0000295
20. Malone GP, Pillow DR, Osman A. The General Belongingness Scale (GBS): assessing achieved belonging. *Pers Individ Dif*. 2012;52(3):311–316. https://doi.org/10.1016/j.paid.2011.10.027
21. Duell N, Steinberg L. Positive risk taking in adolescence. *Child Dev Perspect*. 2019;13(1):48–52. https://doi.org/10.1111/cdep.12310
22. Steinberg L. Risk taking in adolescence: what changes, and why? *Ann N Y Acad Sci*. 2004;1021: 51–58. https://doi.org/10.1196/annals.1308.005
23. Edmondson A. *The Fearless Organization*. New York, NY: John Wiley & Sons; 2018.
24. Lukianoff G, Haidt J. *The Coddling of the American Mind: How Good Intentions and Bad Ideas Are Setting Up a Generation for Failure*. New York, NY: Penguin Audio; 2018.

Firearm Violence Prevention in Peril: A Call to Defend Our Public Safety Infrastructure

Daniel C. Semenza, PhD, Therese S. Richmond, RN, PhD, Sonali Rajan, EdD, Marian E. Betz, MD, MPH, Charles Branas, PhD, Shani A. L. Buggs, PhD, MPH, Stephen Hargarten, MD, MPH, Joseph Richardson, PhD, Frederick P. Rivara, MD, MPH, Ali Rowhani-Rahbar, MD, PhD, Tanya L. Sharpe, PhD, MSW, Daniel W. Webster, ScD, MPH, and Jesenia M. Pizarro, PhD

ABOUT THE AUTHORS

Daniel C. Semenza is with the New Jersey Gun Violence Research Center, Rutgers University, Piscataway, NJ. Therese S. Richmond is with the School of Nursing, University of Pennsylvania, Philadelphia. Sonali Rajan is with the Department of Health Studies and Applied Educational Psychology, Teachers College, Columbia University, New York, NY. Marian E. Betz is with the Department of Emergency Medicine, School of Medicine, University of Colorado School of Medicine, Aurora. Charles Branas is with the Department of Epidemiology, Mailman School of Public Health, Columbia University, New York, NY. Shani A. L. Buggs is with the Centers for Violence Prevention, Department of Emergency Medicine, University of California Davis School of Medicine, Sacramento. Stephen Hargarten is with the Department of Emergency Medicine, Medical College of Wisconsin, Milwaukee. Joseph Richardson is with the Department of African American Studies, University of Maryland, College Park. Frederick P. Rivara is with the Harborview Injury Prevention and Research Center, University of Washington, Seattle. Ali Rowhani-Rahbar is with the Department of Epidemiology, School of Public Health, University of Washington, Seattle. Tanya L. Sharpe is with the Factor-Inwentash Faculty of Social Work, University of Toronto, Toronto, Ontario, Canada. Daniel W. Webster is with the Center for Gun Violence Solutions, Johns Hopkins Bloomberg School of Public Health, Baltimore, MD. Jesenia M. Pizarro is with the School of Criminology and Criminal Justice, Arizona State University, Phoenix.

Firearm-related harm in the United States—including homicides, suicides, and unintentional shootings—has shown meaningful signs of decline in recent years. Roughly 80% of homicides in the United States involve a firearm.[1] In 2024 alone, the national homicide rate fell by more than 16%, marking one of the most significant single-year declines in recent history.[2] This decline followed sustained public investment in violence prevention strategies, including community-based interventions, firearm policy changes, and coordinated public safety initiatives, alongside renewed federal investments in research and surveillance infrastructure.

Critical gains in reducing firearm-related harm are now in jeopardy. Recent federal administrative actions and funding withdrawals threaten to dismantle the foundational infrastructure that undergirds public safety in the United States. These actions encompass the termination of crucial research funding, the curtailment of gun law enforcement, and possible repeal of evidence-informed firearm regulations, all of which pose a direct risk to the public's collective safety and are likely to undermine the progress achieved in recent years. Absent continued intervention, the United States faces a grave risk of backsliding into patterns of preventable violence and inequitable harms.

PROGRESS TOWARD FIREARM VIOLENCE PREVENTION

Firearm violence is a central focus of the nation's broader violence prevention strategy. Between 2021 and 2024, federal, state, and local governments implemented a series of coordinated interventions designed to reduce firearm-related harm. The US Department of Justice launched the Community-Based Violence Intervention and Prevention Initiative, directing substantial resources toward local programs that employed trained community members to prevent shootings and provide support to those at highest risk for violence involvement.

The Bipartisan Safer Communities Act expanded background check requirements to include firearm transfers by anyone selling firearms for profit, provided training and technical assistance for the implementation of extreme risk protection orders, and significantly increased mental health support in K–12 school settings. The legislation allocated $1.6 billion in funding for community-based violence prevention strategies with political support from both sides of the aisle. At the regulatory level, the Bureau of Alcohol, Tobacco, Firearms and Explosives introduced new measures in 2022 to curb the proliferation of unserialized, privately made firearms (also known as "ghost guns") and combat firearm trafficking.

AJPH November 2025, Vol. 115, No. 11

Many of these policy advances were supported by the creation of state and municipal offices of violence prevention across the United States and the expansion of hospital-based violence intervention programs. Collectively, these actions marked a significant step toward institutionalizing a multisector approach to firearm violence prevention, one informed by research and built on sustained partnerships across public health, law enforcement, and community-based organizations. The establishment of the White House Office of Gun Violence Prevention in 2023 further formalized this work by providing a centralized federal office tasked with coordinating gun violence reduction efforts across agencies.

Equally critical to these developments was the revitalization of research capacity at the federal level. After decades of restricted federal funding, both the Centers for Disease Control and Prevention (CDC) and the National Institutes of Health have provided increased support for studies focused on firearm violence prevention.[3] These efforts recognized that firearm violence and its related harms constitute a leading public health challenge, warranting rigorous investigation and sustained investment in solutions. These research investments contributed life-saving insights, a surge of new findings, and the rapid growth of a highly interdisciplinary research field dedicated to addressing firearm violence while respecting the Second Amendment rights of firearm owners. This perspective was reflected in the 2024 advisory issued by United States surgeon general Vivek Murthy, who identified firearm violence as a public health crisis and provided guidance on best practices for prevention and response.

UNRAVELING FEDERAL SUPPORT

Since January 2025, a wide-ranging retrenchment of federal support for firearm violence prevention has taken place. On the first day of the new presidential administration, the White House Office of Gun Violence Prevention was disbanded. The advisory issued by Murthy and its corresponding resources were removed. These decisions were followed by extensive staffing reductions at the CDC, including the near elimination of its Division of Violence Prevention.[4] The cuts had immediate effects across the CDC. For instance, nearly the entire team responsible for maintaining the Division of Injury Prevention's Web-Based Injury Statistics Query and Reporting System received termination notices with the exception of a small suicide prevention unit.[5]

In parallel, the Department of Justice rescinded hundreds of millions of dollars for firearm violence prevention grants, resulting in the abrupt discontinuation of programs serving communities at elevated risk for firearm-related harm. These terminations also targeted victim services grants, shuttering centers that provide vital resources to survivors of violence as well as substance use disorder treatment programs. Both are critical resources to help mitigate the long-term consequences of exposure to violence.[6,7] Federal grants awarded by the National Institutes of Health and the National Science Foundation have been terminated, with limited explanation to affected investigators. Researchers have lost essential funding, forcing the closure of labs and triggering staff layoffs. This abrupt withdrawal of support has had immediate consequences for ongoing studies and has introduced significant uncertainty into the research ecosystem.

These administrative actions have occurred alongside overt political efforts to delegitimize the scientific basis of violence prevention. A small group of members of Congress recently called for a complete ban on federally funded firearm research, echoing the restrictions that effectively halted federal inquiry into firearm violence for more than two decades, resulting in a lost generation of researchers and progress.[8] Simultaneously, firearm regulations previously enacted to better regulate law-breaking firearm dealers have been repealed by the current administration, despite evidence that similar regulations deter illegal firearm trafficking.[9,10] Furthermore, cuts to Medicaid approved by Congress threaten to reduce health care coverage for millions of low- and middle-income households while exacerbating conditions likely to increase violence.[11]

Together, these actions constitute a comprehensive rollback of the federal government's role in preventing firearm-related harm. Before the Biden administration, the responsibility for preventing firearm violence fell largely to individual states for decades in the absence of federal leadership. Given the changes at the federal level, state actions will again become imperative.

The implications of this reversal are far reaching. Firearm violence, including suicide, remains the leading cause of death among children and adolescents and contributes significantly to racial, geographic, and socioeconomic health disparities.[12] Exposure to firearm violence—whether direct, witnessed, or anticipated—is linked to psychological distress, chronic illness, functional impairment, and premature mortality.[13] These harms disproportionately affect communities of color, and firearm suicide places a particularly heavy burden on residents of rural areas.[14] The dismantling of firearm violence prevention systems jeopardizes the capacity of communities across the United States to respond effectively to these risks, and consequently the likelihood of preventable firearm-related harm will almost certainly rise.

SAFETY REQUIRES SYSTEMS

The rapid dismantling of violence prevention infrastructure must be met with a collective and urgent response. Leaders across the medical, scientific, and public health communities must reaffirm the essential role of rigorous research and application of evidence to practice in safeguarding population health. Professional societies, academic institutions, and peer-reviewed journals can serve as critical platforms for articulating the importance of continued investment in prevention infrastructure and for defending the scientific integrity of this field of inquiry.

Firearm violence prevention is not the exclusive domain of any single discipline, nor is it a partisan issue. It is a shared responsibility rooted in public health principles, grounded in empirical evidence, and realized through institutional coordination. Critically, we must resist reverting back to strategies that rely solely on law enforcement and instead prioritize coalition-based approaches that avoid the collateral harms produced by the criminal justice system.[15] The systems that reduce harm—from reducing tobacco-related deaths to creating safer workplaces—operate effectively because they are supported, maintained, and improved over time. The same must be true for firearm violence prevention.

As scholars, we have a responsibility to mentor the next generation of researchers and support early career colleagues, even in a hostile funding environment. We must actively defend the role of science in shaping public safety. That means not only producing high-quality research but also speaking out, publicly and persistently, about the value of firearm violence prevention and the evidence behind it. In moments such as this, sustained scholarly engagement is not just valuable, it is essential.

The recent decline in firearm-related harm demonstrates that strategic, evidence-based interventions can reduce harm and improve public safety. Yet, this progress is contingent on systems—research institutions, public health agencies, law enforcement, community organizations, and federal and state policies—that must be sustained to be effective. Disinvestment from these systems is likely to result in measurable harm, injury, and death.

It is imperative that the nation's public safety infrastructure remain intact and supported. The protection of lives and the prevention of suffering require not only intention but institutional capacity. We must act to ensure that the systems enabling firearm violence prevention are restored and remain a national priority. AJPH

CORRESPONDENCE

Correspondence should be sent to Daniel C. Semenza, PhD, Rutgers University, 405-7 Cooper St, Camden, NJ 08102 (e-mail: daniel.semenza@rutgers.edu). Reprints can be ordered at https://www.ajph.org by clicking the "Reprints" link.

PUBLICATION INFORMATION

Full Citation: Semenza DC, Richmond TS, Rajan S, et al. Firearm violence prevention in peril: a call to defend our public safety infrastructure. *Am J Public Health*. 2025;115(11):1805–1808.

Acceptance Date: June 19, 2025.

DOI: https://doi.org/10.2105/AJPH.2025.308231

ORCID iDs:

Daniel C. Semenza https://orcid.org/0000-0002-3843-9559

Sonali Rajan https://orcid.org/0000-0002-2530-4364

Shani A. L. Buggs https://orcid.org/0000-0003-4538-0206

Ali Rowhani-Rahbar https://orcid.org/0000-0002-2705-4485

Jesenia M. Pizarro https://orcid.org/0000-0002-7468-8640

CONTRIBUTORS

D. C. Semenza wrote the initial draft of the editorial. All of the authors contributed to conceptualization and detailed revision.

ACKNOWLEDGMENTS

The views expressed in this article do not represent those of the institutions with which the authors are affiliated. The authors have written this article in their personal capacity as individual experts in the field.

CONFLICTS OF INTEREST

The authors have no conflicts of interest to disclose.

REFERENCES

1. Kena G, Truman JL. Trends and patterns in firearm violence, 1993–2018. Available at: https://bjs.ojp.gov/content/pub/pdf/tpfv9318.pdf. Accessed October 20, 2024.
2. Lopez E, Boxerman B. Crime trends in US cities. year-end 2024 update. Available at: https://counciloncj.org/crime-trends-in-u-s-cities-year-end-2024-update. Accessed October 20, 2024.
3. Morral AR, Smart R. A new era for firearm violence prevention research. *JAMA*. 2022;328(12):1197–1198.
4. Stone W. With CDC injury prevention team gutted, we will not know what is killing us. Available at: https://www.npr.org/sections/shots-health-news/2025/04/21/nx-s1-5371519/cdc-hhs-injury-prevention-federal-layoffs. Accessed October 20, 2024.
5. Brownlee C. CDC teams that study gun violence and collect data are decimated by layoffs. Available at: https://www.thetrace.org/2025/04/cdc-layoffs-gun-violence-prevention-trump/#:~:text=The%20downsizing%20has%20also%20hit,NIH%20units%20affected%20by%20cuts. Accessed October 20, 2024.
6. Giraldi DM, Swingler S, Kirk DS, Jacoby SF, Melendez-Torres GJ, Kaufman EJ, Humphreys DK. Understanding the broader impacts of non-fatal firearm violence trauma in the United States: a scoping review. Available at: https://www.thelancet.com/journals/lanam/article/PIIS2667-193X(25)00101-2/fulltext. Accessed October 20, 2024.

7. Abba-Aji M, Koya SF, Abdalla SM, Ettman CK, Cohen GH, Galea S. The mental health consequences of interpersonal gun violence: a systematic review. Available at: https://www.sciencedirect.com/science/article/pii/S2666560324000070. Accessed October 20, 2024.
8. Galea S, Branas CC, Flescher A, et al. Priorities in recovering from a lost generation of firearms research. *Am J Public Health.* 2018;108(7):858–860. https://doi.org/10.2105/AJPH.2018.304436
9. Webster DW, Vernick JS, Bulzacchelli MT. Effects of state-level firearm seller accountability policies on firearm trafficking. *J Urban Health.* 2009;86(4):525–537. https://doi.org/10.1007/s11524-009-9351-x
10. Vernick JS, Webster DW, Bulzacchelli MT, Mair JS. Regulation of firearm dealers in the United States: an analysis of state law and opportunities for improvement. *J Law Med Ethics.* 2006;34(4):765–775.
11. Wen H, Hockenberry JM, Cummings JR. The effect of Medicaid expansion on crime reduction: evidence from HIFA-waiver expansions. *J Public Econ.* 2017;154:67–94. https://doi.org/10.1111/j.1748-720x.2006.00097.x
12. Villarreal S, Kim R, Wagner E, Somayaji N, Davis A, Crifasi CK. Gun violence in the United States 2022: examining the burden among children and teens. Available at: https://publichealth.jhu.edu/sites/default/files/2024-09/2022-cgvs-gun-violence-in-the-united-states.pdf. Accessed October 20, 2024.
13. Semenza DC, Kravitz-Wirtz N. Gun violence exposure and population health inequality: a conceptual framework. *Inj Prev.* 2025;31(1):1–8. https://doi.org/10.1136/ip-2023-045197
14. Reeping PM, Mak A, Branas CC, Gobaud AN, Nance ML. Firearm death rates in rural vs urban US counties. *JAMA Surg.* 2023;158(7):771–772. https://doi.org/10.1001/jamasurg.2023.0265
15. Kirk DS, Wakefield S. Collateral consequences of punishment: a critical review and path forward. *Annu Rev Criminol.* 2018;1:171–194. https://doi.org/10.1146/annurev-criminol-032317-092045

Protecting Health Equity Research Among Latinos Who Use Drugs Amid Heightened Immigration Enforcement

Miguel Pinedo, PhD, and Christian Escobar, MEd

ABOUT THE AUTHORS

The authors are with the Department of Kinesiology & Health Education, College of Education, University of Texas at Austin.

See also Coronado et al., p. 1877.

Drawing on four case studies across the United States and the US-Mexico border, Coronado et al. (p. 1877) highlight how the intersection of immigration enforcement and drug policy disrupts harm reduction efforts, undermines trust in public institutions, and impairs the capacity to conduct rigorous health equity research with Latino communities, including those who use drugs. Their work is timely amid the 2025 political climate marked by increasingly punitive immigration policies, intensified anti-immigrant rhetoric, and escalating immigration enforcement actions.[1] In the first half of the year alone, immigration arrests surged by 122%,[2] detentions exceeded 51 000 for the first time since 2019,[3] and the newly reelected Trump administration set an aggressive target of apprehending at least 3000 undocumented immigrants per day, equating to more than 1 million arrests annually.[4]

Despite the rising numbers of detentions and deportations, the majority (72%) of those apprehended have no previous criminal convictions,[5] underscoring the broad and intensified scope of current enforcement practices. Widespread media coverage of large-scale immigration raids in recent months, including images of distressed families, community protests, and violent confrontations with enforcement officials, provides a sobering illustration of the trauma associated with immigration enforcement. Latino communities bear the brunt of immigration enforcement, with enforcement efforts targeting neighborhoods and labor sectors with high concentrations of Latino immigrants.[6] As a result, Latino-origin immigrants represented the majority of immigrants detained and deported over the past two decades.[7] These realities provide important contextual information to better understand and interpret Coronado and colleagues' findings.

The Coronado et al. case studies provide a valuable scientific contribution by documenting how immigration enforcement obstructs public health research on the opioid-overdose crisis affecting Latino communities. This is an urgent public health issue: whereas the first three waves of the opioid-overdose epidemic mostly affected White populations, the current fourth wave is disproportionately affecting Latinos.[8] Opioid-overdose rates among Latinos now surpass those of their White counterparts.[8] Research on risk factors for opioid use, overdose, and drivers of racial/ethnic inequities is urgently needed to inform effective responses to this epidemic.

However, as Coronado et al. document, heightened immigration enforcement poses significant challenges to engaging Latinos who use drugs in research. Fears of detention, deportation, criminalization, and disclosure of sensitive information (e.g., immigration status, substance use history) have hindered recruitment efforts, especially among undocumented immigrants. These fears have also contributed to underuse of treatment and harm reduction services. Strikingly, recruitment barriers have persisted even in San Francisco, California, a well-known sanctuary city that prioritizes the safety of immigrant communities by restricting local law enforcement from enforcing immigration laws or cooperating with immigration enforcement. The persistence of immigration enforcement fears in immigrant-friendly cities highlights the current widespread climate of hostility and criminalization toward immigrant communities. Ultimately, as evident across all four case studies, immigration enforcement weakens community trust and the integrity of research studies and prevention efforts.

Erosion of community trust significantly compromises both health equity research and opioid prevention efforts. The Coronado et al. findings make it clear that failure to capture the experiences of Latinos who use drugs, including undocumented immigrants, limits

AJPH November 2025, Vol. 115, No. 11

our understanding of the evolving overdose crisis and compromises the quality of surveillance and community-based data. With overdose prevention efforts relying heavily on epidemiological surveillance and modeling, maintaining a data infrastructure that reflects the current US population, including Latinos, is essential.

Coronado et al. propose several pragmatic and timely strategies to sustain health equity research with Latino communities during periods of aggressive immigration enforcement. These strategies include strengthening community partnerships, adopting trauma-informed research practices, committing to research and serving those most at risk for criminalization despite logistical challenges, and advocating for legal research protections. These recommendations are timely: a recent Pew Research Center survey revealed that 47% of Latinos worry they or a family member might be deported,[9] and another study showed that 39% of US-born Latino adults have experienced the detention or deportation of a parent or family member.[10] As such, implementing the Coronado et al. recommendations is key to improving equity-focused research and generating the real-time data needed for rapid public health responses.

Beyond research, Coronado and colleagues' findings can also be used to guide public health practice and policy responses to the opioid epidemic, especially during times of limited resources. First, building and maintaining community trust is essential for engaging Latinos in substance use treatment and harm reduction services amid intensified immigration enforcement.[1] Expanding opioid prevention beyond traditional medical settings, such as integrating services within trusted community-based organizations, can help reduce fear and distrust while encouraging use of services. Collaboration with trusted community-based organizations is key to reducing barriers and improving engagement in prevention services.

Second, opioid-overdose prevention, treatment, and harm reduction services must consider the effects of immigration enforcement on substance use. Enforcement-related stressors increase risk of substance misuse and may exacerbate existing racial/ethnic inequities.[10,11] Culturally tailored services that acknowledge these stressors can make services more appealing, increase engagement, and improve outcomes.

Third, a culturally competent public health workforce is critical. Public health professionals working with Latinos who use drugs should understand the emotional, behavioral, and legal consequences of immigration enforcement; be knowledgeable about policies affecting immigrants' rights; and help disseminate guidance on protocols to follow if community members encounter an immigration official.

Finally, policymakers can draw on the Coronado et al. findings to inform policies designed to protect Latino immigrants and people who use drugs, such as limiting police and immigration involvement around opioid-prevention efforts and advocating for reforms that decriminalize immigrants. However, these policy changes remain a challenge under the current anti-immigrant climate, marked by threats to immigrants' rights and safety and funding for health equity research.

In summary, Coronado et al. shed light on the critical need to protect health equity research with Latinos who use drugs. Providing a robust evidence base on the negative effects of immigration enforcement on the opioid epidemic can help inform novel prevention strategies, provide policymakers and advocates with data to advocate for immigration and health policy reforms, and increase use of treatment and harm reduction services to end the opioid crisis. The continued rising rates of opioid use and overdose among Latinos,[8] coupled with increasing anti-immigration policies and rhetoric,[1,11] reinforce the need for high-quality data to guide efforts. The escalation of anti-immigrant sentiment amid the evolving opioid crisis reminds us that the needs of Latinos who use drugs must be centered in research aimed at reducing drug-related harms if health equity is to be achieved. AJPH

CORRESPONDENCE

Correspondence should be sent to Miguel Pinedo, PhD, 2109 San Jacinto Blvd, Stop D3700, Austin, TX 78712-1415 (e-mail: mpinedo@austin.utexas.edu). Reprints can be ordered at https://www.ajph.org by clicking the "Reprints" link.

PUBLICATION INFORMATION

Full Citation: Pinedo M, Escobar C. Protecting health equity research among Latinos who use drugs amid heightened immigration enforcement. *Am J Public Health*. 2025;115(11):1809–1811.

Acceptance Date: August 14, 2025.

DOI: https://doi.org/10.2105/AJPH.2025.308279

ORCID iD:
Miguel Pinedo https://orcid.org/0000-0002-2089-414X

CONTRIBUTORS

The authors contributed equally to this work.

CONFLICTS OF INTEREST

The authors have no conflicts of interest.

REFERENCES

1. Schumacher S, Hamel L, Artiga S, et al. Understanding the US immigrant experience: the 2023 KFF/LA Times survey of immigrants. Available at: https://www.kff.org/racial-equity-and-health-policy/kff-la-times-survey-of-immigrants. Accessed July 29, 2025.

2. Deportation Data Project. ICE data release: September 1, 2023 to late June 2025. Available at: https://deportationdata.org/news/2025-07-15-ICE-release.html. Accessed July 29, 2025.
3. Transactional Records Access Clearinghouse. ICE immigration detention numbers continue to climb. Available at: https://tracreports.org/whatsnew/email.250606.html. Accessed July 25, 2025.
4. Hesson T, Cooke K. ICE's tactics draw criticism as it triples daily arrest targets. Available at: https://www.reuters.com/world/us/ices-tactics-draw-criticism-it-triples-daily-arrest-targets-2025-06-10. Accessed July 24, 2025.
5. Transactional Records Access Clearinghouse. Immigration quick facts: detention and criminal history. Available at: https://tracreports.org/immigration/quickfacts/#detention_nocrim. Accessed July 25, 2025.
6. Magaña-Salgado J. Detention, deportation, and devastation: the disproportionate effect of deportations on the Latino community. Available at: https://www.maldef.org/assets/pdf/Deportation_Brief_MALDEF-NHLA-NDLON.pdf. Accessed July 25, 2025.
7. Pinedo M, Montero-Zamora P, Pasch K, Schwartz S. Immigration policies as political determinants of alcohol and drug misuse among US-born Latinos. *Int J Drug Policy.* 2022;106:103754. https://doi.org/10.1016/j.drugpo.2022.103754
8. Friedman JR, Nguemeni Tiako MJ, Hansen H. Understanding and addressing widening racial inequalities in drug overdose. *Am J Psychiatry.* 2024;181(5):381–390. https://doi.org/10.1176/appi.ajp.20230917
9. Noe-Bustamante L, Im C, Lopez MH. About 1 in 4 US adults worry they or someone close to them could be deported. Available at: https://www.pewresearch.org/short-reads/2025/06/27/about-1-in-4-us-adults-worry-they-or-someone-close-to-them-could-be-deported. Accessed July 25, 2025.
10. Pinedo M. The impact of deportation policies on the substance using behaviors of US-citizen Latinos. *Int J Drug Policy.* 2020;75:102605. https://doi.org/10.1016/j.drugpo.2019.11.013
11. Pinedo M, Valdez CR. Immigration enforcement policies and the mental health of US citizens: findings from a comparative analysis. *Am J Community Psychol.* 2020;66(1–2):119–129. https://doi.org/10.1002/ajcp.12464

Political Decisions, Personal Consequences: Abortion Bans Threaten the Health of All Pregnant People

Diane J. Horvath, MD, MPH

ABOUT THE AUTHOR

Diane J. Horvath is the cofounder and chief medical officer at Partners in Abortion Care, College Park, MD.

See also Nagle et al., p. 1887.

As of July 2025, 12 US states ban abortion at any gestational duration with limited exceptions.[1] Although abortion access was already limited in many states before the Supreme Court's *Dobbs v Jackson Women's Health* decision in June 2022, several of these post-*Dobbs* bans carry criminal penalties, large fines, and potential loss of medical license for clinicians who provide abortions in violation of the law.[2]

Although all of these abortion bans contain language that permits abortions in the case of threat to the life of the pregnant person,[3] in practice, health care providers are left wondering how near death a patient needs to be to receive evidence-based care that will not result in criminal prosecution. Some bans carve out exceptions for care of ectopic pregnancies and the removal of a demised fetus or embryo but do not contain protections for treatment of threatened pregnancy loss where embryonic or fetal cardiac activity may still be present.[3] Clinicians are faced with the impossible choice of risking their livelihood and their freedom if they act and risking harm to patients, medical liability, and moral injury if they do not. The uncertainty and fear of criminal prosecution sowed by these bans have resulted in preventable harm to pregnant people.[4,5]

It is against this backdrop that in this issue of *AJPH* Nagle et al. (p. 1887) examine blood transfusions for pregnancy loss in Texas before and after abortion bans. Their study, which uses blood transfusion related to pregnancy loss as a marker for severe maternal morbidity, is significant for several reasons. It is one of the first studies to quantify the impact of state-level abortion bans on maternal health following the 2022 *Dobbs* decision, which allowed Texas to ban abortion entirely. It includes the periods before Texas Senate Bill 8 in 2021 (the six-week ban) was passed, after *Dobbs* was decided, and between Senate Bill 8 and *Dobbs*. Comparing these time frames allowed the authors to quantify how the six-week ban differed in impact from the subsequent total ban.

The selection of blood transfusions as a marker for severe maternal morbidity is apt. Hemorrhage is the leading cause of maternal death worldwide, accounting for 27% of maternal deaths according to a 2025 World Health Organization analysis.[6] Although life-threatening hemorrhage is more common in the postpartum period than in early pregnancy, significant hemorrhage and the resultant need for transfusion can and does occur earlier in pregnancy, particularly related to pregnancy loss.

Nagle et al. found that there were 50.7 (15.1%) more transfusions than expected during the period following the total abortion ban. This means that significantly more pregnant people experienced severe maternal morbidity and were exposed to the risk of blood transfusions, possibly because of delays in and denials of care.

The American College of Obstetricians and Gynecologists instructs health care providers to manage early pregnancy loss complicated by hemorrhage with urgent surgical uterine evacuation.[7] Notably, the organization does not make a distinction between early pregnancies with and those without cardiac activity when the pregnant person is experiencing a serious hemorrhage. The goal of prompt uterine evacuation after a hemorrhage diagnosis is to quickly empty pregnancy tissue from the uterus to decrease bleeding. Uterine evacuation also aims to prevent additional sequelae such as disseminated intravascular coagulation and the need for transfusion of blood products. Blood transfusion carries its own set of risks, some of which can be life threatening, and results in costs to both the patient and the health care system.

A patient who requires a blood transfusion that could have been prevented with a standard surgical treatment that is available in nearly every hospital is exposed to preventable harm even if they do not experience an adverse transfusion reaction. Abortion bans, even with exceptions, create a climate

AJPH November 2025, Vol. 115, No. 11

of confusion for clinicians and health care facilities. It is not difficult to imagine why a clinician might delay indicated care if they fear loss of license, large fines, or incarceration if someone believes that they have provided an illegal abortion.

This is especially true in states like Texas, whose abortion bans allow both criminal prosecution and civil suits that can be filed by anyone, even if they have no apparent connection to the alleged abortion.[8] The surgical uterine evacuation procedure used to treat early pregnancy loss is identical to the procedure used for induced abortion, and it is very optimistic to expect a nonexpert to understand the difference and appreciate the often complex medical decision-making that occurs when a patient is seriously ill. Although the stated intent of Texas's law is to ban nearly all abortions, which is directly harmful to people who need them, in practice the harm extends to all pregnancy-capable people who might find themselves in a Texas emergency department with any of many health- and life-threatening pregnancy complications that might necessitate urgent treatment to end the pregnancy.

Pregnancy is not a health-neutral event, and we are already in the midst of a maternal health crisis. The US maternal mortality ratio is the worst among economically similar countries,[9] and significant racial disparities exist: in 2023, the maternal mortality rate for Black women was more than three times higher than that for White women.[10] For every one woman who dies because of pregnancy, an additional 100 women will suffer from severe maternal morbidity, with Black women again disproportionately experiencing these adverse pregnancy outcomes at twice the rate of White women.[11] The findings of Nagle et al. empirically demonstrate the harms abortion bans cause to pregnant people, which will likely magnify existing disparities.

Alarmingly, Texas is not the only state with criminal penalties for providing abortion in violation of the law; several states allow sentences up to and including life imprisonment.[2] When legislation disregards evidence-based medicine and disrupts the provision of evidence-informed medical care with the threat of criminal prosecution, it should surprise no one that patients suffer the consequences. AJPH

CORRESPONDENCE

Correspondence should be sent to Diane J. Horvath, MD, MPH, 7305 Baltimore Ave, Suite 107, College Park, MD 20740 (e-mail: dhorvath@partnersclinic.com). Reprints can be ordered at https://www.ajph.org by clicking the "Reprints" link.

PUBLICATION INFORMATION

Full Citation: Horvath DJ. Political decisions, personal consequences: abortion bans threaten the health of all pregnant people. *Am J Public Health*. 2025; 115(11):1812–1813.

Acceptance Date: August 13, 2025.

https://doi.org/10.2105/AJPH.2025.308275

ORCID iD:
Diane J. Horvath https://orcid.org/0009-0002-3938-8578

ACKNOWLEDGMENTS

The author would like to thank Graham Mooney, PhD, for his editing assistance.

CONFLICTS OF INTEREST

The author has no conflicts of interest to disclose.

REFERENCES

1. Guttmacher Institute. Interactive map: US abortion policies and access after Roe. July 23, 2025. Available at: https://states.guttmacher.org/policies?bans=total-abortion-ban. Accessed July 24, 2025.
2. Kaiser Family Foundation. Many states impose a jail sentence for doctors who perform abortions past gestational limits. May 23, 2022. Available at: https://www.kff.org/womens-health-policy/slide/many-states-impose-a-jail-sentence-for-doctors-who-perform-abortions-past-gestational-limits. Accessed July 24, 2025.
3. Felix M, Sobel L, Salganicoff A. A review of exceptions in state abortion bans: implications for the provision of abortion services. June 6, 2024. Available at: https://www.kff.org/womens-health-policy/issue-brief/a-review-of-exceptions-in-state-abortions-bans-implications-for-the-provision-of-abortion-services. Accessed July 24, 2025.
4. Nambiar A, Patel S, Santiago-Munoz P, Spong CY, Nelson DB. Maternal morbidity and fetal outcomes among pregnant women at 22 weeks' gestation or less with complications in 2 Texas hospitals after legislation on abortion. *Am J Obstet Gynecol.* 2022;227(4):648–650.e1. https://doi.org/10.1016/j.ajog.2022.06.060
5. ProPublica. Life of the mother: how abortion bans lead to preventable deaths. September 16, 2024. Available at: https://www.propublica.org/series/life-of-the-mother. Accessed July 29, 2025.
6. Cresswell JA, Alexander M, Chong MYC, et al. Global and regional causes of maternal deaths 2009–2020: a WHO systematic analysis. *Lancet Glob Health.* 2025;13(4):e626–e634. https://doi.org/10.1016/S2214-109X(24)00560-6
7. American College of Obstetricians and Gynecologists' Committee on Practice Bulletins—Gynecology. ACOG Practice Bulletin No. 200: early pregnancy loss. *Obstet Gynecol.* 2018;132(5):e197–e207. https://doi.org/10.1097/AOG.0000000000002899
8. Texas State Law Library. Legal FAQs: is abortion illegal in Texas? June 3, 2025. Available at: https://sll.texas.gov/faqs/abortion-illegal-texas. Accessed July 25, 2025.
9. United Nations Maternal Mortality Estimation Inter-Agency Group. Trends in maternal mortality estimates 2000–2023: estimates by WHO, UNICEF, UNFPA, World Bank Group and UNDESA/Population Division. 2025. Available at: https://www.unfpa.org/publications/trends-maternal-mortality-2000-2023. Accessed July 29, 2025.
10. Hoyert DL. Maternal mortality rates in the United States, 2023. *NCHS Health E-Stats.* 2025. https://doi.org/10.15620/cdc/174577
11. Hailu EM, Maddali SR, Snowden JM, Carmichael SL, Mujahid MS. Structural racism and adverse maternal health outcomes: a systematic review. *Health Place.* 2022;78:102923. https://doi.org/10.1016/j.healthplace.2022.102923

Managing Mental Health Crisis Calls Received by a US Poison Center: A Statewide Collaboration Between the Georgia Poison Center, 911, and 988

Matthew Robert Dernbach, MD, Stephanie Hon, PharmD, Gaylord Lopez, PharmD, Nadine J. Kaslow, PhD, Joseph E. Carpenter, MD, Kevin Tanner, MPA, Aleisha Rucker-Wright, MPA, MA, Dawn Peel, MS, Andrea Corley, MA, Ryan Davis Solis, MA, Tim P. Moran, PhD, Brent W. Morgan, MD, Patrick Filkins, PharmD, Greg Whitaker, Erin Conaway, Brenda Cibulas, APRN, Sophie Arkin, PhD, Desiree Arnold, MBA, and Robert J. Geller, MD

The Georgia Poison Center developed a protocol for managing mental health crisis cases via iterative feedback with Georgia 911–related emergency medical services and Georgia 988–related mental health services. The Georgia Poison Center managed 533 such cases in 2024 (the year of protocol implementation), of which 45 (8.4%) were transferred to 911. Our study demonstrates that emergency services can effectively develop statewide collaborations to improve mental health outcomes and that poison centers have a vital role in national suicide prevention efforts. (*Am J Public Health*. 2025;115(11):1814–1817. https://doi.org/10.2105/AJPH.2025.308229)

AJPH November 2025, Vol. 115, No. 11

Individuals can access mental health crisis and emergency medical services via the 988 and 911 three-digit telephone numbers, respectively.

Poison centers (PCs) manage toxic exposures in patients of all ages. There are currently 53 accredited PCs that support all jurisdictions in the United States. PC staff comprise medical toxicologists (physicians), clinical toxicologists (pharmacists or other nonclinicians), and specialists in poison information (SPIs). Most calls to PCs are handled by SPIs, with toxicologists serving a backup role. Many cases managed by PCs involve intentional overdoses.[1]

INTERVENTION AND IMPLEMENTATION

In 2023, the Georgia Poison Center (GPC), the Georgia Department of Behavioral Health and Developmental Disabilities, the Georgia Crisis and Access Line, the Georgia Emergency Communications Authority, and City of Atlanta 911 collaborated to establish a novel protocol by which GPC callers experiencing mental health crises could be linked to services offered through the Georgia Crisis and Access Line and local 911 centers (referred to as public safety answering points [PSAPs]). We developed the protocol via iterative feedback between stakeholders until consensus was obtained. The GPC developed coding procedures to document calls so that they are countable and searchable.

In developing the mental health crisis protocol, we defined relevant terms, such as, "mental health crisis," "active rescue," and "immediate harm" (Box 1); developed transfer procedures for common cases (Figure A, available as a supplement to the online version of this article at http://www.ajph.org); identified the clinical expertise and limitations of 988 and 911; identified a default PSAP (i.e., City of Atlanta 911) for callers without an identified dispatchable location; and enhanced communication with PSAPs via identification of unpublished "backdoor" telephone numbers (i.e., telephone numbers that ring directly into a PSAP and receive a priority answer), among other elements (Figure A). For this study, we included calls to the GPC for which the subject of the call met the protocol definition of a "mental health crisis." We excluded calls if the caller site or management site was a health care facility.

While managing a mental health crisis, SPIs collected data on demographics, the nature of the mental health crisis, substance exposures, and transfers and

BOX 1— Mental Health Crisis Protocol Definition of Terms: Georgia, 2024

1. Mental health crisis: anyone at elevated risk for harm to self, experiencing suicidality, or exhibiting signs of psychosis or mania, substance use disorder, or developmental disability crisis; examples include (but are not limited to) the following:
   - Patient reports suicidal ideation
   - Patient reports persecutory auditory hallucinations
   - Patient is experiencing emotional distress
   - Patient is seeking substance use treatment
   - Patient is seeking supportive conversation
   - Patient is seeking information on a lethal/toxic dose of a xenobiotic with concern for self-harm purposes without known imminent plan/intent
2. Active rescue: anyone suffering a mental health crisis who is in immediate danger or requiring assistance with clinical decision-making; examples include (but are not limited to) the following:
   - Patient reports suicidal ideation with imminent access to means
   - Patient reports imminent plan to overdose
   - Patient reports an intentional ingestion
   - Patient reports a medical emergency
   - Patient reports being in crisis but refuses to facilitate medical/mental health intervention
3. Immediate harm: anyone suffering a mental health crisis who is a threat to individual or public safety, is observed with or has known access to a dangerous weapon, or is involved in a reported crime requiring some level of investigation; examples include (but are not limited to) the following:
   - Patient reports homicidal ideation
   - Patient is actively causing physical harm to self, others, or property
4. Warm transfer: an instance of the calling operator introducing self and role to the receiving operator, relaying pertinent information, and acknowledging the information transfer
5. Caller: the person who calls and speaks with the poison center
6. Patient: the subject of the mental health crisis call, i.e., the person who is experiencing the mental health crisis
7. Collateral: a third party associated with the patient who may provide reports on the patient, e.g., a patient's parent, spouse, or friend

dispositions. A mental health crisis could be coded as requiring "active rescue" or representing an "immediate harm," both of those criteria, or neither of those criteria. We recorded substance exposures if the subject of the call was exposed to a substance or was contemplating exposure to a substance.

The GPC staff were trained on protocol implementation. The Georgia Department of Behavioral Health and Developmental Disabilities provided the GPC staff with Question, Persuade, Refer Gatekeeper Training, which is evidence-based suicide prevention training for health care workers.[2] The Emory University School of Medicine's Department of Psychiatry and Behavioral Sciences provided peer support stress debriefing training to GPC staff volunteers.

PLACE, TIME, AND PERSONS

The state of Georgia has a population of 10.7 million, with 120 rural and 39 urban counties.[3,4] The GPC has one of the highest call volumes of all PCs in the United States,[5] with a catchment area encompassing the entire state. The Georgia Crisis and Access Line operates Georgia's 988 line. The Georgia Emergency Communications Authority facilitates the operation of individual PSAPs throughout the state. The largest PSAP by call volume in Georgia is City of Atlanta 911. The GPC implemented the protocol on January 1, 2024. We examined data for one year following implementation.

PURPOSE

Although PCs regularly receive calls from individuals experiencing mental health crises,[6] there is variation among PCs in how these calls are managed.[7] Our purpose was to develop and evaluate a protocol for identifying, triaging, and transferring PC callers who are experiencing an active mental health crisis to either emergency medical services (911) or mental health services (988).

EVALUATION AND ADVERSE EFFECTS

We conducted descriptive analyses, finding the number and percentage of cases and median age for mental health crisis cases managed by the GPC between January 1, 2024, and December 31, 2024. Further details regarding the methods we used to analyze crisis call protocol outcomes can be found in Table A (available as a supplement to the online version of this article at http://www.ajph.org).

A prospective analysis of 2024 calls demonstrated that the GPC managed 533 mental health crisis cases, which constituted 0.7% of all exposure cases (i.e., cases in which the subject of the case was a human exposed to a substance) that the GPC managed during that period. Relative to other exposure cases, those experiencing a mental health crisis were older and more likely to be a woman or girl (Table A). Among mental health crisis cases, 103 (19.3%) required active rescue only, 6 (1.1%) had a threat of immediate harm only, and 43 (8.1%) were both. There were 77 (14.4%) mental health crisis cases in which the patient was exposed to a substance before the GPC was called.

Cases could involve exposure to one or more substances. Most mental health crisis cases involved exposure to one substance only (n = 420; 78.8%), but some included up to eight substances. Specific substance category exposures are shown in Table B (available as a supplement to the online version of this article at http://www.ajph.org).

Callers provided a dispatchable location in 392 (73.5%) mental health crisis cases. Forty-five (8.4%) mental health crisis cases were transferred to 911, with an average (interquartile range) call transfer time of three (two to five) minutes. Among those transferred to 911, nine cases were transferred despite patient refusal. Third-party individuals (including cases in which emergency medical services were already en route or on scene) ultimately transported patients to the emergency department in 60 (11.3%) mental health crisis cases. Six (1.1%) cases were transferred to 988. Among transfers to 988, transfer times were identifiable for two patients: one minute for one patient and six minutes for the other.

Implementation of the protocol in 2024 resulted in 50 (9.4%) critical protocol deviations, which involved not calling 911 when otherwise required per the protocol, allowing the patient to go to the emergency department on their own, or having inadequate coding to determine protocol adherence. There were 13 critical protocol deviations in January, and protocol deviations (per crisis case) decreased by about 10% per month, with an overall rate ratio of 0.90 (95% confidence interval = 0.83, 0.98; $P = .01$).

SUSTAINABILITY

Development and implementation of the protocol did not require external funding. The protocol used established emergency services that each have their own funding mechanisms.

The first three months of protocol implementation constituted a pilot period, during which stakeholders refined the protocol and conducted additional staff training. The pilot period also included conversion of the GPC process from a guideline (a practice that staff should follow) to a protocol (a practice that staff must follow); SPI education on implementing the protocol that addressed the nature and purpose of 988; development of a 911 PSAP map that listed "backdoor" telephone numbers and dispatch services; and efforts to raise public awareness about the service. The GPC conducted monthly staff meetings for training and staff feedback on the protocol. Stakeholders also held quarterly interagency meetings to solicit feedback.

Many mental health crisis cases qualified for transfer to 988 but were not transferred. This process and critical protocol deviations can be addressed by ongoing reeducation of SPIs on the protocol and on the roles of 911 and 988. Protocol training did not specifically include cultural sensitivity elements, and there may have been some referral disparities based on race/ethnicity, socioeconomic status, or English language proficiency.

Call routing to the GPC is based on telephone area code, not geographic location; therefore, the GPC received some calls that were misrouted from out of state. Use of Next Generation 911 technology, a PC Federal Communications Commission–based three-digit telephone number (similar to 911 and 988), and geolocating technology may enhance interstate and intrastate implementation of this protocol. Additionally, the development of text-to-chat options may expand the type of caller (e.g., younger patients) and the type of crisis (e.g., domestic violence).

Our triage criteria were relatively conservative regarding transferring to 911, with transfer criteria based predominantly on patient intentionality. Further research should investigate the accuracy of initial exposure reports to determine whether the protocol can be liberalized, for example, determining whether calls can be safely triaged based on the potential lethality of reported exposures. Additional research is needed to assess whether protocol implementation improves long-term patient outcomes, including suicide and self-harm rates, morbidity and mortality, and engagement in aftercare.

PUBLIC HEALTH SIGNIFICANCE

This protocol is a novel, efficacious, and feasible public health intervention for patients experiencing a mental health crisis owing to overdose. Overall, our study demonstrates a vital role for PCs in national suicide prevention efforts.

PCs are already a means of public health toxicosurveillance.[8–10] Our data demonstrate that PCs can also serve as a means of mental health crisis surveillance and infrastructure to collect public health data on mental health crises. SPIs can be trained to collect and document these data in real time while the patient is experiencing an active mental health crisis. PCs can coordinate care for complex cases of repeat overdose for patients who go to multiple health care facilities.[11]

Our study demonstrates that PCs can effectively develop relationships with 911 and 988 services. This protocol, which we implemented at a PC with a relatively large call volume that services the entire state of Georgia, may be translatable to PC and 911–988 collaborations in other states. PCs across the United States manage more than two million exposure cases annually.[5] Scaling up this protocol for use in other PCs can potentially affect tens of thousands of patients in mental health crisis annually. AJPH

ABOUT THE AUTHORS

Matthew Robert Dernbach, Joseph E. Carpenter, Tim P. Moran, and Brent W. Morgan are with the Department of Emergency Medicine, Emory University School of Medicine, Atlanta, GA. Stephanie Hon, Gaylord Lopez, and Patrick Filkins are with the Georgia Poison Center, Atlanta. Nadine J. Kaslow and Sophie Arkin are with the Department of Psychiatry and Behavioral Sciences, Emory University School of Medicine. Kevin Tanner is with the Georgia Department of Behavioral Health and Developmental Disabilities, Atlanta. Aleisha Rucker-Wright and Greg Whitaker are with the Georgia Emergency Communications Authority, Atlanta. Dawn Peel, Erin Conaway, and Brenda Cibulas are with the Division of Behavioral Health, Georgia Department of Behavioral Health and Developmental Disabilities. Andrea Corley is with Behavioral Health Link, Atlanta, GA. Ryan Davis Solis and Desiree Arnold are with City of Atlanta 911, Atlanta, GA. Robert J. Geller is with the Department of Pediatrics, Emory University School of Medicine.

CORRESPONDENCE

Correspondence should be sent to Matthew Robert Dernbach, Department of Emergency Medicine, Emory University School of Medicine, 50 Hurt Plaza SE, Suite 600, Atlanta, GA 30303 (e-mail: mrdernbach@carilionclinic.org). Reprints can be ordered at https://www.ajph.org by clicking the "Reprints" link.

PUBLICATION INFORMATION

Full Citation: Dernbach MR, Hon S, Lopez G, et al. Managing mental health crisis calls received by a US poison center: a statewide collaboration between the Georgia Poison Center, 911, and 988. *Am J Public Health.* 2025;115(11):1814–1817.

Acceptance Date: June 18, 2025.

DOI: https://doi.org/10.2105/AJPH.2025.308229

ORCID iDs:

Matthew Robert Dernbach https://orcid.org/0000-0002-5907-0914

Gaylord Lopez https://orcid.org/0009-0009-0470-835X

Nadine J. Kaslow https://orcid.org/0000-0003-0775-8597

Joseph E. Carpenter https://orcid.org/0000-0001-5487-6671

Andrea Corley https://orcid.org/0009-0006-1583-5512

Tim P. Moran https://orcid.org/0000-0003-0425-1256

Patrick Filkins https://orcid.org/0009-0001-8785-699X

Erin Conaway https://orcid.org/0009-0000-4486-8571

Robert J. Geller https://orcid.org/0000-0002-1578-1087

CONTRIBUTORS

M. R. Dernbach conceptualized and designed the study, analyzed the data, and drafted the article. M. R. Dernbach, S. Hon, G. Lopez, N. J. Kaslow, J. E. Carpenter, K. Tanner, A. Rucker-Wright, D. Peel, A. Corley, R. D. Solis, B. W. Morgan, P. Filkins, G. Whitaker, E. Conaway, B. Cibulas, S. Arkin, D. Arnold, and R. Geller designed the study and reviewed the article. T. P. Moran analyzed the data and reviewed the article.

ACKNOWLEDGMENTS

Results were presented at the 2025 Poison Center Leadership Meeting, New Orleans, LA, and at the 2024 North American Congress of Clinical Toxicology, Denver, CO.

The authors would like to thank the following individuals for their assistance with this study: Britni Overall and Alison Jones (Georgia Poison Center); Malika Bey, Cassandra Price, and Dustin Infinger (Division of Behavioral Health, Georgia Department of Behavioral Health and Developmental Disabilities); Katie Cossette, Kelly Parry, and Anna Bourque (Georgia Crisis and Access Line, Georgia Department of Behavioral Health and Developmental Disabilities); Amy Ramsey and Skylar Whitaker (Georgia Emergency Communications Authority); Cliveita Brown, MPA (Department of Emergency Medical Services, Grady Memorial Hospital); and Stephanie Medina (City of Atlanta 911).

CONFLICTS OF INTEREST

The authors do not have any actual or potential conflicts of interest pertaining to this study.

HUMAN PARTICIPANT PROTECTION

The Emory University institutional review board (IRB) deemed this study to be public health practice and therefore exempt from full IRB review and oversight (STUDY00009459).

REFERENCES

1. Farah R, Cole RJ, Holstege CP. Increasing severity of medical outcomes and associated substances in cases reported to United States poison centers. *Clin Toxicol (Phila).* 2024;62(4):248–255. https://doi.org/10.1080/15563650.2024.2337897
2. Stephan W. Training poison specialists with QPR to improve care for suicidal callers [meeting abstract A294]. North American Congress of Clinical Toxicology (NACCT) 2023. *Clin Toxicol (Phila).* 2023;61(suppl 2):143. https://doi.org/10.1080/15563650.2023.2233835
3. US Census Bureau. 2020 Decennial census: Georgia. April 2020. Available at: https://data.census.gov/profile/Georgia?g=040XX00US13. Accessed April 22, 2025.
4. State Office of Rural Health, Georgia Department of Community Health. Georgia rural counties. August 2021. Available at: https://dch.georgia.gov/document/document/georgia-rural-counties-map/download. Accessed April 22, 2025.
5. Gummin DD, Mowry JB, Beuhler MC, et al. 2023 Annual report of the National Poison Data System (NPDS) from America's Poison Centers: 41st annual report. *Clin Toxicol (Phila).* 2024;62(12):793–1027. https://doi.org/10.1080/15563650.2024.2412423
6. Fitchette B. The ethics of referral and intervention with non-life threatening suicide attempts by overdose of medication and ingestion of harmful substances. *Omega (Westport).* 1996;33(3):179–191. https://doi.org/10.2190/06GR-2KFX-YYEA-NJ2A
7. Davis A, Allegro J. Use of tabletop simulation to develop a guideline for triaging adult callers at imminent risk for harm to self or others [meeting abstract A167]. North American Congress of Clinical Toxicology (NACCT) 2024. *Clin Toxicol (Phila).* 2024;62(suppl 2):84. https://doi.org/10.1080/15563650.2024.2370671
8. Friedman LS. Real-time surveillance of illicit drug overdoses using poison center data. *Clin Toxicol (Phila).* 2009;47(6):573–579. https://doi.org/10.1080/15563650902967404
9. Spiller HA, Griffith JR. The value and evolving role of the US Poison Control Center System. *Public Health Rep.* 2009;124(3):359–363. https://doi.org/10.1177/003335490912400303
10. Carpenter JE, Chang AS, Bronstein AC, et al. Identifying incidents of public health significance using the National Poison Data System, 2013–2018. *Am J Public Health.* 2020;110(10):1528–1531. https://doi.org/10.2105/AJPH.2020.305842
11. Lemon S, Banerji S. A case of extreme repeat APAP exposure: 83 overdoses in 1 person within a 21-month span [meeting abstract A280]. North American Congress of Clinical Toxicology (NACCT) 2024. *Clin Toxicol (Phila).* 2024;62(suppl 2):142. https://doi.org/10.1080/15563650.2024.2370671

Falling Further Over the US Safety Net Benefits Cliff After COVID-19

Vickie M. Mays, PhD, MSPH, and Michelle Sarah Livings, PhD, MPH

ABOUT THE AUTHORS

Vickie M. Mays is with the Department of Psychology and the Department of Health Policy & Management, Fielding School of Public Health, University of California, Los Angeles. Michelle Sarah Livings is with the Department of Health Sciences, Rutgers University-Camden, Camden, NJ.

See also COVID-19 Benefits Cliff, pp. 1821–1867.

After the declaration of COVID-19 as a public health emergency in the United States in early 2020, private health insurers and health care providers were given leeway from regulations and provided innovative risk reduction care approaches through online portals and increased access to telehealth services. This modernized service delivery, particularly for those with barriers to health care access, and reduced public contact with an infectious agent. Furthermore, the public health emergency declaration paved the way for federal waivers or modifications in safety net programs such as Medicare, Medicaid, and the Children's Health Insurance Program.[1]

Congress passed a number of bills to provide health and welfare benefits, such as the Families First Coronavirus Response Act[2]; the Coronavirus Aid, Relief, and Economic Security Act[3]; the American Rescue Plan Act[4]; the Inflation Reduction Act[5]; and the Consolidated Appropriations Act.[6] However, almost all COVID-19-related legislation had expired by 2023, when COVID-19 was no longer a US public health emergency. The safety net expansions implemented by the US federal government during the COVID-19 public health emergency to reduce infections, protect socially vulnerable populations, and maintain a level of economic stability were removed.

The federal eviction moratorium ended in August 2021, followed by the Coronavirus Aid, Relief, and Economic Security Act moratorium on foreclosures in September 2021.[7] The expanded Child Tax Credit achieved a record low child poverty rate in 2021; after this expansion expired at the end of 2021, the child poverty rate more than doubled in 2022.[8] The longest-lasting safety net expansions implemented during the COVID-19 pandemic—the Supplemental Nutrition Assistance Program (SNAP) emergency allotments and continuous coverage for Medicaid beneficiaries—ended in spring 2023.[9] The payment pause on student loans ended in September 2023, and millions of individuals were already past due on payments by January 2024.[10] The ending of these expansions has created benefits cliffs with a range of repercussions, particularly among socially vulnerable populations.

This special section of *AJPH* presents a collection of five articles that incorporate different research approaches and

Continued on page 1819...

HISTORY CORNER

25 YEARS AGO

State Welfare Reform Policies and Declines in Health Insurance

Others have reported the chronological relationship between welfare reform, declines in Medicaid, and increases in uninsurance. What this analysis adds to those observations is an indication that policies deterring TANF enrollment may contribute to these changes. . . . The problem may also derive from the philosophic shift regarding governmental support for the poor, and particularly for poor women and children, that underlies the PRWORA. Enrollment in other government benefit programs, such as food assistance, has also declined during this same time period, even as requests for emergency food assistance across the country have increased sharply. Governmentally subsidized childcare was the only program that received additional funds, in order to enable women receiving TANF to comply with workfare requirements, and transitional childcare was extended to women losing TANF, so that they might work. However, despite widespread recognition of lack of childcare, there has been poor uptake of this benefit. We speculate that the message communicated to the poor is the undifferentiated one that, in general, benefit programs are no longer available, although, of course, many factors are at work in such complex social phenomena.

From *AJPH*, June 2000, p. 906

cover various aspects of the postpandemic benefits cliffs. As new benefits cliffs are looming in the wake of the current political determinants of health in the United States, this timely collection of articles gives some insights into the consequences of legislation that erodes foundational safety net programs such as Medicare, Medicaid, and SNAP.

In "Children's Insurance Stability and Coverage Inequities During the COVID-19 Continuous Coverage Provisions" (p. 1848), Eliason et al. investigate changes in children's public health insurance coverage during the continuous coverage provisions under the Families First Coronavirus Response Act, which froze Medicaid disenrollment nationally by offering enhanced federal fund matching to states that ensured continuous coverage for Medicaid beneficiaries. The authors analyze data from the Medical Expenditure Panel Survey, comparing 2015 to 2019 (pre-COVID-19) with 2020 to 2021 (during COVID-19). Although this study does not look past the end of the Families First Coronavirus Response Act in April 2023, the authors conclude that continuous eligibility policies reduce insurance churning and noncoverage among children. They estimate that more than 6 million children likely lost public health insurance coverage after this benefits cliff, foreshadowing what may come from the safety net reductions of the 2025 legislative actions.

In "Expansion of the Earned Income Tax Credit for Young Adults in 2021 and Mental Health of US Home Renters" (p. 1858), Ali and Lyu examine mental health among young adult homeowners and renters using 2021 to 2023 Behavioral Risk Factor Surveillance System data. They compare the periods before and after the enactment of the American Rescue Plan Act in March 2021, which expanded the Earned Income Tax Credit for childless adults for one year and extended eligibility to young adults 19 to 24 years of age for the first time. Their results suggest that federal antipoverty measures are beneficial to mental health and well-being, especially for cost-burdened individuals such as young adult renters. This insight comes at a time in which the United States faces increased mental health challenges for younger populations including school disruptions, climate change, and immigration stresses.

In "Lived Experiences of Families Navigating Safety Net Expansions and Retractions During the Pandemic: A Qualitative Study" (p. 1836), Fernández-Viña et al. examine the experiences of low-income California families throughout the COVID-19-related safety net expansions and retractions. Drawing on semistructured interviews, the authors identify main themes such as "the end of SNAP [emergency allotments] exacerbated food insecurity" and "administrative burdens created barriers to safety net participation." The authors highlight the unmet needs that the COVID-19-related safety net addressed. However, new and returning administrative burdens that result in public benefits being more difficult to access, such as additional eligibility requirements, may increase stress among individuals and families already on the fringes of economic survival.

Related to one of the themes featured by Fernández-Viña et al., Bitler and Schanzenbach explore the effects of the end of SNAP emergency allotments in "Pandemic-Era Increases in SNAP Benefits Reduced Food Insufficiency" (p. 1821). Using SNAP quality control administrative data and food insufficiency data from the Census

Continued on page 1820...

HISTORY CORNER

36 YEARS AGO

The Impact of Medicaid on Physician Use by Low-Income Children

The preceding analysis has shown that Medicaid coverage increases access to office-based physicians, within the low-income population. The results obtained in this study suggest that previous studies which focus on the general population may obscure the effect of Medicaid on physician use by low-income children. Another important effect of Medicaid was on the number of visits among those with at least one visit. By lowering the relative price of a visit, Medicaid children made more visits than uninsured children, but not compared to privately insured children. These results are particularly important in light of recent Congressional initiatives allowing states to expand Medicaid eligibility to low-income children through age eight with incomes up to 100 percent of the federal poverty line, and infants under age one with incomes up to 185 percent of the federal poverty line.

From *AJPH*, September 1989, p. 1224

Household Pulse Survey, the authors find that the reduction in benefits after SNAP emergency allotments ended was related to higher rates of food insufficiency among most adult age groups. Their analysis also suggests that increased SNAP benefits reduce food insufficiency. As both food insufficiency and food insecurity are associated with increased chronic disease risk[11] and poor mental health,[12] the increase in food insufficiency after the end of SNAP emergency allotments is likely contributing to other US health crises.

Finally, in "Pandemic-Related Funding Termination and Structural Drivers of Inequities: A Case Study of a *Promotores/as*-Focused Community-Based Organization" (p. 1824), LeBrón et al. investigate the effects of the postpandemic benefits cliffs on individuals, families, and community-based organizations (CBOs) working with vulnerable communities. CBOs received substantial funding from federal COVID-19 relief and recovery programs, allowing for increased staffing and programming; however, that governmental funding ended. The LeBrón et al. study highlights the experiences of promotores (community health workers) working with a midsized California CBO during COVID-19; in California, Latines are still experiencing excess COVID-19 mortality, particularly among immigrants.[13,14] The authors illustrate that losses of pandemic-related governmental funding to support CBOs jeopardized the stability and good work of these organizations at a time when marginalized populations and communities are still suffering from the aftershocks of COVID-19.

There is precedent for providing continuous safety net benefits when a pandemic has ongoing negative health and economic impacts. Such precedents are often driven by public health needs and are in the service of containment, reduction, or elimination of a public health epidemic. For example, although the overall rate of HIV/AIDS in the United States has dramatically decreased, a number of socially vulnerable populations are still disproportionately affected. Congressional legislation and federal funding continue to stay in place in such forms as the Ryan White HIV/AIDS Program, the Minority HIV/AIDS Fund, and the Ending the HIV Epidemic in the US initiative, among others.

Sadly, what we learn from history repeating itself is the extent to which presidential administrations—with their contrasting social, economic, and cultural worldviews—emerge as the factor that most markedly affects public health infectious disease policies. This special section presents scientific and CBO perspectives on post-COVID-19 benefits cliffs. Yet, the political climate and voting and election results will determine the future of US safety net policies: whether we lose more benefits or ensure the best public health policies for our most vulnerable residents. AJPH

CORRESPONDENCE

Correspondence should be sent to Michelle Sarah Livings, PhD, MPH, Armitage Hall 420, 311 N 5th St, Camden, NJ 08102 (e-mail: michelle.livings@rutgers.edu). Reprints can be ordered at https://www.ajph.org by clicking the "Reprints" link.

PUBLICATION INFORMATION

Full Citation: Mays VM, Livings MS. Falling further over the US safety net benefits cliff after COVID-19. *Am J Public Health*. 2025;115(11):1818–1820.

Acceptance Date: August 11, 2025.

DOI: https://doi.org/10.2105/AJPH.2025.308272

ORCID iD:

Michelle Sarah Livings https://orcid.org/0000-0002-8529-1614

CONTRIBUTORS

The authors contributed equally to this editorial.

CONFLICTS OF INTEREST

The authors have no potential or actual conflicts of interest to disclose.

REFERENCES

1. Cubanski J, Kates J, Tolbert J, Guth M, Pollitz K, Freed F. What happens when COVID-19 emergency declarations end? Implications for coverage, costs, and access. Available at: https://www.kff.org/coronavirus-covid-19/issue-brief/what-happens-when-covid-19-emergency-declarations-end-implications-for-coverage-costs-and-access. Accessed July 11, 2025.
2. Moss K, Dawson L, Long M, et al. The Families First Coronavirus Response Act: summary of key provisions. Available at: https://www.kff.org/coronavirus-covid-19/issue-brief/the-families-first-coronavirus-response-act-summary-of-key-provisions. Accessed August 13, 2025.
3. Moss K, Wexler A, Dawson L, et al. The Coronavirus Aid, Relief, and Economic Security Act: summary of key health provisions. Available at: https://www.kff.org/coronavirus-covid-19/issue-brief/the-coronavirus-aid-relief-and-economic-security-act-summary-of-key-health-provisions. Accessed August 13, 2025.
4. 117th Congress. American Rescue Plan Act of 2021 (HR 1319). Available at: https://www.congress.gov/bill/117th-congress/house-bill/1319. Accessed August 13, 2025.
5. 117th Congress. Inflation Reduction Act of 2022 (HR 5376). Available at: https://www.congress.gov/bill/117th-congress/house-bill/5376. Accessed August 13, 2025.
6. 117th Congress. Consolidated Appropriations Act, 2023 (HR 2617). Available at: https://www.congress.gov/bill/117th-congress/house-bill/2617. Accessed August 13, 2025.
7. Haas J, Rangel J, Garnham JP, Hepburn P. Preliminary analysis: eviction filing trends after the CDC moratorium expiration. Available at: https://evictionlab.org/updates/research/eviction-filing-trends-after-cdc-moratorium. Accessed July 9, 2025.
8. Hughes J. Lapse of Expanded Child Tax Credit led to unprecedented rise in child poverty. Available at: https://itep.org/lapse-of-expanded-child-tax-credit-led-to-unprecedented-rise-in-child-poverty-2023. Accessed July 9, 2025.
9. Center on Budget and Policy Priorities. Timeline: understanding the impact of the end of the public health emergency and COVID-19 waivers on SNAP households. Available at: https://www.cbpp.org/research/food-assistance/understanding-the-impact-of-the-end-of-the-public-health-emergency-and. Accessed July 9, 2025.
10. US Government Accountability Office. When the student loan payment pause ended, did borrowers pay? Available at: https://www.gao.gov/blog/when-student-loan-payment-pause-ended-did-borrowers-pay. Accessed July 9, 2025.
11. Weaver LJ, Fasel CB. A systematic review of the literature on the relationships between chronic diseases and food insecurity. *FNS*. 2018;9(5):519–541. https://doi.org/10.4236/fns.2018.95040
12. Nagata JM, Ganson KT, Whittle HJ, et al. Food insecurity and mental health in the US during the COVID-19 pandemic. *Am J Prev Med*. 2021;60(4):453–461. https://doi.org/10.1016/j.amepre.2020.12.004
13. Riley AR, Chen YH, Matthay EC, et al. Excess mortality among Latino people in California during the COVID-19 pandemic. *SSM Popul Health*. 2021;15:100860. https://doi.org/10.1016/j.ssmph.2021.100860
14. California Department of Public Health. COVID-19 age, race, and ethnicity data. Available at: https://www.cdph.ca.gov/Programs/CID/DCDC. Accessed July 16, 2025.

Pandemic-Era Increases in SNAP Benefits Reduced Food Insufficiency

Marianne Bitler, PhD, and Diane Whitmore Schanzenbach, PhD

ABOUT THE AUTHORS

Marianne Bitler is with the Department of Economics, University of California, Davis, and the National Bureau of Economic Research, Cambridge, MA. Diane Whitmore Schanzenbach is with the McCourt School of Public Policy, Georgetown University, Washington, DC, and the National Bureau of Economic Research, Cambridge, MA.

See also COVID-19 Benefits Cliff, pp. 1818–1867.

At its peak during COVID-19 and afterward, the Supplemental Nutrition Assistance Program (SNAP) served one in eight Americans, helping them to purchase food. Just as it had done during previous recessions, SNAP expanded the number of people served as families newly fell on hard times and needed assistance from the safety net. Building on lessons from prior recessions, during COVID-19, Congress authorized several temporary emergency provisions that made SNAP more responsive to the economic downturn, including the suspension of work requirements, administrative flexibilities that reduced the need for in-person contact with state caseworkers, an across-the-board benefit increase, and substantially increased benefit levels through a provision called Emergency Allotments (EAs). When EAs ended, average benefit levels fell by over 35%, from about $475 per month to about $290.

Usually, researchers have used variation in SNAP participation along the extensive margin—comparing outcomes for those who receive benefits to those who do not—to estimate the impact of SNAP on outcomes such as food insufficiency. The changes implemented during COVID-19 allowed us to provide new evidence on the relationship between benefit levels and outcomes. We used the drop in SNAP benefits resulting from the ending of EAs, first in selected states and then nationally, to estimate how food insufficiency responds to changes in benefit levels.

Under typical circumstances, SNAP benefits decline as family income increases. Families with no income (such as after allowable deductions under the program for housing, medical care, and child care) receive the maximum SNAP benefit for their family size. This maximum benefit amount is based on the cost of the US Department of Agriculture's "Thrifty Food Plan," and was $509 per month for a family of three at the onset of COVID-19 in 2020. As family incomes rise, SNAP benefits are reduced by about 30 cents for each extra dollar families have, until their income is high enough that they are no longer eligible for SNAP.

EAs increased a family's SNAP benefits to the maximum benefit amount. If the difference between the family's typical SNAP benefit and the maximum benefit was less than $95, then they received a $95 increase, ensuring that the lowest-income families also received additional benefits. EAs were $95 for about half of SNAP participants, increasing benefits by 30% on average (with increases ranging between 8% and 59%). Some higher-income SNAP recipients who typically receive relatively modest benefits had increases that were several times their normal benefit amount. For example, 19% of SNAP households typically receive $100 or less in benefits. Among these families, their typical benefits average $45 per month, and EAs added $265 per month.

Nationwide, EAs were eliminated after the payments made in February 2023. Prior to this, 16 states chose to end their EA payments early.[1] Idaho was the first to end EA payments in May 2021, and Indiana was the last state to terminate EAs early (in June 2022). We used this variation and a quasi-experimental, difference-in-differences analytic approach to measure the impact of the sizable reduction in SNAP benefit levels at the end of the COVID-19 period on food insufficiency.

To measure the effects of the end of EAs on benefits, we analyzed SNAP Quality Control administrative data spanning July 2021 through September 2023. These data contain detailed information on participating families' demographics, income from all sources, and benefit levels, and are nationally representative.[2] Measures of food insufficiency over the same period were drawn from the Census Household Pulse Survey, a quick response data set collected by the Census Bureau to track the effects of COVID-19 on family well-being and economic resources over time. The Pulse included a question asking respondents about the food available to them over the prior seven days. If they reported that they "sometimes" or "often" did not have enough to eat over the past week,

AJPH November 2025, Vol. 115, No. 11

we coded them as having food insufficiency. Following Bauer et al.,[3] we limited the Pulse analysis to those with incomes below 130% of the poverty threshold to align with SNAP eligibility rules.

We used differences-in-differences analysis to compare outcomes before and after a policy change, such as the end of EAs in states making the policy change, and then used a control group of states that did not experience this policy change to provide a counterfactual "what would have happened in the treatment states had they not experienced the policy change." Our difference-in-differences regressions included controls for the state of residence and the timing of the survey, to account for time-invariant state-specific factors and time-varying national factors such as other COVID-19 policies or changes in national economic conditions. We estimated eight separate regressions in each data set, grouping the data by respondent's age and the presence of children in their households.

Overall, we found that SNAP benefits declined across all groups when EAs ended, with declines ranging from an average of $125 per month among those aged 18 to 34 years without children to an average of $267 per month among those aged 35 to 49 years with children. When we combined all of the households' monthly resources from earnings, other income, and SNAP benefits, resources declined on average between 7% and 16% (depending on the group) when EAs ended. The corresponding increase in food insufficiency measured in the Pulse ranged from small and not statistically significant (for younger, childless respondents) to a 23% rise (from 30% to 37%, among respondents aged 50 to 64 years with children).

Figure 1 displays our findings, by group, of the impacts of the termination of EAs. The horizontal axis represents the average decline in total household resources, and the vertical axis shows the change in food insufficiency. The size of the circles corresponds to the share of the SNAP population in each group, and the line fits a weighted least squares regression to these averages. Groups that experienced larger declines in resources also had larger increases in food insufficiency.

This evidence suggests that increased benefit levels reduced food insufficiency, complementing findings from other pandemic-era programs showing reduced food insufficiency from increased resources. For example, food insufficiency was reduced by Pandemic

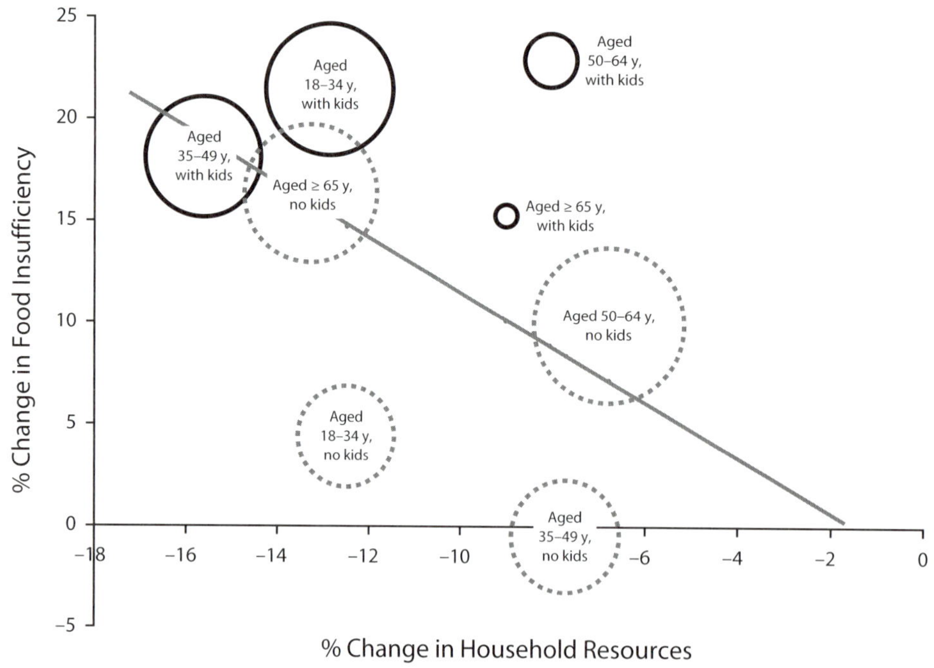

FIGURE 1— Change in Food Insufficiency vs Change in Resources After SNAP Emergency Allotment Payments Ended: United States, 2020–2023

Note. SNAP = Supplemental Nutrition Assistance Program. The size of the circles corresponds to the share of the SNAP population in each group, and the line fits a weighted least squares regression to these averages. Percentage change in household resources on the horizontal axis was measured using SNAP Quality Control data, July 2021 to September 2023. Percentage change in food insufficiency on the vertical axis was measured using Census Household Pulse Survey, weeks 13 to 60 (August 19–31, 2020 through July 26–August 7, 2023).

Electronic Benefits Transfer payments that provided food benefits to replace missed school meals during school closures,[3] and by the expanded Child Tax Credit in 2021.[4] Other work has also found that food insufficiency increased after states' early termination of EAs[5] and declined when a different pandemic-era SNAP policy increased maximum SNAP benefits by 15% across the board.[6]

Although SNAP EAs were only a temporary boost during COVID-19, we can use them to learn about the relationship between benefit levels and food insufficiency—a relationship that is important to understand but previously has been difficult to study. In 2021, unrelated to COVID-19, the Thrifty Food Plan on which SNAP benefit levels are based was updated for the first time in decades. As a result, SNAP benefits were increased by an average of 21%. If the same relationship holds as we found in Figure 1, we predict that this national policy reduced food insufficiency by over 5%.

The passage of the recent "One Big Beautiful Bill Act" made major changes in SNAP's funding, eligibility, and administrative rules. Although there is still too much uncertainty to predict the law's likely impacts on food insufficiency, evidence certainly suggests that reducing safety net benefits will negatively affect food insufficiency. AJPH

CORRESPONDENCE

Correspondence should be sent to Marianne Bitler, UC Davis Department of Economics, 1 Shields Ave, Davis, CA 95616 (e-mail: bitler@ucdavis.edu). Reprints can be ordered at https://www.ajph.org by clicking the "Reprints" link.

PUBLICATION INFORMATION

Full Citation: Bitler M, Schanzenbach DW. Pandemic-era increases in SNAP benefits reduced food insufficiency. *Am J Public Health*. 2025;115(11): 1821–1823.

Acceptance Date: August 13, 2025.

DOI: https://doi.org/10.2105/AJPH.2025.308274

ORCID iD:
Marianne Bitler https://orcid.org/0000-0002-5425-401X

CONTRIBUTORS

M. Bitler and D. W. Schanzenbach contributed equally to the conceptualization, drafting, writing, and final approval. D. W. Schanzenbach conducted the analysis.

CONFLICTS OF INTEREST

Neither author has any conflicts of interest to report.

REFERENCES

1. Schanzenbach DW. The impact of SNAP emergency allotments on SNAP benefits and food insufficiency. Institute for Policy Research Rapid Research Report. 2023. Available at: https://www.ipr.northwestern.edu/documents/reports/ipr-rapid-research-report-snap-emergency-allotments-impact-27-january-2023.pdf. Accessed August 22, 2025.
2. Cunnyngham K. Reaching those in need: estimates of state Supplemental Nutrition Assistance Program participation rates in 2020. 2023. Available at: https://fns-prod.azureedge.us/sites/default/files/resource-files/snap-participation-2020-final-report.pdf. Accessed August 22, 2025.
3. Bauer L, Ruffini K, Schanzenbach DW. The effects of lump-sum food benefits during the COVID-19 pandemic on spending, hardship, and health. *J Public Econ*. 2024;240:105269. https://doi.org/10.1016/j.jpubeco.2024.105269
4. Parolin Z, Ananat E, Collyer SM, Curran M, Wimer C. *The Initial Effects of the Expanded Child Tax Credit on Material Hardship*. Cambridge, MA: National Bureau of Economic Research; 2021. NBER Working Paper 29285.
5. Dasgupta K, Plum A. *Termination of SNAP Emergency Allotments, Food Sufficiency, and Economic Hardships*. Washington, DC: Board of Governors of the Federal Reserve System; 2023. Finance and Economics Discussion Series 2023-046.
6. Jackson KE, Chiang AY, Hamad R. The association of increased SNAP benefits during COVID-19 with food insufficiency and anxiety among US adults: a quasi-experimental study. *Public Health Nutr*. 2024; 27(1):e186. https://doi.org/10.1017/S1368980024001447

Pandemic-Related Funding Termination and Structural Drivers of Inequities: A Case Study of a *Promotores/as*-Focused Community-Based Organization

Alana M. W. LeBrón, PhD, MSc, Melina Michelen, MPH, Patricia J. Cantero, PhD, Gloria Itzel Montiel, PhD, Loreta Ruiz, BA, Kory Razaghi, MS, MBA, Laura Pantoja, Josefina Jimenez, Marisela Ramirez, America Bracho, MD, MPH, CDE, and John Billimek, PhD

See also COVID-19 Benefits Cliff, pp. 1818–1867.

AJPH November 2025, Vol. 115, No. 11

During the COVID-19 pandemic, governmental agencies expanded safety net programs to ameliorate profound economic suffering. However, structural challenges excluded many low-income, immigrant, and racially minoritized communities, deepening inequities. *Promotores/as* and community-based organizations (CBOs), whose models focus on addressing structural drivers of inequities, were vital to communities navigating these challenges.

This analytic essay examines how terminating pandemic-related funding strained CBOs and the communities they serve. Through a case study of a midsized *promotores/as* model CBO, we analyze practice-based qualitative and quantitative data, alongside a qualitative study of COVID-19 *promotores/as* models. Findings illuminate a dual postpandemic benefits cliff. As pandemic benefits expired, individuals once again faced the economic hardships that had been temporarily alleviated. Simultaneously, heightened demands on CBOs, along with reduced funding and resources, threatened their ability to meet community needs.

Findings indicate the importance of coalition-building for structural transformation and governmental and nongovernmental support of *promotores/as* models and CBOs to promote health equity. (*Am J Public Health*. 2025;115(11):1824–1835. https://doi.org/10.2105/AJPH.2025.308154)

The COVID-19 pandemic (henceforth, "pandemic") disproportionately affected historically and contemporarily disenfranchised communities, such as low-income communities, immigrant communities, and communities of color (henceforth, "minoritized communities") in the United States.[1–4] Racial/ethnic inequities in COVID-19 mortality widened between 2020 and 2021.[5] Inequities in wealth, employment, and health care worsened, with higher unemployment rates and slower recovery for Black and Latiné communities compared with White communities, highlighting the structural nature of inequities.[3] Housing insecurity also surged, with communities of color experiencing more rent difficulties and evictions.[3] Furthermore, school closures deepened achievement gaps and increased childcare and nutrition challenges.[3]

US federal, state, and local agencies mobilized to meet this unprecedented need, expanding Supplemental Nutrition Assistance Program (SNAP) benefits to unemployed and low-income individuals or households, increasing the child tax credit and Medicaid expansions, and implementing moratoria on evictions, foreclosures, and student loans.[6] While this expanded safety net reflected governmental efforts to meet unprecedented need, minoritized communities experienced substantial barriers to accessing resources, including explicit exclusions and bureaucratic barriers.[7,8] Governmental and health organizations recognized their own gaps in reaching and meeting these significant needs and acknowledged reliance on community health workers (CHWs) and community-based organizations (CBOs) to widen their reach during the pandemic.[9,10]

Building on their roles in addressing structural inequities, CBOs accountable to minoritized communities accompanied residents to address social, economic, and health-related needs worsened by the pandemic.[11–13] For example, CBOs raised awareness about the expansion of safety net programs in the pandemic and accompanied residents in navigating these safety nets. CBOs also engaged in systems change, such as leveraging their collaborations with governmental agencies (e.g., health departments, school districts) and nonprofit organizations (e.g., faith-based organizations, CBOs) to elevate community-level experiences of social, economic, and health inequities and to raise awareness of the benefits and barriers of safety net programs.[14] In addition, CBOs and grassroots initiatives developed mutual aid systems to address communities' unmet needs.[15,16]

PANDEMIC-SPECIFIC EXPANSION OF FUNDING AND COLLABORATION

From the early months of the pandemic, the scope and scale of CBO efforts expanded rapidly because of a sudden and substantial influx of federal funding to state and local governments. In addition to substantial safety net expansions directly allocated to individuals by the federal government, the American Rescue Plan Act (ARPA) delivered direct and flexible aid to more than 30 000 state, local, Tribal, and territorial governments through State and Local Fiscal Recovery Funds (SLFRF) to support a strong and equitable response and recovery.[17] Around 1500 state and local agencies budgeted $11.8 billion in SLFRF projects addressing public health needs, many in collaboration with CBOs. The Centers for Disease Control and Prevention (CDC) COVID-19 Health Disparities grants[18] brought an additional $2.25 billion to state and local governments for similar purposes. Programs including the National Institutes of Health (NIH) Community Engagement Alliance Against COVID-19 Disparities,[19] NIH Rapid Acceleration of Diagnostics–Underserved Populations,[20] and the Office of Minority Health Community Programs to Improve Minority Health[21] introduced funds to catalyze collaboration between academic institutions, CBOs, and state and local governments.

Federal funding passed through state and local governments to CBOs in the form of contracts and subawards to leverage CBOs' long-standing work addressing structural drivers of inequities to take leadership in the pandemic response. CBOs utilized expanded contracts to continue to directly support residents and advocate for policy and programmatic interventions. Collaboration across CBOs and between CBOs and governmental agencies (e.g., health departments, school districts) grew to unprecedented levels.[22] The rapid initiation and expansion of local government contracts with CBOs required CBOs to hire, train, and deploy staff quickly to operate at an expanded scope for pandemic response and recovery.

DUAL POSTPANDEMIC BENEFITS CLIFF IMPACTS

The expiration of federal funding and benefits, as well as expanded CBO funding, culminating in the December 2024 obligation deadline to use or return SLFRF funds,[23] has affected individuals and CBOs simultaneously. As pandemic relief programs and benefits expired, economic hardships quickly resurfaced. For instance, in mid-December 2020, 38% of US adults reported struggling to cover usual household expenses (e.g., food, housing, car payments, medical bills, student loans); this figure decreased to 29% by September–October 2021.[24] However, by February 2024, 36% of adults were again experiencing these difficulties, back to the same levels as the middle of the pandemic.[25] In addition, in 2023, overall and child poverty rates were substantially higher than in 2020 or 2021, when poverty levels were down to historic lows since 1967, given temporary pandemic relief measures.[26] Limited research has investigated the dual postpandemic benefits cliff: impacts on individuals, families, and communities, and impacts on CBOs who work alongside minoritized communities. CBOs are essential sources of community support, yet they face significant funding challenges.[27]

The purpose of this essay is to examine the impact of the postpandemic benefits cliff on a midsized CBO, Latino Health Access (LHA), that has long worked to address structural drivers of health inequities, experienced increased demands for services, and, subsequently, experienced decreased funding with the postpandemic benefits cliff. LHA applies a CHW or *promotores/as* (henceforth, "*promotores/as*") model. *Promotores/as* are trusted community members who integrate their lived experiences and health-related training to accompany residents in addressing unmet needs and build relationships and strategies to transform structural inequities that produce health inequities.[28] LHA's model is based on *promotores/as* providing navigation support and accompaniment of community members to understand and organize to overcome structural barriers to health, often involving multiple points of contact and long-term relationships.[14] This study integrates an analysis of data from practice-based sources, a qualitative study of COVID-19 *promotores/as* models, and insights from health services and public health scholars collaborating with LHA.

METHODS

This case study drew upon multiple data sources (Appendix A, available as a supplement to the online version of this article at https://ajph.org). First, we examined practice-based evidence from LHA, including (1) a thematic analysis[29] of a focus group discussion (October 2024; n = 5) with *promotores/as* and support staff (e.g., coordinators, directors) regarding the postpandemic benefits cliff, (2) a trend analysis of 2021 to 2023 evaluation data (e.g., outreach, contacts, services provided) and discussions with the evaluation and finance departments, and (3) a trend analysis of 2018/2019 to 2023 contracts and grants data (e.g., revenue, outreach). Second, we leveraged qualitative data from the CATALYST (Community Activation to TrAnsform Local sYSTems) Study of COVID-19 health equity *promotores/as* models, drawing on interviews and focus group discussions with LHA *promotores/as* (n = 10) conducted in 2023.[30] CATALYST followed a flexible coding approach, which involves indexing transcripts according to major discussion topics, maintaining analytical memos to document data-driven insights, and identifying relevant indices and attributes for further in-depth analysis.[31]

RESULTS

In the sections that follow, we describe the prepandemic, pandemic, and postpandemic contexts shaping CBO and community experiences.

Promotores/as in a Prepandemic Context

Since 1993, LHA, a midsized CBO, has partnered with communities to address structural drivers of health inequities and foster health, equity, and sustainable change through services, consciousness-raising, and civic participation.[32] Based in Santa Ana, California, a predominantly Latiné, immigrant, and low-income community, LHA's primary service area covers Orange County, California.[33] Before the pandemic, LHA's *promotor/a* model focused on raising awareness and accompanying residents to address the structural drivers of health, including departments focused on (1) chronic disease prevention and management, (2) mental health and emotional wellness, and (3) civic engagement and advocacy (e.g., voter engagement, housing counseling). A core group of 61 *promotores/as* facilitated programs and reached 9562 unduplicated participants (2018). LHA's expertise and model of addressing structural drivers and participants' immediate needs through *promotor*-led services, while building community capacity to engage in policy, systems, and environmental change, set the foundation for a rapid expansion of the number of *promotores/as* who would respond to the pandemic.

LHA practices a continuum of participation through the *promotores/as* model, starting with direct services and support and progressing to leadership roles through training and volunteer opportunities. This structure builds a pool of community leaders for future hiring and provides career pathways for *promotores/as* to advance while staying connected with residents,[34] which became an important infrastructure for pandemic response.

Pandemic-Related Contracts

Before the pandemic, LHA relied primarily on foundations for funding, accounting for 63% and 58% of total revenue in 2018 and 2019, respectively, compared with only 4% and 16%, respectively, from government grants in those 2 years (Figure 1).

As the pandemic unfolded, LHA experienced massive and rapid workforce and revenue growth. LHA's total revenue more than tripled from 2018 to 2020 and quadrupled by 2021 (Figure 2a and 2b). By 2020, LHA's total staff grew 2.5 times relative to 2018 and 2019, with the number of CHWs employed increasing by 2.7 times in the same interval (Figure 2b). This workforce growth reflected a shift in the traditional composition of LHA's *promotores/as'* demographics (e.g., predominantly female, Latina, Spanish-speaking) to include male *promotores* involved in peer campaigns and younger (college-aged) bilingual staff in the call center.

LHA's rapid growth was primarily attributable to a 30-fold increase in governmental funding from 2018 to 2020, and a nearly 57-fold increase from 2018 to 2021, almost entirely attributable to federal COVID-19 relief and recovery programs. During this period,

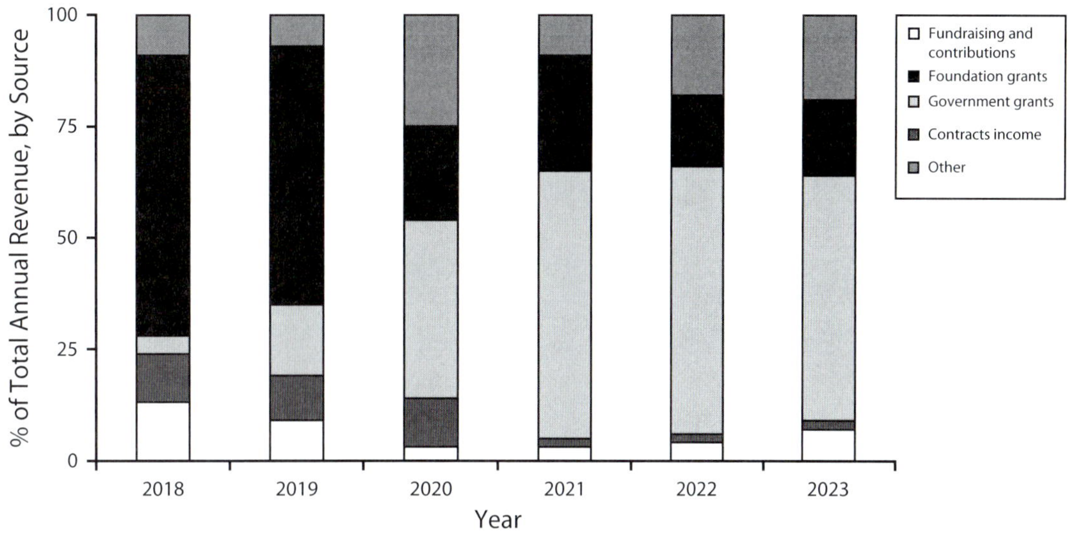

	2018	2019	2020	2021	2022	2023
Fundraising and contributions	13%	9%	3%	3%	4%	7%
Foundation grants	63%	58%	21%	26%	16%	17%
Government grants	4%	16%	40%	60%	60%	55%
Contracts income	11%	10%	11%	2%	2%	2%
Other	9%	7%	25%	9%	18%	19%

FIGURE 1— **Changes in Funding Mix at Latino Health Access: Orange County, CA, 2018–2023**

Note. Values are the percentage of total revenue represented by each funding source for a given year.

foundation grants that represented the majority of revenue in 2018 to 2019 remained relatively stable in absolute terms, fluctuating between 82% and 169% of 2018 levels in 2020 to 2023. This combination of rapidly increasing staffing, substantial growth in governmental funding, and modest increases in foundation funding meant that LHA was now primarily supported by governmental funding to sustain operations, increasing from 4% of LHA's revenue in 2018 to 60% by 2021. This led to a shift in contracting and increased mechanisms for fiscal compliance. Among the administrative changes, LHA hired a director of compliance and additional finance department staff (e.g., grants manager, accounting staff).

This pattern left LHA vulnerable to sudden decreases in governmental funding as federal COVID-19 spending decreased. In 2022, as some governmental grants ended, total revenue decreased as fast from 2021 levels (−21% year-over-year) as it increased from 2020 to 2021 (+23% year-over-year). With this decreased revenue, total staffing decreased by 28% and the number of CHWs employed dropped by 37%. Declines in governmental funding and total revenue continued into 2023 and are likely to deepen after the final appropriations from ARPA expired in December 2024 (Figure 2a and 2b). While increased support enabled LHA to strengthen its foundational approach, the loss of funding could jeopardize these advancements, highlighting the urgent need for sustained resources to address structural drivers of health inequities.

Dual Postpandemic Benefits Cliff

This section describes how LHA is applying pandemic-related knowledge and transformations, with a focus on how pandemic funding and the postpandemic benefits cliff affect individual, household, and community-level well-being and position and constrain community health equity efforts, drawing on data from interviews and focus groups (Box 1).

Initial response. In June 2020, LHA received its first 6-month contract from the local health department, doubling its budget. This funded 60 additional *promotores/as*, training LHA's staff in delivering COVID-19 information, managing the call center, developing outreach materials, and conducting a countywide outreach

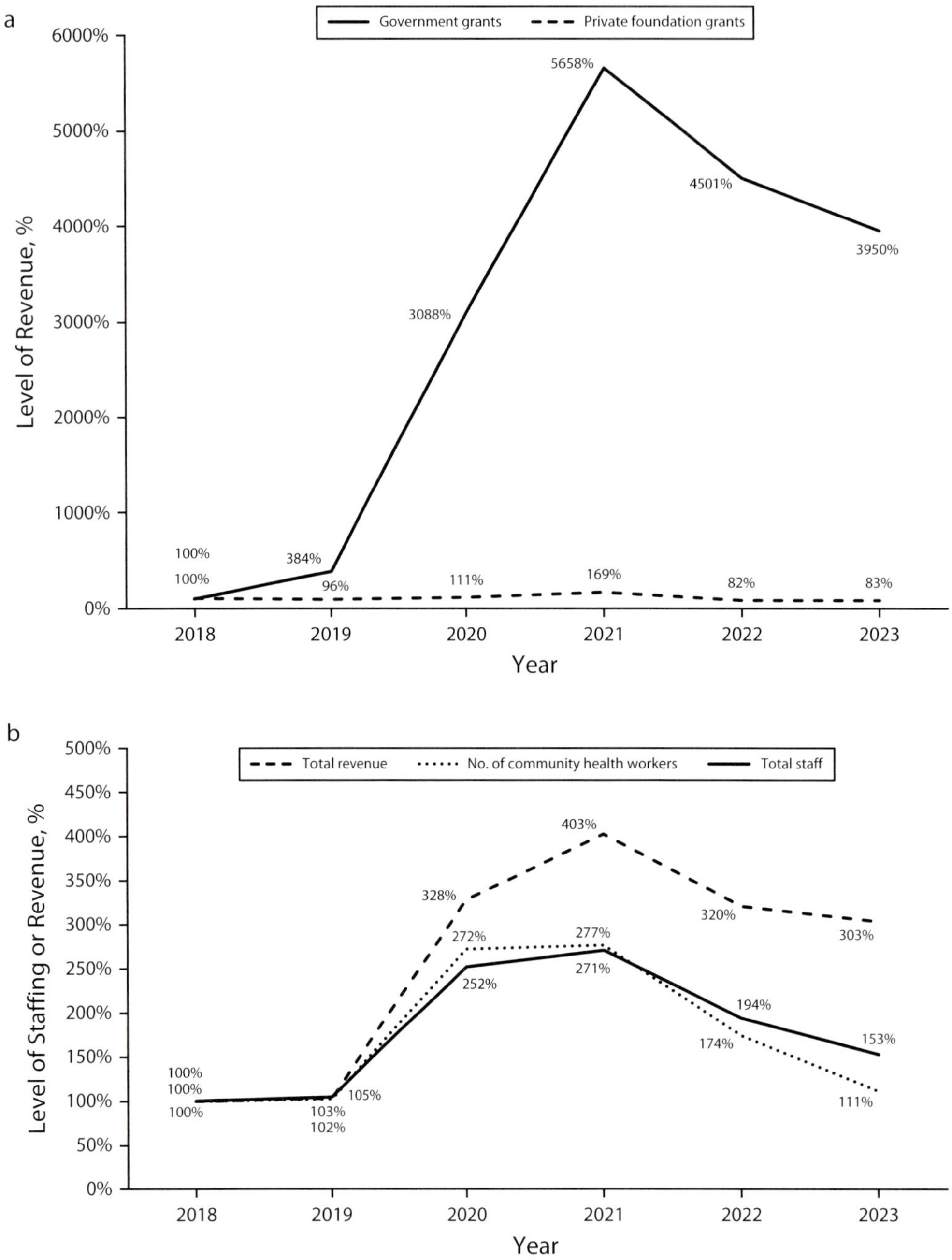

FIGURE 2— **Changes in Latino Health Access Levels of (a) Revenue by Source and (b) Staffing and Total Revenue: Orange County, CA, 2018–2023**

Note. All values reported are levels normalized to 2018 levels (100% = 2018 level of revenue or staffing): (a) changes in levels of grants revenue, by source; (b) changes in staffing (total and community health worker staffing) and in total revenue.

and information campaign. Importantly, *promotores/as* conducted community outreach in person—complying with pandemic requirements—to deliver personal protective equipment, food, and information via one-on-one outreach (in-person, telephone). *Promotores/as* noted that their years-long model uniquely positioned them to connect with residents despite pandemic restrictions, economic suffering, and virus transmission concerns and build upon their existing framework to respond nimbly to pandemic-related challenges. One *promotor/a* recalled, "It was a time for the organization and *promotoras* to mature and to respond. . . . The next day, we were already making calls."

Public health issues. Although the pandemic was declared over in May 2023,[35] sequelae remain, including economic inequities, housing insecurity, worsened mental well-being, and stigma, in addition to other interconnected and worsening crises, such as racial, environmental, and climate injustices.

In speaking of current needs, one *promotor/a* shared,

> We've also seen a massive migration . . . they have a lot of needs, including

BOX 1— Major Themes and Illustrative Quotes From *Promotoras/es* Navigating Pandemic Funding and the Benefits Cliff: Orange County, CA, 2018–2023

Theme	Illustrative Quotes
Initial response	"Work was being done based on a routine, on a habit that we already had from what we were already observing in the neighborhood. But this pandemic accelerated all of that. It took 100% more to bring more resources, to bring more services, to get closer to families. It increased the speed, on our end. And on the part of the families, to find the resources. But also on the part of the allies. On the part of these foundations, on the part of those groups that have the resources to accelerate the speed so that the resources reach the families. To get together, let's say, so that that was possible. . . . the pandemic came to bring us together, but to think quickly. Think fast. Act fast. Right? Learning things we didn't know, but learning and doing at that time." –CATALYST interview participant
Public health issues	"Mental health has increased a lot too. There are more people in a mental health crisis situation and with mental health diagnoses that often have the wrong information about their own diagnosis." –*Promotores/as* benefits cliff discussion "Even though there's no longer a COVID-19 emergency, we still see the impact, we still see the consequences of COVID-19 [that] allowed us to learn about mental health, stigma, and substance use, as well as strengthen our programs." –*Promotores/as* benefits cliff discussion
Services and programs	"For example, the Healthy Family [program] disappeared. And it was a good help for many families. Right? So things like those that people have gone through causes a lot of mistrust. And the one who is offering it is the *promotor*. Then we are terrified of putting our faces and then have it not happen later. That fear, because it costs a lot to gain the trust of the community." –CATALYST interview participant "Support groups, including one for grief, were reduced. From 12 groups, only 4 remained. Another one that went away is the support group for men. Also, the assistance to the community was cut, because even if there were some help, there was still a lot of need in the community and some community members are still suffering from the loss." –*Promotores/as* benefits cliff discussion
Training, learning opportunities, and career pathways for *promotores/as*	"I think that another barrier we also had is that many new people came to the team. Something positive is that LHA has been present and training *promotores/as* for many years, but there were also a lot of new people who were being asked to have the skills and responses of a *promotores/as* who had been working for 20 years . . . or for 15 years. . . . And it was like, I'll transmit all my thoughts to you." –CATALYST focus group participant "The training for COVID [Contact] Tracer was very extensive, very good. It was easy because you had to be focused because it was online, and I had never taken any online courses before. So, you have to be there, paying attention, taking notes." –CATALYST interview participant
Partnerships	"The work and collaboration with other organizations—organizations come and they know that participants come here, and they bring gift cards to participants, etc. community power will continue [to] grow." –*Promotores/as* benefits cliff discussion "The deep awareness that this is not going to change unless we all move together." –*Promotores/as* benefits cliff discussion

Continued

BOX 1— Continued

Theme	Illustrative Quotes
Advocacy and accompaniment	"The pandemic lifted the curtain so that . . . with hard numbers [we could] demonstrate what really is happening in the community in terms of SDOH [social determinants of health] that are impacting our community." –*Promotores/as* benefits cliff discussion "And I think that was a very big barrier when we had to ask to put it [testing platforms] in Spanish. How is it that I have to advocate for something to be in Spanish? We had to ask them not to ask for health insurance. Those requests are a form of aggression, right? If I don't speak, if I don't raise my voice, they won't realize, or they won't do anything. So I think that was a great barrier for me, and it was one of the things that surprised me the most about the deployment of the government during the pandemic and the access to all resources during the pandemic." –CATALYST focus group participant
Funding initiatives	"I would say that I would like the grants to support the reality more, right? Because many times the grants, they come out, 'Well, I'm going to give you so much money to run this group.' And, to run a group, you need 2 hours to get to the participants, 2 hours to prepare the topic, and 2 hours to run the group. But then in the grant they only pay you 3, right? So it's okay, we survive, yes. The payment is not going to be the same as what you have to pay a nurse . . . , but neither can you proletarianize by making us laborers, right? Of the system. I think it puts organizations, especially like LHA that are nonprofits, in such a difficult situation. And to the *promotoras* because when your boss tells you, 'Well, you have 3 paid hours here,' but you see that the workload is actually another 2, that's why I told you about how the heart gets conquered, and the heart is very weak. It says, 'Oh, but for the group that they are paying me for 3 hours to turn out well, I am going to work 5.' And no, that's where the 'for now' comes from, all this comes from, so I think that the granters should sit down with the nonprofit organizations and tell them, 'Really, how long are you taking to do this job?' And let me not be extravagant but try to find a middle ground, right?" –CATALYST focus group participant "Emotional wellness support groups—there's an effort to sustain them, but without funds, so we stretch funds here and there. For example, [in] an arts and craft support group, they recycle and find materials, and sometimes the participants sell their crafts." –*Promotores/as* benefits cliff discussion

Note. CATALYST = Community Activation to TrAnsform Local sYSTems; LHA = Latino Health Access.
Source. Group discussion about postpandemic benefits cliff with LHA *promotores/as* and CATALYST study interviews and focus group discussions with LHA *promotores/as*.

> housing. Immigration processes are so long, right now we are living [in] an economic situation that is affecting everyone. Community members have to have other jobs—so many situations that we don't have enough resources to help.

Another *promotor/a* described how the pandemic contributes to continued unemployment and economic precarity:

> [N]ow families who come to me . . . right now [2024] when the pandemic is affecting, participants are talking about job loss, if they were sick, they didn't return, and they call to ask for help, and that help is no longer there.

Services and programs. LHA's services and programs continue to experience a high demand, including from residents who learned about and worked with *promotores/as* during the pandemic. The growth of LHA's *promotor* model during the pandemic and collaborations with schools enabled about 3.3 billion outreach messages and contacts in 2021 (mostly social media; Table 1). Despite outreach messages decreasing by 95% in 2022 and nearly 99% in 2023, direct outreach remained high, as *promotores/as* facilitated access to testing and vaccination, with direct outreach increasing by 26% from 2021 to 2022. At their peak, LHA served 94 097 unique individuals in 2021, while this reach declined by 52% in 2022 and nearly 84% in 2023. This translated to a 39% and 54%, respectively, decrease in services provided in 2022 and 2023 relative to 2021 (502 090 services). Services included, for example, navigation support, such as accompanying residents to address barriers to testing, contact tracing, and vaccination; food

TABLE 1— Latino Health Access Services Delivered: Orange County, CA, 2021–2023

	2021, No.	2022, No.	2023, No.	2021–2022 Percent Change	2021–2023 Percent Change
Overall services					
Outreach messages[a]	3 321 311 415	159 288 492	39 883 937	−95	−99
Direct outreach	783 562	989 907	808 375	26.3	3.2
Unduplicated people served	94 097	44 909	15 272	−52	−84
Services provided	502 090	304 767	228 896	−39	−54
Specific services delivered					
Financial assistance, $	5 414 378.55	1 299 816.82	0	−76	−100
Navigation services	300 386	121 118	63 279	−60	−79
COVID-19 testing and vaccination clinics cohosted in the community	39 744	2 201	13	−94	−100
Linkages to and administration of COVID-19 vaccines	40 962	899	79	−98	−100
Linkages to and administration of COVID-19 tests	43 109	8 928	2 082	−79	−95
Boxes of food distributed	32 897	29 953	28 090	−9	−15

Source. Latino Health Access Evaluation Department, 2024.
[a]Refers to social media outreach as well as the school district's automated outreach to parents.

distribution; and distributing financial assistance—all of which declined precipitously in 2022.

Promotores/as explained: "People may have come in from COVID-19 or the foodbank, but they keep coming back because they got to know us." Consistent with work before and during the pandemic, *promotores/as* continue to accompany residents to navigate and overcome structural barriers to accessing services that are overburdened and systematically exclude low-income, immigrant communities. One *promotor/a* explained,

> *Promotoras* still need to navigate systems. We now have CalOptima [county Medicaid provider], but CalOptima is saturated. There are waitlists. Even when CalOptima is available for people with or without status, CalOptima is saturated. . . . *Promotores* have to continue to help community members navigate, especially around mental health.

Indeed, in LHA's model, accompaniment and navigation support are core to helping residents access and use services.[28] While navigational services, or "high touch" approaches were high in 2021, reflecting actions taken by *promotores/as* to reduce or eliminate barriers to receive tests and vaccines, these were reduced drastically after funding cuts (Table 1). Nonetheless, direct outreach continued increasing.

To meet continued demand, *promotores/as* and residents creatively strategized to sustain programs that governments and foundations previously recognized and supported as essential. For example, funding to support emotional wellness initiatives has substantially declined, yet mental health needs remain enormous. One *promotor/a* shared how they sustain their efforts: "Emotional wellness [staff] organized to give at least $5/each pay period, accepted clothing donations (sell to organization that pays per pound) to pay for hotels, food for participants."

Pandemic-related *promotor/a* and organizational capacity-building efforts created conditions for LHA to expand to provide contracted services for which *promotor/a* services have become reimbursable through health insurance providers and public health agencies. One *promotor/a* explained, "Creating capacity at this time, it also allowed us to contract ourselves to provide other services around mental health, food, and housing. Now, what we're doing is applying that knowledge we learned during the pandemic." Capacity-building, training, and scaling the *promotor* model during the pandemic, as well as LHA's extensive outreach to reach the most vulnerable individuals in the community, laid the foundation and built LHA's resume to pursue larger contracts.

Training, learning opportunities, and career pathways for promotores/as. The pandemic created new learning, training, and apprenticeship opportunities for *promotores/as*; expanded their workforce; and opened pathways for career advancements. One *promotor/a* explained that trainings facilitated outreach efforts: "We were able to expand our work by learning technology." To meet local needs, LHA expanded its *promotor/a* workforce through hiring and increasing current staff from part-time to full-time roles, which created economic opportunities for those greatly impacted by the pandemic. One *promotora* shared, "We have employed a lot of community residents" and "[the pandemic] allowed us to generate jobs for people who were already close to us." Others explained that the expansion of the *promotor/a* workforce and funding contributed to creating career pathways for *promotores*. One *promotor/a* described,

> We have achieved new positions (lead *Promotor/a*, *promotor/a* coordinator), increased pathways for community-based volunteering, and this has allowed us to strengthen the quality of work for each department, and the community is supporting and increasing their consciousness about advocacy and enhancing the *promotor/a* model.

LHA has since launched the Promotor Learning Institute, focused on identifying and meeting capacity-building needs within LHA and co-designing and co-leading trainings to external organizations, which present a revenue-generating opportunity.

During the pandemic, the credibility of *promotores/as* increased alongside their respect from traditional institutions, as evidenced by more organizations working with *promotores/as*.[9,36] This increased respect influenced medical reimbursement policies[37,38] that now include *promotores/as* as providers and other initiatives seeking better compensation for *promotores/as*.[39]

Partnerships. LHA built or deepened partnerships and collaboration during the pandemic, which positioned them to call upon those partnerships to creatively address emerging safety net gaps, such as loss of access to services because of ineligibility after the pandemic benefits cliff. One *promotor/a* explained that when community members face barriers to access, *promotores/as* accompany them through alternate solutions: "[T]his has allowed us to be creative to say, 'These people no longer qualify for services because we're not in the pandemic emergency anymore, but we can leverage the community health centers.'" In addition, while COVID-19 vaccine coverage for uninsured individuals ended, California expanded Medicaid for income-eligible individuals, regardless of immigration status. *Promotores/as* refer participants to enrollment services, invite enrollers to come to LHA to directly connect with community members, and support community members to overcome barriers to navigating Medicaid coverage. Even in direct services, *promotores/as* foster an understanding and approach of the need for collective action and bring people together and move them along a spectrum of participation.

However, some collaborations were scaled back or ended as pandemic funding ended. One *promotor* reflected on a cycle of collaboration with the local health department:

> [CBO director] got in contact with authorities of the County Health Department, and they decided together that . . . the office didn't know exactly how to work with the Latino community, so they ask[ed] [CBO] to take care of it. They started to hire people; to get them prepared and we started in July, and it ended when the county funds were gone.

Advocacy and accompaniment. LHA's model of community mobilization to transform the conditions that produce health inequities continues, using similar communication and power-building tools. One *promotora* described, "[V]olunteer work has not stopped. We can see this in the food bank, in our meetings. There's an organization that's going to sell pozole [traditional Mexican stew] to help knock [on] doors for a ballot measure." *Promotores/as* also described how residents continue to practice the *promotor* model by accompanying and supporting others, such as "taking food to individuals who are homebound without the necessary resources." These mechanisms for volunteering and participation continue to build community power to problem solve, track data and experiences, and identify issues and pathways for advocacy.

LHA has been a leader in advocacy for equitable funding structures for *promotores/as*, especially as the model has gained national recognition. In California, there has been a movement to integrate *promotores/as* into clinical settings. LHA has advocated to retain its community-based roots and to grow the career ladder so that *promotores/as* can be recognized and funded as a career. The success of these programs relies on adequate funding and living wages to support *promotores/as* and CBOs.

LHA has been in collaborative spaces to inform resource allocation, to elevate the focus on structural factors, and to center community experiences. One *promotor/a* explained, "[T]he openness of the public health systems to listen to these numbers has also allowed us to advocate at the local and state level. It allowed LHA to have evidence at a community-wide level to show what we've been advocating for a long time." LHA played a pivotal role in leading the Latinx Health Equity Coalition, which was crucial for delivering services and organizing advocacy efforts. Various population health collaborations are now harnessing their collective power to collaborate and advance equity in the postpandemic landscape.

Funding initiatives. While the structural determinants of health inequities have not changed since the pandemic, we are experiencing a dual postpandemic benefits cliff: residents are contending with the loss of pandemic-related benefits, and CBOs and *promotores/as* accompany residents to address significant issues (e.g., housing, economic) without robust governmental funding. One *promotor/a* described the inequitable allocation of funding: "[For the] system and government, [a] small percentage in the California budget is for housing, but a lot is for the jail systems. [T]oo [long] waitlist for housing, systems are no longer working, none of them. Education, judicial systems, economic crisis." *Promotores/as* work in the context of insufficient funding for programming, worsened by the loss of the pandemic safety net, particularly mental health. The benefits cliff directly impacts funding *promotores/as*, as one shared:

> One of the problems that prevent the possibility of hiring more people is financing right? The *promotores* have to get paid well, a fair and dignified salary with benefits. And that costs money. And if there is no financing, it won't be valued. So, it is very important that the government institutions think about the needs of the *promotores*. Your role, which is the means and most efficient tool to be in contact with the community and know their needs.

DISCUSSION

The pandemic exposed the imperative for the government to fund essential needs, including health care, food, services, and housing. It also underscored the importance of collaborating with CBOs to apply a health equity focus; reduce bureaucratic barriers to accessing resources, wide-scale testing, vaccination, and quarantine support; and disburse funds to frontline CBOs and *promotores/as*. The governmental response demonstrated the capability of acting efficiently to meet community needs.

However, similar to governmental responses to past epidemics (e.g., AIDS, tuberculosis), the government's declaration of the pandemic's end reflects a focus on treating the pandemic as a clinical emergency, rather than a social emergency. This prioritizes the well-being of middle- and upper-class Americans while overlooking the continued social and health risks for minoritized communities. These risks existed before the pandemic but were amplified by the pandemic and continue to compound alongside other inequities (e.g., HIV, lead). The pandemic heightened public awareness of health inequities and their structural causes, our interconnectedness, and societal vulnerability. However, the political will of governmental and foundation decision-makers has shifted, as evidenced by reduced community-level funding to address the structural drivers of health inequities and a return to highly bureaucratic processes (e.g., extensive grant proposals) to access funding. Health and governmental organizations should increase contracts with CBOs and leverage *promotores/as'* deep community knowledge and expanded scope of services, representing a structural shift with potential to ameliorate the benefits cliff effects and address the structural drivers of health inequities.

Promotores/as were ready to respond to community needs in real time, bringing courage and commitment to their on-the-ground efforts and their ready understanding of the structural drivers of health inequities. Major achievements include increased visibility of *promotores/as* models and funding to address housing inequities. Legacies of *promotores/as* models include increased community awareness, power, and mobilization. We need to build community-level and neighborhood-level person-powered infrastructures to prepare communities for climate, environmental, health, economic, and social crises that are on the rise.

PUBLIC HEALTH IMPLICATIONS

This case study indicates that the dual postpandemic benefits cliff affects individuals, households, and communities who experience social, economic, and health injustices. Many of the pandemic's social, economic, and health legacies and inequities remain. At LHA, the *promotor/a* model is affected by 2 overarching features of the postpandemic benefits cliff: the loss of pandemic benefits for individuals and households and the loss of pandemic funding to support CBOs and *promotores/as* in accompanying residents to address their needs and transform the conditions that affect health inequities. At stake is the reach and depth of community engagement and power building, the strength of partnerships, *promotores/as'* connection to and elevation of community experiences, and the sustainability of CBOs accountable to minoritized communities. Local, state, and national preparedness, along with sustained and adequately funded collaborations with *promotores/as*-focused CBOs, are particularly important for future and increasingly frequent public health threats, including governmental mistrust, economic downturns, low vaccination rates, and emerging public health crises (e.g., bird flu, measles). AJPH

ABOUT THE AUTHORS

Alana M. W. LeBrón is with the Department of Health, Society, and Behavior in the Joe C. Wen School of Population & Public Health and the Department of Chicano/Latino Studies in the School of Social Sciences, University of California, Irvine. Melina Michelen is with the Department of Health, Society, and Behavior in the Joe C. Wen School of Population & Public Health, University of California, Irvine. Gloria I. Montiel is with AltaMed Health Services Corporation, Los Angeles, CA. Patricia J. Cantero, Loreta Ruiz, Kory Razaghi, Laura Pantoja, Marisela Ramirez, Josefina Jimenez, and America Bracho are with Latino Health Access. John Billimek is with the Department of Family Medicine, in the School of Medicine, University of California, Irvine.

CORRESPONDENCE

Correspondence should be sent to Alana M. W. LeBrón, PhD, MSc, University of California, Irvine, Joe C. Wen School of Population & Public Health, 856 Health Sciences Quad, Irvine, CA 92697-3957 (e-mail: alebron@uci.edu). Reprints can be ordered at https://ajph.org by clicking the "Reprints" link.

PUBLICATION INFORMATION

Full Citation: LeBrón AMW, Michelen M, Cantero PJ, et al. Pandemic-related funding termination and structural drivers of inequities: a case study of a *promotores/as*-focused community-based organization. *Am J Public Health*. 2025;115(11): 1824–1835.

Acceptance Date: April 9, 2025.

DOI: https://doi.org/10.2105/AJPH.2025.308154

ORCID iDs:

Alana M. W. LeBrón https://orcid.org/0000-0003-0964-4673

Melina Michelen https://orcid.org/0000-0003-3659-7788

Gloria Itzel Montiel https://orcid.org/0000-0003-2540-1487

CONTRIBUTORS

A. M. W. LeBrón, M. Michelen, and J. Billimek led the writing and revisions of the article. All authors conceptualized the article, contributed ideas, and critically edited, revised, and approved the final version of this article.

ACKNOWLEDGMENTS

Research reported in this National Institutes of Health (NIH) Rapid Acceleration of Diagnostics Underserved Populations (RADx-UP) publication was supported by the NIH Loan Repayment Program; the Diverse Institution Faculty Development Fellowship Supplement project, which is supported by the Health Resources and Services Administration of the US Department of Health and Human Services under grant 5-UE7-MC26282-10–National Maternal and Child Health Workforce Development Center Cooperative Agreement; California Department of Public Health (California Collaborative for Pandemic Recovery and Readiness Research); National Institute on Minority Health and Health Disparities (U01MD017433); Center for Population, Inequality, and Policy and the Center for Liberation, Anti-Racism, and Belonging, University of California, Irvine; University of California, Irvine, Interim COVID-19 Research Recovery Program; Wen School of Population & Public Health, University of California, Irvine; and Department of Chicano/Latino Studies, School of Social Sciences, University of California, Irvine.

The authors wish to thank *promotores/as* and staff at Latino Health Access for informing and guiding the analysis of the impact of the postpandemic benefits cliff for our communities and for the work of *promotores/as* models. We extend our gratitude to Alejandra Chavez for their support in gathering data for this report, the *promotores/as* involved in data collection, the data entry staff, managers, and the evaluation and finance teams responsible for tracking, standardizing, and analyzing vast amounts of data, especially throughout the challenges of the pandemic. We are also immensely grateful to all *promotores/as* whose involvement and discussions about this issue made this work possible. We express our gratitude to advocates promoting health and racial equity and to the individuals who shared their stories, resilience, and aspirations, shaping the essence of this work. Special recognition is extended to the University of California, Irvine, students in the VoiCES lab whose commitment, enthusiasm, and assistance greatly facilitated our research efforts and significantly contributed to the success of this project. We also acknowledge the representatives of University of California, Irvine, Wen School of Population & Public Health for their support and collaboration.

Note. The content is solely the responsibility of the authors and does not necessarily represent the official views of the funders.

CONFLICTS OF INTEREST

The authors have no conflicts of interest to declare.

HUMAN PARTICIPANT PROTECTION

Study protocols were approved by the University of California, Irvine's institutional review board in 2020 (UCI IRB 1272).

REFERENCES

1. Shen AK, Hughes Iv R, DeWald E, Rosenbaum S, Pisani A, Orenstein W. Ensuring equitable access to COVID-19 vaccines in the US: current system challenges and opportunities: analysis examines ensuring equitable access to COVID-19 vaccines. *Health Aff (Millwood)*. 2021;40(1):62–69. https://doi.org/10.1377/hlthaff.2020.01554
2. Webb Hooper M, Nápoles AM, Pérez-Stable EJ. COVID-19 and racial/ethnic disparities. *JAMA*. 2020;323(24):2466–2467. https://doi.org/10.1001/jama.2020.8598
3. Tai DBG, Shah A, Doubeni CA, Sia IG, Wieland ML. The disproportionate impact of COVID-19 on racial and ethnic minorities in the United States. *Clin Infect Dis*. 2021;72(4):703–706. https://doi.org/10.1093/cid/ciaa815
4. Williamson EJ, Walker AJ, Bhaskaran K, et al. Factors associated with COVID-19-related death using OpenSAFELY. *Nature*. 2020;584(7821):430–436. https://doi.org/10.1038/s41586-020-2521-4
5. Singh GK, Lee H. Widening disparities in COVID-19 mortality and life expectancy among 15 major racial and ethnic groups in the United States, 2020–2021. *J Racial Ethn Health Disparities*. 2025;12(2):1323–1332. https://doi.org/10.1007/s40615-024-01966-6
6. Cloud LK, Moran-McCabe K, Platt E, Prood N. A chronological overview of the federal, state, and local response to COVID-19. *Temple University Legal Studies Research Paper Forthcoming*. Published online July 31, 2020. Available at: https://ssrn.com/abstract=3675780. Accessed August 23, 2024.
7. Bernstein H, Gonzalez D, Echave P, Guelespe D. Immigrant families faced multiple barriers to safety net programs in 2021. Urban Institute. 2022. Available at: https://www.urban.org/sites/default/files/2022-11/Immigrant%20Families%20Faced%20Multiple%20Barriers%20to%20Safety%20Net%20Programs%20in%202021.pdf. Accessed August 23, 2024.
8. Gonzalez D, Bernstein H, Karpman M, Kenney GM. Mixed-status families and immigrant families with children continued avoiding safety net programs in 2023. Urban Institute. 2024. Available at: https://www.urban.org/sites/default/files/2024-08/Mixed-Status-Families-and-Immigrant-Families-with-Children-Continued-Avoiding-Safety-Net-Programs-in-2023.pdf. Accessed October 1, 2024.
9. Morey BN, Michelen M, Phan M, et al. Structural supports and challenges for community health worker models: lessons from the COVID-19 response in Orange County, California. *SSM Qual Res Health*. 2025;7:100510. https://doi.org/10.1016/j.ssmqr.2024.100510
10. County of Orange Social Services Agency. *Annual Conditions of Children in Orange County Report*. 2023. Available at: https://ssa.ocgov.com/about-us/news-publications/COCR. Accessed March 10, 2025.
11. Evans D, Norrbom C, Schmidt S, Powell R, McReynolds J, Sidibe T. Engaging community-based organizations to address barriers in public health programs: lessons learned from COVID-19

vaccine acceptance programs in diverse rural communities. *Health Secur.* 2023;21(suppl 1):S17–S24. https://doi.org/10.1089/hs.2023.0017

12. Wong JA, Yi SS, Kwon SC, Islam NS, Trinh-Shevrin C, Đoàn LN. COVID-19 and Asian Americans: reinforcing the role of community-based organizations in providing culturally and linguistically centered care. *Health Equity.* 2022;6(1):278–290. https://doi.org/10.1089/heq.2021.0124
13. Shen AK, Browne S, Srivastava T, Kornides ML, Tan ASL. Trusted messengers and trusted messages: the role for community-based organizations in promoting COVID-19 and routine immunizations. *Vaccine.* 2023;41(12):1994–2002. https://doi.org/10.1016/j.vaccine.2023.02.045
14. Montiel GI, Cantero PJ, Montiel I, Moon K, Nawaz S. Commentary: rebuilding with impacted communities at the center: the case for a civic engagement approach to COVID-19 response and recovery. *Fam Community Health.* 2021;44(2):81–83. https://doi.org/10.1097/FCH.0000000000000294
15. Carstensen N, Mudhar M, Munksgaard FS. 'Let communities do their work': the role of mutual aid and self-help groups in the Covid-19 pandemic response. *Disasters.* 2021;45(suppl 1):S146-S173. https://doi.org/10.1111/disa.12515
16. Michelen M, Lopez Galeana B, Zárate S, et al. "Each one of us did the best we could for the community, while also supporting each other": community residents' perspectives on community health worker (CHW) response during the COVID-19 pandemic—a community science worker-led qualitative study. *BMC Public Health.* 2025;25(1):1269. https://doi.org/10.1186/s12889-025-22497-7
17. Office of Recovery Programs. American Rescue Plan Two Years In: The American Rescue Plan Act's Historic Investments in a Stronger Economic Future. Washington, DC: US Department of Treasury; 2023.
18. Centers for Disease Control and Prevention. CDC announces $2.25 billion to address COVID-19 health disparities in communities that are at high-risk and underserved. 2021. Available at: https://archive.cdc.gov/www_cdc_gov/media/releases/2021/p0317-COVID-19-Health-Disparities.html. Accessed October 1, 2024.
19. Mensah GA, Johnson LE, Zhang X, et al. Community Engagement Alliance (CEAL): a National Institutes of Health program to advance health equity. *Am J Public Health.* 2024;114(suppl 1):S12–S17. https://doi.org/10.2105/AJPH.2023.307476
20. Pérez-Stable EJ, Hodes RJ, Schwetz TA. An NIH response to COVID-19 that engages communities and scientists. *Am J Public Health.* 2022;112(suppl 9):S844. https://doi.org/10.2105/AJPH.2022.307118
21. US Department of Health and Human Services Office of Minority Health. Notice of Funding Opportunity: Minority Leaders Development Program Opportunity Number: MP-CPI-21-008. Available at: https://apply07.grants.gov/apply/opportunities/instructions/PKG00267812-instructions.pdf. Accessed August 24, 2024.
22. Chen AT, Smith DO, Ojikutu BO, Auerbach J. The community as a full partner: a new model for public health: article examines strengthening US public health by shifting toward greater community engagement and leadership. *Health Aff (Millwood).* 2024;43(6):805–812. https://doi.org/10.1377/hlthaff.2024.00033
23. Rochford P, Bauer J, Wallace M. What to know about the 2024 end-of-year ARPA obligation deadline. July 18, 2024. Available at: https://www.nlc.org/article/2024/07/18/what-to-know-about-the-2024-end-of-year-arpa-obligation-deadline. Accessed August 24, 2024.
24. Center on Budget and Policy Priorities. The COVID-19 economy's effects on food, housing, and employment hardships. 2022. Available at: https://www.cbpp.org/sites/default/files/8-13-20pov.pdf. Accessed August 24, 2024.
25. US Census Bureau. QuickFacts: Santa Ana City, California. Available at: https://www.census.gov/quickfacts/fact/table/santaanacitycalifornia/PST045223. Accessed August 24, 2024.
26. Center on Budget and Policy Priorities. Analyzing the Census Bureau's 2023 poverty, income, and health insurance data. September 12, 2024. Available at: https://www.cbpp.org/blog/analyzing-the-census-bureaus-2023-poverty-income-and-health-insurance-data. Accessed August 24, 2024.
27. Petchel S. COVID-19 makes funding for health and social services integration even more crucial. *Health Affairs Forefront.* April 14, 2020. https://doi.org/10.1377/forefront.20200413.886531
28. Montiel GI, Moon KJ, Cantero PJ, et al. *Queremos transformar comunidades*: incorporating civic engagement as an equity strategy in promotor-led COVID-19 response efforts in Latinx communities. *Harvard Journal of Hispanic Policy.* 2021; 33:79–101.
29. Saunders CH, Sierpe A, Von Plessen C, Coproduction Laboratory, et al. Practical thematic analysis: a guide for multidisciplinary health services research teams engaging in qualitative analysis. *BMJ.* 2023;381:e074256. https://doi.org/10.1136/bmj-2022-074256
30. LeBrón AMW, Michelen M, Morey B, et al. Community Activation to TrAnsform Local sYSTems (CATALYST): a qualitative study protocol. *Int J Qual Methods.* 2024;23:16094069241284217. https://doi.org/10.1177/16094069241284217
31. Michelen M, Phan M, Zimmer A, et al. Practical qualitative data analysis for public health research: a guide to a team-based approach with flexible coding. *Int J Qual Methods.* 2024;23:1–16. https://doi.org/10.1177/16094069241289279
32. Latino Health Access. The promotor model. Available at: https://www.latinohealthaccess.org/what-we-do-overview#promotores-council. Accessed September 30, 2024.
33. California Immigrant Data Portal. Indicator: foreign born: California has been home to immigrants for generations. Available at: https://immigrantdataca.org/indicators/foreign-born?geo=07000000000669000. Accessed October 1, 2024.
34. Bracho A, Lee G, Giraldo GP, De Prado RM. *Recruiting the Heart, Training the Brain: The Work of Latino Health Access.* Oakland, CA: Hesperian Health Guides; Latino Health Access; 2016.
35. Centers for Disease Control and Prevention. End of the federal COVID-19 public health emergency (PHE) declaration. Available at: https://archive.cdc.gov/www_cdc_gov/coronavirus/2019-ncov/your-health/end-of-phe.html. Accessed September 24, 2024.
36. Rodriguez NM. Community health workers in the United States: time to expand a critical workforce. *Am J Public Health.* 2022;112(5):697–699. https://doi.org/10.2105/AJPH.2022.306775
37. California Hospital Association. Medi-Cal Coverage of community health worker (CHW) services is effective July 1, 2022. July 11, 2022. Available at: https://calhospital.org/medi-cal-coverage-of-community-health-worker-services-effective-july-1. Accessed January 21, 2025.
38. Connecticut Health Foundation. 50-state scan of Medicaid payment for community health workers. Available at: https://www.cthealth.org/publication/50-state-scan-of-medicaid-payment-for-community-health-workers. Accessed March 27, 2025.
39. Colvin CJ, Hodgins S, Perry HB. Community health workers at the dawn of a new era: 8. Incentives and remuneration. *Health Res Policy Syst.* 2021; 19(suppl 3):106. https://doi.org/10.1186/s12961-021-00750-w

Lived Experiences of Families Navigating Safety Net Expansions and Retractions During the Pandemic: A Qualitative Study

Nicole Fernández-Viña, MPH, Lia C. H. Fernald, PhD, MBA, Rita Hamad, MD, PhD, Kaitlyn E. Jackson, MPH, and Wendi Gosliner, DrPH, RD

See also COVID-19 Benefits Cliff, pp. 1818–1867.

Objectives. To understand the experiences of families with low income in California with pandemic safety net support expansions and retractions, including barriers to program access.

Methods. Using open-ended questions, we explored the self-reported experiences of pandemic-era safety net expansions and expirations between January and June 2023 among a group of caregivers of young children (n = 44). We used the Immersion-Crystallization technique to analyze the data, creating a codebook and identifying themes as they emerged.

Results. We identified 4 main themes, including appreciation for safety net expansions, varied experiences because of the timing of supports, challenges meeting basic needs after expirations, and administrative burdens significantly impairing program access.

Conclusions. The study themes highlighted how expansions to policies like the Child Tax Credit and Supplemental Nutrition Assistance Program improved food and housing security, and that unpredictable benefits, although appreciated, also added stress.

Public Health Implications. State and federal policymakers should consider the poverty reduction and food and housing security benefits of expansions to pandemic-era supports that have expired when crafting future policy. They should pay special attention to addressing administrative barriers to reduce poverty-related health inequities. (*Am J Public Health*. 2025;115(11):1836–1847. https://doi.org/10.2105/AJPH.2025.308201)

AJPH November 2025, Vol. 115, No. 11

The US social safety net is a combination of federal, state, and local-level programs aimed at supporting families by enhancing economic security to improve well-being. In response to the hardships of the COVID-19 pandemic, US safety net policies were expanded to combat the economic upheaval that exacerbated food, housing, and general insecurity during this period.[1–3] For example, monthly Supplemental Nutrition Assistance Program (SNAP, formerly known as food stamps) allotments increased for most participants, while the Special Supplemental Nutrition Program for Women, Infants, and Children (WIC, which provides food and nutrition education for qualifying pregnant and postpartum women and children younger than 5 years) modified in-person requirements for services. In this same timeframe, the Pandemic Electronic Benefits Transfer (P-EBT) program provided emergency nutrition benefits to eligible schoolchildren when schools closed and meal access became more difficult, and the Child Tax Credit (CTC) was increased and provided advanced monthly payments during July through December 2021.[1,4–7]

There were significant benefits of safety net program modifications during this period, including vast reductions in child poverty and growing evidence of improved adult mental health and food security.[8–10] Yet most program modifications were temporary and expired by 2023, when the public health emergency was deemed to have ended. Subsequently, a growing literature is examining the health implications of these often abrupt "benefit cliffs," although quantitative studies often struggle to disentangle individual program effects given the confluence of program changes.[11–13]

Our study fills a crucial gap in the existing scientific literature, examining the lived experiences of families with safety net support programs during the pandemic, including barriers to access and experiences with the termination of expanded benefits. Through qualitative interviews with caregivers of young children in California in early 2023, this qualitative study aimed to illuminate firsthand experiences, allowing for a deeper and nuanced understanding of the experiences and challenges these families faced, which is critical to improving the US public health and policy response.

METHODS

We conducted 44 semistructured qualitative interviews as part of the Assessing California Communities' Experiences with Safety Net Supports (ACCESS) Study, a 2-wave longitudinal study of California caregivers with children, who at baseline were eligible for the Earned Income Tax Credit (the largest US poverty alleviation policy). Full study details have been described previously and in the Appendix (available as a supplement to the online version of this article at http://www.ajph.org).[14,15]

Sample selection for this qualitative substudy is shown in Figure 1. A subset of 83 participants were randomly selected from the original ACCESS study sample (n = 497) to complete the qualitative interview during their follow-up interview between January and June 2023. This subsample was confirmed to be representative of the overall ACCESS sample by race, ethnicity, tax filing status, and language spoken. Forty-four of the 83 randomized participants completed the qualitative interview, and 39 were lost to follow-up (Figure 1).

The semistructured qualitative interview guide was developed by the research team and is shown in Box 1. Qualitative interviewers were trained by W. G. to conduct neutral and objective interviews. The original interview guide, implemented from January to March 2023, included questions about caregivers' experiences with COVID-19 safety net program expansions. Because of the expiration of many pandemic safety net program expansions during the study period, the interview guide was updated in April 2023 to include questions about caregivers' experiences with the termination of P-EBT and SNAP expansions. See the online Appendix for additional methods.

RESULTS

Most caregivers (72%) resided in southern California, 73% had less than a college education, and 45% identified as Latino/Hispanic, 32% as Black, 9% as White, and 14% as Other (Table 1). Median income was $22 610 in 2021. The demographic characteristics of our study sample were generally representative of the original ACCESS study (Table A, available as a supplement to the online version of this article at http://www.ajph.org).

Our qualitative analysis revealed 4 main themes and 6 subthemes presented below and in Box 2. Box 2 is designed with thematic categories and corresponding participant quotes to provide an organized display of key

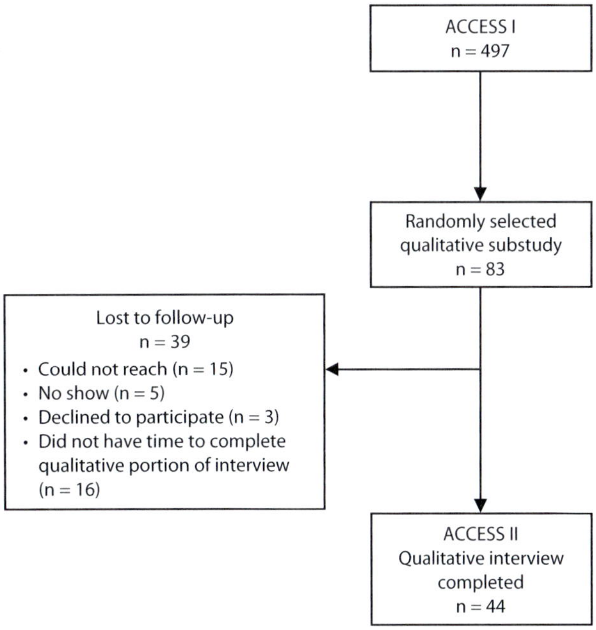

FIGURE 1— Sample Selection Flow Chart: ACCESS Study, California, January–June 2023

Note. ACCESS = Assessing California Communities' Experiences with Safety Net Supports.

BOX 1— Semi-Structured Qualitative Interview Guide: ACCESS Study, California, January–June 2023

Question No.	Semi-Structured Questions
	Original Semi-Structured Interview Guide (January–March 2023)
Pandemic-specific: asked to all interviewees	
1	Over the course of the pandemic, can you talk about any challenges you faced in getting enough food or the kinds of foods you wanted to feed your family?
2	Can you talk about whether or how any safety net programs like stimulus checks, SNAP, WIC, EITC, the Child Tax Credit, P-EBT, school meals, unemployment, Medi-Cal, and TANF helped you and your family meet your food and nutrition needs? [If participant responded affirmatively] What made these programs helpful in meeting your food and nutrition needs? What else might have helped you and your family more to meet food and nutrition needs?
3	During the pandemic, what made it most difficult to secure enough of the kinds of food that you wanted? [If participant responded affirmatively] Do these difficulties persist currently?
4	Thinking more broadly about support programs during the COVID-19 pandemic, such as the ones mentioned above like EITC, SNAP, TANF, Unemployment Insurance, etc., how did you first hear about these types of programs?
5	Were you familiar with changes made to programs like SNAP, WIC, P-EBT, TANF, Medi-Cal during the pandemic? [If participant responded affirmatively] Which changes were the most helpful for you and your household and why? Which program changes were most challenging for you? Did your feelings about participating in these programs change over the course of the pandemic, if so, why?
6	Some programs during the pandemic were routine and predictable such as SNAP, while others like the stimulus checks and P-EBT were unpredictable. Can you describe your experience receiving predictable and unpredictable support during the pandemic? Would you say one type of support was more valuable than the other? [If participant responded affirmatively] Can you talk about what made that true for you?
7	What programs do you wish you had used or applied for but did not? What are the reasons why you have not taken advantage of relief?
8	How did use of these programs impact your decisions about childcare or work?
9	How would you say receiving assistance from these programs impacted your physical health? Your mental health? Your child's/children's health?
Monthly CTC-specific: asked to interviewees who reported receiving the monthly CTC	
10	You received monthly Child Tax Credit payments from July through December 2021. How did you feel about receiving these monthly CTC payments? How did these payments affect you and your family?
11	How did you feel when the monthly CTC payments stopped after December 2021? How did losing the monthly CTC payments impact food security and your ability to feed your children?
12	The CTC provided advance payments monthly, in addition to lump sum payments given to eligible recipients with their tax return. Did you prefer lump sums or monthly benefits? Why?
	Updated Semi-Structured Interview Guide (April–June 2023)
SNAP/P-EBT–specific: asked to interviewees who reported receiving SNAP/P-EBT	
13	Some programs during the pandemic were routine and predictable such as SNAP, while others like P-EBT were unpredictable. Can you describe your experience receiving predictable and unpredictable support during the pandemic? Would you say one type of support was more valuable than the other? [If participant responded affirmatively] Can you talk about what made that true for you?
14	There are lots of news media reports about long lines at food pantries since benefits have gone down. We know a lot of families, especially with school getting out, are struggling to have enough of the kinds of foods they want to eat. Can you talk a little bit about what this experience has been like for you?
15	How have these changes impacted the way your family eats?
16	How have these changes impacted your ability to eat the kinds of foods you want yourself/family to eat?
17	How have these changes impacted the way you get food, for example the types of stores you shop at or the other places you get food?
18	Overall, what would you say these changes will mean to you and your family?
19	Can you tell me what you know about changes to P-EBT?
20	We've heard that there is a lot of confusion about P-EBT benefits. Do you have any thoughts about how this program could be most useful to you or to families like yours?
21	How would you like to get information about the program? How do you think information could be most effectively shared?
22	P-EBT was canceled in April, and then it was recently announced that P-EBT will be extended starting in July. Can you tell me what it means for your family that you will get P-EBT in July? Has the gap in time from when school ended and the time you get P-EBT created any challenges for your family?

Continued

BOX 1— Continued

Question No.	Semi-Structured Questions
23	Thinking about the timing and amount of money you'll get from P-EBT, how well do you think this will support your family's food needs? Is there a way the program could be more supportive?

Note. Questions from the Updated Semi-Structured Interview Guide replaced all but Question 6 (renumbered as Question 13) from the Original Semi-Structured Interview Guide. ACCESS = Assessing California Communities' Experiences with Safety Net Supports; CTC = Child Tax Credit; EITC = Earned Income Tax Credit; P-EBT = Pandemic-Electronic Benefits Transfer; SNAP = Supplemental Nutrition Assistance Program; TANF = Temporary Assistance for Needy Families; WIC = Special Supplemental Nutrition Program for Women, Infants, and Children.

themes, ensuring a direct representation of participant voices.

Theme 1

Theme 1, "COVID-19 Safety Net Program Expansions Reduced Perceived Stress and Enhanced Feelings of Food and Housing Security," captures caregivers' reflections on how safety net program expansions allowed them to worry less about meeting their basic needs. As one caregiver said,

> These programs can be the difference between survival and literally death for people and for children . . . you are giving them foundational things to survive upon . . . a house, food . . . some sense of security. (Participant 1, aged 35–50 years, Latinx/Hispanic, income $3000)

Furthermore, caregivers often called out how particular safety net programs provided support.

TABLE 1— Characteristics of Study Participants: ACCESS Study, California, January–June 2023

Characteristics	Study Sample (n = 44), No. (%) or Median (IQR)	Lost to Follow-Up (n = 39), No. (%) or Median (IQR)	ACCESS II (n = 380), No. (%) or Median (IQR)
Age, y	30 (21–48)	35 (21–49)	32 (21–50)
Income in 2021, $	22 610 (0–87 171)	20 141 (0–49 320)[a]	27 177 (0–94 765)
Female	42 (95)	39 (100)	362 (95)
Race/ethnicity			
Latinx/Hispanic	20 (45)	26 (67)	209 (55)
Non-Hispanic Black	14 (32)	7 (18)	84 (22)
Non-Hispanic White	4 (9)	1 (3)	44 (12)
Other[b]	6 (14)	5 (13)	43 (11)
Education			
High school or less	13 (30)	17 (44)	100 (26)
Some college/vocational/associate's	19 (43)	16 (41)	185 (49)
Bachelor's or higher	12 (27)	6 (15)	93 (25)
Adults in home			
1	20 (45)	16 (41)	114 (30)
2	14 (32)	15 (38)	178 (47)
≥ 3	10 (23)	8 (20)	88 (23)
Children in home			
1	16 (36)	13 (33)	85 (22)
2	14 (32)	4 (10)	145 (38)
≥ 3	14 (32)	22 (56)	148 (39)

Note. IQR = interquartile range. Data drawn from the qualitative substudy of the Assessing California Communities' Experiences with Safety Net Supports (ACCESS) Study.
[a]Income in 2019.
[b]Other race/ethnicity included 1 American Indigenous/Alaska Native and 5 who identified as multiple race categories.

BOX 2— Overview of Qualitative Themes, Subthemes, and Interview Quotations: ACCESS Study, California, January–June 2023

Theme	Subtheme	Interview Quotations
Theme 1. COVID-19 safety net program expansions reduced perceived stress and enhanced feelings of food and housing security.		"Every month I was not worrying about paying my insurance or my cell phone . . . or . . . if my car needed repairs, I was able to get that done. . . . It was greatly beneficial for my family." (Participant 3, aged 25–34 years, White, income $30 000)
		"With that help [SNAP] at least I felt like I could buy something. I had access to buy things for my children to eat, and even though I owed rent, I knew at least my kids weren't going to go without food." (Participant 4, aged 35–50 years, Latinx/Hispanic, income $18 000)
		"The P-EBT was more food on the table. It was extra even more so it was so helpful. And like you, you asked questions earlier about, you know, are you able to get the type of food you want? And yes, we were." (Participant 5, aged 35–50 years, Black, no income reported)
Theme 2. Predictable pandemic safety net supports (e.g., SNAP) were universally appreciated, while more infrequent supports (e.g., stimulus checks) were both appreciated and a source of anxiety and challenge.	2a. Predictable safety net supports alleviated perceived stress and facilitated planning and budgeting.	"Well, the predictable like you could plan for, like, okay, I get my benefits on the 10th and I could plan, like with the different sale ads, like where I was going to go to maximize like my use of them." (Participant 2, aged 35–50 years, White, income $27 000)
		"Uh, well, knowing helped me budget better, know how to plan meals better, shop better, because I knew that on this day I was getting this amount. And that was for sure more valuable." (Participant 7, aged 25–34 years, Black, income $18 000)
		"[SNAP] helps you manage your finances a lot better. . . . It definitely decreases anxiety and all these other nasty feelings. It lets you live a little bit when you're left on survival mode." (Participant 8, aged 25–34 years, Latinx/Hispanic, no income reported)
	2b. Unpredictable support created challenges and uncertainty, provoking anxiety.	"The unpredictable support. Um, sometimes made me anxious because I didn't know if I was eligible for it or if I was eligible when it would come." (Participant 9, aged 25–34 years, Black, income $24 000)
		"The stimulus. . . . It was always like, when am I going to get it? When am I going to get it? When am I going to get it?" (Participant 5, aged 35–50 years, Black, no income reported)
		"Having a nonscheduled assistance arrive, it's a benefit, but sometimes it's also anxiety striking because you have to figure out how to maneuver, you know, that's like problem solving." (Participant 10, aged 25–34 years, Black, income $57 000)
	2c. Still, unpredictable support was appreciated.	"It was like something I wasn't expecting . . . because before I did try to call and see if I was able to get it, but they said no. . . . And then when I got it, I was really, really surprised." (Participant 18, aged 35–50 years, Latinx/Hispanic, income $4000)
		"The pandemic-EBT was like a pleasant surprise, right? When you don't rely on it to come, when you're not expecting it to come. And then it comes sometimes, right when you need it. So that was a little helpful." (Participant 12, aged 25–34 years, Other, no income reported)
		"For whatever reason, any time I got a stimulus check or a P-EBT card, I really needed it. Like I was just like, I don't know how much longer I can be creative. And then it showed up. So yeah, that felt divine. . . . I was grateful every time for sure. . . . Every little bit helps." (Participant 13, aged 35–50 years, Black, income $51 000)

Continued

BOX 2— Continued

Theme	Subtheme	Interview Quotations
Theme 3. Termination of pandemic emergency P-EBT and SNAP benefits exacerbated food insecurity.		"Especially with the inflation going up on groceries, it's been more challenging to actually be able to get the same amount of food in the same quality. So oftentimes you have junk food that is cheaper than fresh food or organic food. . . . And that obviously has its own effects on mental health and physical health. So I think that the loss of that extra stipend is detrimental to my household . . . " (Participant 12, aged 25–34 years, Other, no income reported)
		". . . [the decrease in benefits] changed the food stores we go to . . . because healthy foods are more expensive and it means that they're trying to have us lean more toward unhealthy foods, which means we're spending more to try to keep our kids in that more healthy area of getting the right nutrition. . . . It just means that sometimes I have to go to food banks, I'm restricted financially and sometimes I'll go without eating to make sure my kids do. They don't miss a meal. I will." (Participant 16, aged 25–34 years, White, no income reported)
		"So when I was getting the P-EBT, we had a little bit more room to shop at like Ralphs or Albertsons. So now I'm back at like Superior or Food for Less, you know, and you really got to watch stuff in those stores . . . like watch their expiration date, things of that nature because, you know, it's cheap food. So I think more so like the quality of where I purchase my groceries, um, has been hit hard . . ." (Participant 20, aged 25–34 years, Other, income $25 000)
Theme 4. Administrative burdens created challenges in seeking and receiving help from safety net supports.	4a. Compliance costs created obstacles to accessing and utilizing safety net supports.	"I have to get recertified, so I know I'm going to go through this whole headache again. . . . But it's just the whole process of paperwork, you know?" (Participant 21, aged 35–50 years, Other, income $14 000)
		"They could have helped more families without asking all these questions . . . without all this bring me this, bring me that . . . there were a lot of people who became unemployed . . . so they shouldn't have asked so much of the families . . ." (Participant 4, aged 35–50 years, Latinx/Hispanic, income $18 000)
		"And I'm, you know, literate enough to go through the application process. . . . But I know that what a privilege that is. You know, and like I said, I've seen people mistreated. I've seen people disorganized, not have the paperwork, not have the patience to stand in line like all of those things." (Participant 13, aged 35–50 years, Black, income $51 000)
	4b. Psychological costs when seeking and receiving help from safety net supports.	"We had a lot of difficulties, because my husband lost his job and he didn't have a stable job and so when one goes to apply and takes all the documentation, it's really embarrassing . . . the man who helped us with this SNAP application was asking, "Oh, your husband isn't working? Why isn't he working?" like, questions that are very personal . . ." (Participant 4, aged 35–50 years, Latinx/Hispanic, income $18 000)
		"The people there, they're not trained to treat people like humans. They pretty much are trained to treat them like a file. . . . I'm a single mom with 2 kids. And instead of humanizing me, I'm just a case. I'm a file." (Participant 14, aged 25–34 years, Black, no income reported)
		"Anything that you needed done, it was like you had to fight for it. You had to go through something. . . . People expect you to, how can I say this right? Kiss their behind just to get the help, you know? And if you make a mistake or, you know, you don't turn in something that needs to be turned in, they'll dock your money." (Participant 14, aged 25–34 years, Black, no income reported)

Continued

BOX 2— Continued

Theme	Subtheme	Interview Quotations
	4c. Learning costs when applying for and receiving P-EBT because of a lack of clarity and communication from the program.	"There was going to be a new . . . I think P-EBT 3.0 or something like that. . . . I'm not sure if we're going to get a new card or how does that work? There's not really any type of outreach, I feel, to really inform parents in terms of what's going on." (Participant 23, aged 25–34 years, Black, income $24 000)
		"The Social Services department should be in charge of announcing or sending a flyer. Because it's just unclear. So something more clear, like a flyer or extra information, that can help us understand." (Participant 19, aged 35–50 years, Latinx/Hispanic, income $25 000)
		"They should have, I don't know, announced [P-EBT ending] on their website because I do have a portal for the website . . . they should at least put it like on a bulletin." (Participant 24, aged 25–34 years, Latinx/Hispanic, income $400)

Note. ACCESS = Assessing California Communities' Experiences with Safety Net Supports; P-EBT = Pandemic-Electronic Benefits Transfer; SNAP = Supplemental Nutrition Assistance Program. Reported income has been rounded to preserve confidentiality. For additional supporting interview quotations by theme, please see Table B in the Appendix (available as a supplement to the online version of this article at http://www.ajph.org).

Caregivers felt that the monthly CTC payments alleviated many of the pressures associated with affording basic living expenses, including worrying less about affording monthly expenses like cell phone and insurance payments, as well as less stress around unexpected payments like car repairs. Others reported that the monthly CTC provided relief when many were experiencing pandemic-related unemployment and job loss. One caregiver cited it as the reason they were able to afford rent at a time when they were struggling to find work cleaning businesses and houses because of pandemic-related lockdowns:

> [monthly CTC] could go towards where I was living at the time . . . that's almost half the rent. . . . So that helped a lot. (Participant 2, aged 35–50 years, White, income $27 000)

Additionally, caregivers noted that SNAP and P-EBT expansions were particularly helpful for affording food during the pandemic. The SNAP emergency allotments allowed caregivers to feed their families throughout the month, in contrast to their typical experience of benefits falling short. The expanded SNAP benefits also ensured that children did not go hungry when household income needed to be directed to pay rent. Caregivers also felt that P-EBT was particularly important to their children's food security because it provided specific funding to feed children during pandemic-related school closures, to compensate for loss of access to school meals:

> When my kids were home and not eating at least one meal per day at school . . . [P-EBT] helped us to have food, so that they could eat all day like they used to. (Participant 3, aged 25–34 years, White, income $30 000)

Theme 2

Theme 2, "Predictable Pandemic Safety Net Supports (e.g., SNAP) Were Universally Appreciated, While More Infrequent Supports (e.g., Stimulus Checks) Were Both Appreciated and a Source of Anxiety and Challenge," illustrates caregivers' varied experiences with the timing of safety net supports.

Subtheme 2a. Predictable safety net supports alleviated perceived stress and facilitated planning and budgeting. Caregivers spoke positively about benefits that arrived on an expected schedule, and several emphasized that the predictability of certain supports allowed them to budget and plan more effectively, giving them greater control over their decision-making when purchasing groceries. Some described planning the dates of benefit disbursals with sale ads and coupons to be able to maximize their use of the extra funds. Caregivers noted that the ability to budget offered by these consistent benefits reduced perceived stress, including alleviating some of the anxieties associated with living on a tight budget:

> [I]f you don't know how you're going to pay for groceries the next month,

> that's an incredibly stressful situation. . . . I think consistency is hugely important . . . I mean, pure and simple. There's the ability to budget. (Participant 1, aged 35–50 years, Latinx/Hispanic, income $3000)

Subtheme 2b. Unpredictable support created challenges and uncertainty, provoking anxiety. Notably, safety net supports that came inconsistently often contributed to perceptions of stress among caregivers. Caregivers expressed that the unclear eligibility criteria and uncertainty regarding benefit distribution made navigating these support systems more challenging. Some reflected that the anticipation of waiting for these supports' arrival provoked feelings of worry and fear about when and whether they might receive the benefit:

> It was difficult to not know if they were ever going to send me like the checks that everybody was getting. . . . So I was like, scared. (Participant 6, aged 25–34 years, Latinx/Hispanic, no income reported)

In addition, receiving benefits at random became a source of labor, with some describing the experience of keeping track of when benefits were arriving akin to holding a managerial position:

> Unpredictable was uncertainty or trying to figure out or manage things. . . . So it was like a manager role. (Participant 11, aged 35–50 years, Black, no income reported)

Subtheme 2c. Still, unpredictable support was appreciated. Despite perceived feelings of stress around unpredictable support, caregivers felt deeply grateful. They reported that the unpredictable nature of stimulus checks and P-EBT made them a welcome surprise, reporting that these types of benefits seemed to arrive when they were most needed:

> The unpredictable was like the hidden blessing . . . like, oh my gosh. Wait, hold on. Where'd this money come from? (Participant 14, aged 25–34 years, Black, no income reported)

Theme 3

Theme 3, "Termination of Pandemic Emergency P-EBT and SNAP Benefits Exacerbated Food Insecurity," captures caregivers' reports that the termination of SNAP emergency allotments and P-EBT made it significantly more challenging to purchase adequate and nutritious food for their families. This change, coupled with rising grocery costs driven by inflation, forced many to alter their shopping and eating habits to be able to continue affording food. Several talked about how the reduction in benefits forced them to choose less healthy and nutritious foods for their families:

> [W]e will eat less healthy, because buying vegetables is so expensive right now . . . the junk food is cheaper than the healthy food, but as a parent you can't give your kids junk food. (Participant 19, aged 35–50 years, Latinx/Hispanic, income $25 000)

Additionally, caregivers talked about the dilemma between choosing unhealthy options and exceeding their budget and described the negative impacts these food choices had on both mental and physical well-being. Caregivers described concerns about the types of grocery stores they could afford to go to and the poor quality of perishable items there, sometimes resorting to using food banks and skipping meals to ensure that their children could continue to eat.

Theme 4

Theme 4, "Administrative Burdens Created Challenges in Seeking and Receiving Help From Safety Net Supports," describes caregivers' experiences of administrative burdens when applying for and receiving help from safety net supports.

Subtheme 4a. Compliance costs created obstacles to accessing and utilizing safety net supports. Caregivers expressed frustration with the costs involved in accessing safety net supports. They described application and renewal processes, often filled with too many questions and paperwork, as a headache. Others felt that these processes demanded too much from individuals already facing significant challenges:

> It's just like a lot of . . . government. They want documentation, they want all this stuff . . . it makes it harder for a person . . . because they're vulnerable already. (Participant 21, aged 35–50 years, Other, income $14 000)

Similarly, long wait times were noted as a source of frustration and a barrier to accessing help. When talking about utilizing safety net supports, one caregiver mentioned that the distribution of P-EBT cards was particularly annoying and created additional work for parents:

> The P-EBT is every time they give you money, it's a new card. It's annoying. . . . It makes you not even want to use it. (Participant 22, aged 35–50 years, Other, income $19 000)

Subtheme 4b. Psychological costs when seeking and receiving help from safety net supports. Although these were not particularly prominent findings mentioned across multiple interviews, a handful of caregivers spoke about feelings of embarrassment during the application process, perceiving the questions as invasive. One person described the experience as dehumanizing, characterizing it as a constant battle for necessary support:

> It was very stressful to receive [help], to just be human, like a human in need of help . . . you weren't nobody, you weren't nothing and your problems didn't matter. And you would literally have to fight, stress, email . . . just to get something approved. (Participant 14, aged 25–34 years, Black, no income reported)

Others spoke about the stress they experienced when communicating with customer service agents, citing poor communication and lack of information as significant issues:

> The person who was assisting me, she gave me an ultimatum. As in like . . . if this document is not turned in, your benefits will not be renewed. . . . And that was like a huge stressor . . . me and my daughter rely on this. . . . So the lack of information is pretty much the downfall. (Participant 8, aged 25–34 years, Latinx/Hispanic, no income reported)

Subtheme 4c. Learning costs when applying for and receiving P-EBT because of a lack of clarity and communication from the program. Caregivers widely agreed that poor communication about P-EBT made it confusing to access and use the program. They highlighted difficulties in understanding the application process, how to use the benefits, and when to expect disbursements:

> I think that some more education needs to be sent out to the community . . . there were families that they didn't know how to get it, how to apply for it . . . (Participant 20, aged 25–34 years, Other, income $25 000)

Additionally, caregivers voiced frustration over the absence of updates on future rounds of P-EBT, emphasizing the need for better communication through texts, phone calls, and other methods:

> I had no idea [P-EBT was ending]. You're the first one to tell me that. . . . I mean, put it on a billboard. (Participant 16, aged 25–34 years, White, no income reported)

DISCUSSION

This qualitative study aimed to explore the experiences of families with low income in California with pandemic safety net support expansions and retractions, including barriers to program access. Our findings identified 2 key areas of barriers, including the structure of the supports and the administrative burdens the systems imposed upon recipients. The study also captured the importance of the safety net supports in facilitating housing and food security, and the challenges people experienced when the pandemic enhancements ended. Overall, we found that the additional supports and flexibilities of the pandemic safety net helped to alleviate perceived stress for recipients, particularly when the supports were relatively consistent and predictable. However, the retractions of the safety net supports exacerbated perceived stress.

Furthermore, we found that administrative burdens, including compliance, psychological, and learning costs, created barriers to safety net participation. These costs of participation included frustrations with application and renewal processes, embarrassment related to participation, and confusion because of limited information and communication. Given the potential for safety net supports to alleviate perceived stress and enhance food and housing security, addressing the administrative burdens is essential for optimizing the public health benefits of safety net supports. Few qualitative studies have explored this area, and the qualitative nature of this study allows for a deeper and nuanced understanding of the experiences of people accessing safety net supports, particularly during a dynamic and challenging period.

One of the novel findings of this study was that the timing and consistency of benefits played a crucial role in caregivers' experiences, affecting their sense of security and overall well-being. Although earlier studies indicated that stimulus checks were associated with reduced likelihood of anxiety and depressive symptoms,[16,17] we found that the delays and uncertainty surrounding unpredictable forms of support also had the opposite effect, adding anxiety as families struggled to determine how to incorporate these sporadic funds into financial plans. In contrast, predictable benefits fostered feelings of stability, empowering families to plan and budget. Although any financial assistance was appreciated, our findings suggest that irregular support can also create feelings of instability and challenge, underscoring the importance of delivering aid in a consistent and predictable manner to enhance resilience among people struggling to meet basic needs. This resonates with prior findings that less frequently disbursed benefits can lead to riskier health behaviors compared with more frequent benefits, perhaps as a coping mechanism to deal with stress.[18] Moreover, although families were grateful for unpredictable benefits, prior research shows that regular monthly payments are more effective in reducing childhood poverty rates than lump sum payments.[19] In sum, there are tradeoffs between providing routine supports to families during a crisis and providing sporadic supports to stimulate the economy. This study, in combination with prior research, suggests that when poverty alleviation and well-being are the desired outcomes, dependable, regularly distributed benefits offer enhanced support.

One of the other novel findings of this study is the significant administrative burdens participants encountered when seeking assistance from safety net programs. Previous research has found that administrative burdens not only hinder access to safety net supports, but they may also lead to adverse health consequences through increased stress associated with navigating complex bureaucratic systems.[20,21] Our study adds to this literature by specifically focusing on pandemic-era dynamic policy shifts. Several caregivers expressed frustration with extensive paperwork and long wait times (i.e., compliance costs), as well as negative interactions with customer service representatives (i.e., psychological costs). Prior research found that, among households with young children, loss of benefits because of missing eligibility deadlines was common, and 4 in 10 households experienced a temporary loss of SNAP benefits because of missed recertification deadlines.[22] Another prior study documented the perceived stress that SNAP participants experienced during a federal government shutdown that affected benefit distribution and led to experiences of poor customer service and inadequate communications between SNAP agencies and their participants.[23] Many caregivers struggled to access P-EBT—reporting not knowing how to access or use benefits and feeling unsure of when they would receive them—which led to considerable frustration. Research has identified the patchwork experiences families had with P-EBT based on the schools their students attended; some received P-EBT automatically whereas others missed out on these automatic benefits, placing the burden of application on parents.[24,25] These challenges underscore the need for programs to simplify application and renewal processes, consider needs that may arise during a crisis, and ensure that people experiencing disruptions and economic challenges can effectively access the benefits they need. For example, in 2021, the Internal Revenue Service automatically deposited monthly CTC benefits into the bank accounts of eligible individuals who had filed a tax return in the prior 2 years. This new system increased uptake of the CTC relative to prior years and other similar tax credits.[26] However, families who had not recently filed taxes similarly missed out on the automatic distribution and had to apply separately.

We also explored the role of pandemic safety nets in mitigating food and housing insecurity, providing relief, and reducing perceived stress for families with low income. The study was well positioned to capture what people experienced when these benefits expired, as data collection was underway when the pandemic expansions ended. Our findings indicated that pandemic safety net supports significantly improved food and housing security. This is consistent with literature highlighting CTC, SNAP, and P-EBT as essential supports to families navigating pandemic-related hardships. For example, the expanded CTC was shown to reduce depressive and anxiety symptoms among low-income adults, and increased SNAP benefits in January 2021 were estimated to prevent 850 000 cases of food insufficiency weekly.[8–10] Additionally, P-EBT, especially when combined with other programs, significantly supported children's access to food.[27]

Furthermore, we found that the termination of certain safety net program expansions increased perceived stress and food insecurity among the caregivers we interviewed. Many of the caregivers we spoke with emphasized that although these programs were vital for short-term relief, the reduction of benefits felt premature, leaving many still grappling with the lingering effects of the pandemic, including inflation, particularly rising grocery prices.[13] These findings are consistent with previous research indicating that the expiration of monthly CTC payments resulted in a 25% increase in household food insufficiency compared with the period just before their expiration, and trends signaling large reductions in child poverty in 2021 were later reversed, with rates climbing back to 12.4% in 2022 and 13.7% in 2023.[28,29] In states where SNAP emergency allotments ended early, food insufficiency and financial hardships were exacerbated, with SNAP recipients experiencing a 21% increase in both food insufficiency and child food insufficiency.[11,12] Additionally, in states where these allotments expired later in March 2023, food insufficiency increased by 8%, and food pantry use and difficulty paying for household expenses increased by 2%.[30] Compounding these issues, in 2023, SNAP benefits were found to be insufficient to cover the cost of a modestly priced meal plan in most of the United States, underscoring the urgent need for continued support as families face continued challenges.[31]

PUBLIC HEALTH IMPLICATIONS

This study highlights the critical needs the social safety net can help address, as well as the unintended health effects of program modifications and benefit cliffs during periods of crisis and beyond. The study findings highlight the need to design and modify safety net policies to maximize the ability of participants to access benefits and thereby reduce worry, which enhances well-being and health equity among marginalized families. Additionally, our study highlights an important challenge related to the distribution of benefits during a crisis: it found that consistent benefits provided security and were perceived to be more consistently helpful than intermittent benefit distributions that, though helpful, also added to perceptions of chaos and stress. Providing reliable, adequate, relatively easy-to-access safety net supports appears to enhance participants' feelings of safety and security, improving food security and perceptions of well-being, both of which are associated with better health. Future efforts to modify the social safety net to improve public health should consider these important factors. AJPH

ABOUT THE AUTHORS

Nicole Fernández-Viña and Lia C. H. Fernald are with the Division of Community Health Sciences, School of Public Health, University of California, Berkeley. Rita Hamad and Kaitlyn E. Jackson are with the Department of Social & Behavioral Sciences, Harvard School of Public Health, Boston, MA. Wendi Gosliner is with the Nutrition Policy Institute, University of California, Division of Agriculture and Natural Resources, Oakland, CA.

CORRESPONDENCE

Correspondence should be sent to Nicole Fernández-Viña, University of California, Berkeley School of Public Health, 2121 Berkeley Way West, Berkeley, CA 94704 (e-mail: nfvina@gmail.com). Reprints can be ordered at http://www.ajph.org by clicking the "Reprints" link.

PUBLICATION INFORMATION

Full Citation: Fernández-Viña N, Fernald LCH, Hamad R, Jackson KE, Gosliner W. Lived experiences of families navigating safety net expansions and retractions during the pandemic: a qualitative study. *Am J Public Health*. 2025;115(11):1836–1847.

Acceptance Date: May 18, 2025.

DOI: https://doi.org/10.2105/AJPH.2025.308201

ORCID iDs:

Nicole Fernández-Viña https://orcid.org/0009-0004-7018-093X

Lia C. H. Fernald https://orcid.org/0000-0003-1555-4607

Rita Hamad https://orcid.org/0000-0003-0730-4077

Kaitlyn E. Jackson https://orcid.org/0000-0002-5154-1494

CONTRIBUTORS

N. Fernández-Viña and W. Gosliner designed analysis and analysis tools. L. C. H. Fernald, K. E. Jackson, and R. Hamad contributed to analysis tools and analysis design. N. Fernández-Viña and W. Gosliner analyzed and interpreted data, and L. C. H. Fernald, K. E. Jackson, and R. Hamad contributed to interpretation of results. N. Fernández-Viña drafted the original manuscript and L. C. H. Fernald, W. Gosliner, K. E. Jackson, and R. Hamad reviewed and edited the manuscript. All authors approved the final version of the manuscript.

ACKNOWLEDGMENTS

This work was funded by the Robert Wood Johnson Foundation, the Tipping Point Foundation, the University of California Office of the President, and the Berkeley Population Center at the University of California Berkeley (National Institute for Child Health and Human Development of the National Institutes of Health, award no. 5T32HD101364).

The authors thank Zoe Varner for her contributions to data collection and Ayla Malefakis for her contributions to data analysis.

CONFLICTS OF INTEREST

The authors have no conflicts of interest to disclose.

HUMAN PARTICIPANT PROTECTION

All study protocols were approved by the California Committee for the Protection of Human Subjects and the institutional review board of the University of California, Berkeley.

REFERENCES

1. Jackson KE, Yeb J, Gosliner W, Fernald LCH, Hamad R. Characterizing the landscape of safety net programs and policies in California during the COVID-19 pandemic. *Int J Environ Res Public Health*. 2022;19(5):2747. https://doi.org/10.3390/ijerph19052747
2. Baicker K. How much safety did the social safety net provide during the COVID-19 pandemic? *JAMA Health Forum*. 2023;4(10):e234237. https://doi.org/10.1001/jamahealthforum.2023.4237
3. Bitler M, Hoynes H, Whitmore Schanzenbach D. *The Social Safety Net in the Wake of COVID-19*. Cambridge, MA: National Bureau of Economic Research; 2020. National Bureau of Economic Research Working Paper Series.
4. US Dept of Agriculture. SNAP COVID-19 emergency allotments guidance. Food and Nutrition Service. 2023. Available at: https://www.fns.usda.gov/snap/covid-19-emergency-allotments-guidance. Accessed September 9, 2024.
5. California Dept of Social Services. Pandemic EBT. 2023. Available at: https://www.cdss.ca.gov/home/pandemic-ebt. Accessed September 24, 2024.
6. Pandemic Oversight. Update: three rounds of stimulus checks. See how many went out and for how much. Making sense of COVID-19 relief spending and programs. 2023. Available at: https://www.pandemicoversight.gov. Accessed September 9, 2024.
7. Internal Revenue Service. How the expanded 2021 Child Tax Credit can help your family. 2021. Available at: https://www.irs.gov/newsroom/how-the-expanded-2021-child-tax-credit-can-help-your-family. Accessed September 4, 2024.
8. Batra A, Jackson K, Hamad R. Effects of the 2021 Expanded Child Tax Credit on adults' mental health: a quasi-experimental study. *Health Aff (Millwood)*. 2023;42(1):74–82. https://doi.org/10.1377/hlthaff.2022.00733
9. Jackson KE, Chiang AY, Hamad R. The association of increased SNAP benefits during COVID-19 with food insufficiency and anxiety among US adults: a quasi-experimental study. *Public Health Nutr*. 2024;27(1):e186. https://doi.org/10.1017/S1368980024001447
10. Bryant A, Follett L. Hunger relief: a natural experiment from additional SNAP benefits during the COVID-19 pandemic. *Lancet Reg Health Am*. 2022;10:100224. https://doi.org/10.1016/j.lana.2022.100224
11. Dasgupta K, Plum A. *Termination of SNAP Emergency Allotments, Food Sufficiency, and Economic Hardships*. Washington, DC: Board of Governors of the Federal Reserve System; 2023. Finance and Economics Discussion Series 2023-046.
12. Richterman A, Roberto CA, Thirumurthy H. Associations between ending Supplemental Nutrition Assistance Program emergency allotments and food insufficiency. *JAMA Health Forum*. 2023;4(8):e232511. https://doi.org/10.1001/jamahealthforum.2023.2511

13. Blanchard OJ, Bernanke BS. *Unpacking the Causes of Pandemic-Era Inflation in the US*. Cambridge, MA: National Bureau of Economic Research; 2023. National Bureau of Economic Research Working Papers.
14. Mooney AC, Jackson KE, Hamad R, Fernald LCH, Hoskote M, Gosliner W. Experiences of distress and gaps in government safety net supports among parents of young children during the COVID-19 pandemic: a qualitative study. *BMC Public Health*. 2023;23(1):1099. https://doi.org/10.1186/s12889-023-16037-4
15. Hamad R, Gosliner W, Brown EM, et al. Understanding take-up of the Earned Income Tax Credit among Californians with low income. *Health Aff (Millwood)*. 2022;41(12):1715–1724. https://doi.org/10.1377/hlthaff.2022.00713
16. Chu L, Teng L. Does stimulus check payment improve people's mental health in the COVID-19 pandemic? Evidence from US Household Pulse Survey. *J Ment Health Policy Econ*. 2022;25(4):133–142. Available at: http://www.icmpe.org/test1/journal/issues/v25i4toc.html. Accessed August 18, 2025.
17. Tsai J, Huang M, Montgomery AE, Elbogen EB. Receipt, spending, and clinical correlates of the economic impact payment among middle- and low-income US adults. *Psychiatr Serv*. 2021;72(12):1377–1384. https://doi.org/10.1176/appi.ps.202100001
18. White JS, Basu S. Does the benefits schedule of cash assistance programs affect the purchase of temptation goods? Evidence from Peru. *J Health Econ*. 2016;46:70–89. https://doi.org/10.1016/j.jhealeco.2016.01.005
19. Hamilton C, Wimer C, Collyer S, Sariscsany L. *Monthly Cash Payments Reduce Spells of Poverty Across the Year*. New York, NY: Center of Poverty and Social Policy, Columbia University; 2022. Poverty & Social Policy Brief.
20. Herd P, Moynihan DP. *Administrative Burden: Policymaking by Other Means*. New York, NY: Russell Sage Foundation; 2019.
21. Herd P, Moynihan D. *How Administrative Burdens Can Harm Health. Health Affairs Health Policy Brief*. 2020. https://doi.org/10.1377/hpb20200904.405159
22. Kenney EL, Soto MJ, Fubini M, Carleton A, Lee M, Bleich SN. Simplification of Supplemental Nutrition Assistance Program recertification processes and association with uninterrupted access to benefits among participants with young children. *JAMA Netw Open*. 2022;5(9):e2230150. https://doi.org/10.1001/jamanetworkopen.2022.30150
23. Gosliner W, Chen WT, Johnson C, et al. Participants' experiences of the 2018–2019 government shutdown and subsequent Supplemental Nutrition Assistance Program (SNAP) benefit disruption can inform future policy. *Nutrients*. 2020;12(6):1867. https://doi.org/10.3390/nu12061867
24. Acciai F, Ohri-Vachaspati P, Yedidia MJ. Schools' participation in the community eligibility provision affects students' receipt of emergency benefits during the COVID-19 pandemic. *Nutrients*. 2022;14(22):4919. https://doi.org/10.3390/nu14224919
25. Cadenhead JW, McCarthy JE, Nguyen TTT, Rodriguez M, Koch PA. Qualitative study of participation facilitators and barriers for emergency school meals and pandemic electronic benefits (P-EBT) in an urban setting during COVID-19. *Nutrients*. 2022;14(16):3358. https://doi.org/10.3390/nu14163358
26. Jackson KE, Gosliner W, Fernald LCH, Fernandez-Viña N, Hamad R. Take-up and awareness of 2021 Child Tax Credit expansion: continuing barriers to health equity. *Ann Epidemiol*. 2025;109:59–64. https://doi.org/10.1016/j.annepidem.2025.06.015
27. Kenney EL, Walkinshaw LP, Shen Y, et al. Costs, reach, and benefits of COVID-19 pandemic electronic benefit transfer and grab-and-go school meals for ensuring youths' access to food during school closures. *JAMA Netw Open*. 2022;5(8):e2229514. https://doi.org/10.1001/jamanetworkopen.2022.29514
28. Bovell-Ammon A, McCann NC, Mulugeta M, Ettinger de Cuba S, Raifman J, Shafer P. Association of the expiration of Child Tax Credit advance payments with food insufficiency in US households. *JAMA Netw Open*. 2022;5(10):e2234438. https://doi.org/10.1001/jamanetworkopen.2022.34438
29. Trisi D. *Expiration of Pandemic Relief Led to Record Increases in Poverty and Child Poverty in 2022*. Washington, DC: Center on Budget and Policy Priorities; 2024.
30. Wells W, Jackson K, Leung CW, Hamad R. Food insufficiency increased after the expiration of COVID-19 emergency allotments for SNAP benefits in 2023. *Health Aff (Millwood)*. 2024;43(10):1464–1474. https://doi.org/10.1377/hlthaff.2023.01566
31. Waxman E, Gupta P. SNAP benefits remained too low to help families afford food in 2023. 2024. Available at: https://www.urban.org/sites/default/files/2024-05/SNAP-Benefits-Remained-Too-Low-to-Help-Families-Afford-Food-in-2023.pdf. Accessed September 21, 2024.

Children's Insurance Stability and Coverage Inequities During the COVID-19 Continuous Coverage Provisions

Erica L. Eliason, PhD, MPH, Aditi Vasan, MD, MSHP, and Daniel B. Nelson, MD, MPP

See also COVID-19 Benefits Cliff, pp. 1818–1867.

AJPH November 2025, Vol. 115, No. 11

Objectives. To explore the association between the March 2020 Families First Coronavirus Response Act (FFCRA) Medicaid disenrollment freeze during the COVID-19 public health emergency (PHE) and children's insurance coverage by family income, race/ethnicity, and language.

Methods. We used 2015 to 2021 US Medical Expenditure Panel Survey data, comparing monthly coverage for publicly insured children before (2015–2019) and during (2020–2021) the PHE. Outcomes included continuous public coverage, private coverage, no coverage, total months of public coverage, and total number of uninsured months. We estimated weighted multivariable linear regression models with a PHE period indicator.

Results. The PHE was associated with an increase in continuous public coverage among children of 4.2% percentage points, reduced transitions to private coverage (−2.3 percentage points) and no insurance (−1.9 percentage points), and increases in months of public coverage. The largest continuous public coverage improvements were among children from families with incomes between 200% and 399% of the federal poverty level (FPL), non-Hispanic White children, and Hispanic children.

Conclusions. The FFCRA improved children's public coverage continuity, particularly among children from families with incomes between 200% and 399% of the FPL, non-Hispanic White children, and Hispanic children, who may face coverage loss with disenrollment resuming. (*Am J Public Health*. 2025;115(11):1848–1857. https://doi.org/10.2105/AJPH.2024.307900)

Continuous insurance coverage is necessary to ensure access to health care for children, who are more likely to miss critical well-child visits, vaccines, preventive service visits, and sick care visits when they are uninsured or experiencing gaps in coverage.[1,2] Stable medical care access is especially important in childhood, as increased childhood insurance coverage can have long-term consequences in terms of reducing hospitalizations, disability, and mortality.[3,4] There are long-standing inequities in children's health insurance coverage and coverage adequacy, with low-income children and children of color more likely to be uninsured and to experience insurance "churning" (transitions between coverage types or periods of coverage and no coverage).[5,6]

The particular importance of continuous coverage for children has been recognized in the form of policy action to improve children's insurance stability, including state-level policy options that allow children to maintain consistent Medicaid or Children's Health Insurance Program (CHIP) coverage even if there are short-term changes in their eligibility.[7] These policies have been found to increase children's coverage stability and improve child health outcomes.[8]

To promote access to care during the COVID-19 public health emergency (PHE), the Families First Coronavirus Response Act (FFCRA) incentivized continuous coverage for all Medicaid beneficiaries through the offering of enhanced federal matching funds.[9] As all states chose to participate in this enhanced federal match, Medicaid disenrollment was nationally frozen for all enrollees for the duration of the policy, starting March 18, 2020, and continuing through at least April 1, 2023. Research has shown that continuous eligibility under the FFCRA is associated with increased monthly Medicaid enrollment among children,[10,11] with mixed findings on children's consistent public coverage enrollment.[12,13] No previous research to our knowledge has included an in-depth examination of how changes in coverage stability under the FFCRA vary according to children's demographic characteristics. Our aim in this study was to examine changes in coverage among publicly insured children during the FFCRA continuous coverage provisions based on children's income, race and ethnicity, and language.

METHODS

We used full-year consolidated files from the 2015 to 2021 Medical Expenditure Panel Survey (MEPS), a nationally representative panel survey that includes monthly health insurance coverage for all respondent household members, including children, for 2 calendar years. As continuous eligibility under the FFCRA was implemented in March 2020, we limited our sample population to children aged 18 years or younger who were enrolled in public insurance as of March of each survey year.

Variables

Outcomes of interest in this study included children's continuous public coverage enrollment, transitions to private coverage, transitions to no insurance, total months of enrollment in public coverage, and total months of no insurance, measured from April through December of each survey year. Continuous public coverage enrollment was measured through consistent reporting of public insurance each month, including coverage through Medicaid or CHIP. Coverage transitions were defined as changes from public coverage to private coverage or to no insurance coverage occurring any time between April and December. Coverage changes were considered transitions only if respondents reported no longer being enrolled in public coverage. Total months of public coverage enrollment and no insurance were measured as the total nonconsecutive number of months of public coverage or no insurance (0–9 months).

We considered children's demographic characteristics including age in years and sex (measured only as female or male), family income as a percentage of the federal poverty level according to the US Department of Health and Human Services' Poverty Guidelines (FPL; < 100%, 100%–199%, 200%–399%, or ≥ 400%), race and ethnicity (non-Hispanic Asian or Pacific Islander, non-Hispanic Black, Hispanic, non-Hispanic Indigenous or other, and non-Hispanic White), interview language (English only, Spanish, or other), nativity (born in the United States or outside the United States), and family size. We included race and ethnicity as proxies for racism and discrimination that individuals in minoritized groups might experience when accessing health insurance. In households interviewed in Spanish, interviews were conducted in Spanish only or a combination of Spanish and English.

There were no missing data among the variables, as MEPS employs methods to edit and impute variables to address missing data (Appendix Table A, available as a supplement to the online version of this article at http://www.ajph.org).[14] Nativity status was categorized as unknown for fewer than 1% of respondents.

Statistical Analysis

We calculated weighted demographic characteristics of the sample population and coverage outcomes before (2015–2019) and during (2020–2021) the PHE. To measure changes in enrollment during the FFCRA, we estimated unadjusted and adjusted linear probability models using an indicator for the PHE period (2020–2021) as our primary exposure. Adjusted models controlled for child's age and sex, family income, race/ethnicity, interview language, nativity, family size, and year fixed effects. To examine changes in coverage inequities, we conducted stratified analyses by family income (for children in families with incomes below 100% of the FPL, 100%–199% of the FPL, and 200%–399% of the FPL), by children's race and ethnicity (non-Hispanic Black, Hispanic, and non-Hispanic White), and by interview language (for children in families interviewed in English only or in Spanish).

We applied survey weights to all of our analyses, and these weights were divided by the number of study years so that they were generalizable to population estimates over the average annual periods in our study.[15] Weights for each panel were adjusted to reflect independent population totals.[14] The use of survey weights accounted for the complex survey design through adjustment for factors such as stratification, clustering, oversampling, and nonresponse.[16] Standard errors estimated from the complex multistage survey design were used for the main models.

Supplemental Analysis

In addition to analyzing coverage changes before and during the PHE, we calculated unadjusted and adjusted annual trends in coverage to examine yearly changes in children's public coverage continuity and insurance churning. In our primary analyses, we estimated standard errors by adjusting for the complex survey design; we also conducted a sensitivity analysis estimating overall models with standard errors clustered at the individual respondent level. Given that respondents are surveyed for 2 consecutive calendar years and report their insurance status for each month, clustering at the individual level accounted for the nonindependence of observations from the same respondent within and across survey years. Finally, we conducted exploratory analyses in stratified models for non-Hispanic Asian or Pacific Islander children and non-Hispanic Indigenous or other children because we lacked sufficient power to include them in the primary stratified analyses.

RESULTS

Our study sample included 28 405 MEPS respondents aged 18 years or younger, representing a weighted total of 30 161 655 children nationally. Children with public insurance coverage during March 2015 to 2021 were an average of 9.2 years old and were approximately evenly split between female (49.5%) and male (50.5%; Table 1). The highest shares of children in the sample were from families with incomes below 100% (36.2%) and 100% to 199% (35.8%) of the FPL. Hispanic children were the largest racial/ethnic group within the sample (36.9%), followed by non-Hispanic White children (32.5%), non-Hispanic Black children (20.1%), children who were non-Hispanic Indigenous or other (6.4%), and children who were non-Hispanic Asian or Pacific Islander (4.1%). Most children were from families interviewed in English only (79.6%); 19.5% were from families interviewed in Spanish only or a combination of Spanish and English. A large majority of children in the sample (96.3%) were born in the United States. The mean family size of children in the sample was 4.5 persons.

Demographic characteristics were generally consistent among children in the sample before and during the PHE, with no meaningful changes with respect to sex, race and ethnicity, interview language, nativity, or mean family size. Fewer children in the sample during the PHE were from families with incomes below 100% of the FPL (33.4% during the PHE, 37.3% before the PHE), whereas higher percentages were from families with incomes that were 200% to 399% of the FPL (25.4% during the PHE, 22.0% before the PHE).

There were significant changes in children's coverage stability during the PHE, with a 4.2-percentage-point (95% confidence interval [CI] = 1.7, 6.7) increase in public coverage stability in adjusted models, from a baseline of 90.2% of children with continuous enrollment in public coverage before the PHE (Table 2). The PHE was associated with decreases in insurance churning among children, with a 2.3-percentage-point (95% CI = −4.3, −0.2) decrease in transitions to private coverage from a baseline of 6.2% of children before the PHE and a 1.9-percentage-point (95% CI = −3.3, −0.5) decrease in transitions to no insurance from a baseline of 3.6% of children before the PHE. These coverage changes resulted in an increase in the total months of public coverage enrollment by 0.2 months (95% CI = 0.0, 0.3) from an average of 8.6 months before the PHE and no significant changes in total months of no insurance.

Before the PHE, baseline levels of continuous public coverage enrollment were lowest among children from families with incomes that were 200% to 399% of the FPL (85.1%), non-Hispanic White children (89.6%), and children interviewed in English (89.7%; Figure 1; Appendix Tables C and D, available as supplements to the online version of this article at http://www.ajph.org). In stratified adjusted models, the largest increases in public coverage continuity were among children from families with incomes that were 200% to 399% of the FPL (8.4 percentage points; 95% CI = 1.3, 15.5), non-Hispanic White children (6.1 percentage points; 95% CI = 0.8, 11.3), and Hispanic children (5.8 percentage points; 95% CI = 2.1, 9.5). Children from families with incomes that were 100% to 199% of the FPL and children from families interviewed in English exhibited smaller gains in public coverage continuity.

Almost all subgroups with increases in public coverage continuity during the PHE also exhibited significant declines in transitions to private insurance. The exception was children from families with incomes that were 200% to 399% of the FPL.

Correspondingly, children with family incomes that were 200% to 399% of the FPL exhibited the largest reductions in no insurance during the PHE (5.3 percentage points; 95% CI = −10.0, −0.7, from a pre-PHE baseline level of 7.8%). Hispanic children also exhibited significant reductions in lack of

AJPH November 2025, Vol. 115, No. 11

TABLE 1— Demographic Characteristics of Children Enrolled in Public Coverage in March 2015–2021, Before and During the COVID-19 Public Health Emergency (PHE): United States

Demographic Characteristic	Overall (n = 28 405; Weighted n = 30 161 655)	Before PHE (2015–2019; n = 22 405; Weighted n = 21 641 410)	During PHE (2020–2021; n = 6000; Weighted n = 8 520 244)
Age, y, mean (95% CI)	9.2 (9.1, 9.2)	9.1 (9.0, 9.1)	9.4 (9.3, 9.6)
Sex, % (95% CI)			
Female	49.5 (48.7, 50.2)	49.1 (48.2, 50.0)	50.4 (48.8, 52.0)
Male	50.5 (49.8, 51.3)	50.9 (50.0, 51.8)	49.6 (48.0, 51.2)
Family income, % of FPL, % (95% CI)			
< 100	36.2 (35.5, 36.9)	37.3 (36.5, 38.1)	33.4 (32.0, 34.9)
100–199	35.8 (35.1, 36.6)	36.1 (35.2, 36.9)	35.2 (33.6, 36.7)
200–399	23.0 (22.3, 23.7)	22.0 (21.2, 22.8)	25.4 (23.9, 27.0)
≥ 400	5.0 (4.6, 5.5)	4.7 (4.2, 5.1)	6.0 (5.1, 6.9)
Race/ethnicity, % (95% CI)			
Non-Hispanic Asian or Pacific Islander	4.1 (3.8, 4.4)	3.9 (3.6, 4.3)	4.5 (3.8, 5.4)
Non-Hispanic Black	20.1 (19.6, 20.7)	20.4 (19.7, 21.0)	19.6 (18.3, 20.9)
Hispanic	36.9 (36.2, 37.6)	36.5 (35.7, 37.3)	37.9 (36.4, 39.4)
Non-Hispanic Indigenous or other	6.4 (6.0, 6.8)	6.5 (6.1, 7.0)	5.9 (5.1, 6.7)
Non-Hispanic White	32.5 (31.7, 33.3)	32.6 (31.8, 33.5)	32.2 (30.6, 33.8)
Interview language, % (95% CI)			
English only	79.6 (79.1, 80.1)	79.8 (79.2, 80.4)	79.1 (77.9, 80.2)
Spanish[a]	19.5 (19.0, 20.0)	19.3 (18.7, 19.9)	20.0 (18.9, 21.2)
Other	0.9 (0.7, 1.1)	0.9 (0.7, 1.0)	0.9 (0.6, 1.4)
Nativity, % (95% CI)			
Born in the United States	96.3 (96.0, 96.6)	96.1 (95.8, 96.4)	96.6 (95.9, 97.2)
Born outside the United States	3.5 (3.3, 3.8)	3.6 (3.3, 3.9)	3.3 (2.7, 4.0)
Unknown	0.2 (0.1, 0.3)	0.3 (0.2, 0.4)	0.0 (0.0, 0.1)
Mean family size, no., mean (95% CI)	4.5 (4.5, 4.6)	4.6 (4.5, 4.6)	4.5 (4.5, 4.6)

Note. CI = confidence interval; FPL = federal poverty *level (according to the US Department of Health and Human Services' Poverty Guidelines)*. Data were derived from an analysis of 2015–2021 Medical Expenditure Panel Survey full-year consolidated files.
[a]Includes interviews conducted in Spanish only and interviews conducted in a combination of Spanish and English.

insurance (−3.7 percentage points; 95% CI = −7.0, −0.4, during the PHE from the pre-PHE baseline level of 2.7%). Despite having the largest reductions in transitions to no insurance during the PHE among the subgroups, children from families with incomes that were 200% to 399% of the FPL did not exhibit significant decreases in total months of no insurance. Hispanic children did exhibit a small but statistically significant decline in total months uninsured (−0.1 months; 95% CI = −0.2, −0.0; Figure 2; Appendix Table C).

Annual adjusted and unadjusted trends revealed larger changes in continuous public coverage enrollment and transitions to private coverage in 2021 than in 2020, with relatively consistent decreases in transitions to no insurance during the PHE (Appendix Figures A and B, available as supplements to the online version of this article at http://www.ajph.org). Sensitivity analyses incorporating alternative standard errors clustered at the respondent level showed consistent significant increases in public coverage and decreases in private coverage and no insurance transitions, along with significant decreases in total months of no insurance overall (−0.1 months; 95% CI = −0.1, −0.0; Appendix Table B, available as a supplement to the online version of this article at http://www.ajph.org).

In exploratory analyses among non-Hispanic Asian or Pacific Islander children, we found significant decreases in continuous public coverage enrollment during the PHE, although these estimates were sensitive to covariates (Appendix Table C). We found no

TABLE 2— Estimates of Changes in Children's Public Coverage Continuity and Insurance Churning During the COVID-19 Public Health Emergency (PHE): United States, 2015–2021

Outcome	Before PHE (2015–2019)	During PHE (2020–2021)	Unadjusted Difference	Adjusted Difference
Continuous public coverage enrollment, % (95% CI)	90.2 (89.4, 91.0)	93.6 (92.2, 94.7)	3.4 (1.9, 4.9)	4.2 (1.7, 6.7)
Transition to private coverage, % (95% CI)	6.2 (5.6, 6.8)	4.2 (3.3, 5.3)	−2.0 (−3.2, −0.8)	−2.3 (−4.3, −0.2)
Transition to no insurance, % (95% CI)	3.6 (3.1, 4.1)	2.2 (1.6, 3.0)	−1.4 (−2.2, −0.5)	−1.9 (−3.3, −0.5)
Total months enrolled in public coverage, no. (95% CI)	8.6 (8.6, 8.6)	8.7 (8.7, 8.8)	0.1 (0.1, 0.2)	0.2 (0.0, 0.3)
Total months uninsured, no. (95% CI)	0.2 (0.2, 0.2)	0.2 (0.1, 0.2)	−0.1 (−0.1, 0.0)	−0.1 (−0.2, 0.0)

Note. CI = confidence interval. Data were derived from an analysis of 2015–2021 Medical Expenditure Panel Survey full-year consolidated files. The sample size was 28 405 (weighted n = 30 161 655). The model was adjusted for child's age and sex, family income, race/ethnicity, interview language, nativity, family size, and year fixed effects.

evidence of significant changes in coverage among non-Hispanic Indigenous or other children in exploratory analyses.

DISCUSSION

Using nationally representative survey data on monthly health insurance coverage among children who had public coverage during March 2015 to 2021, we found that continuous Medicaid eligibility during the COVID-19

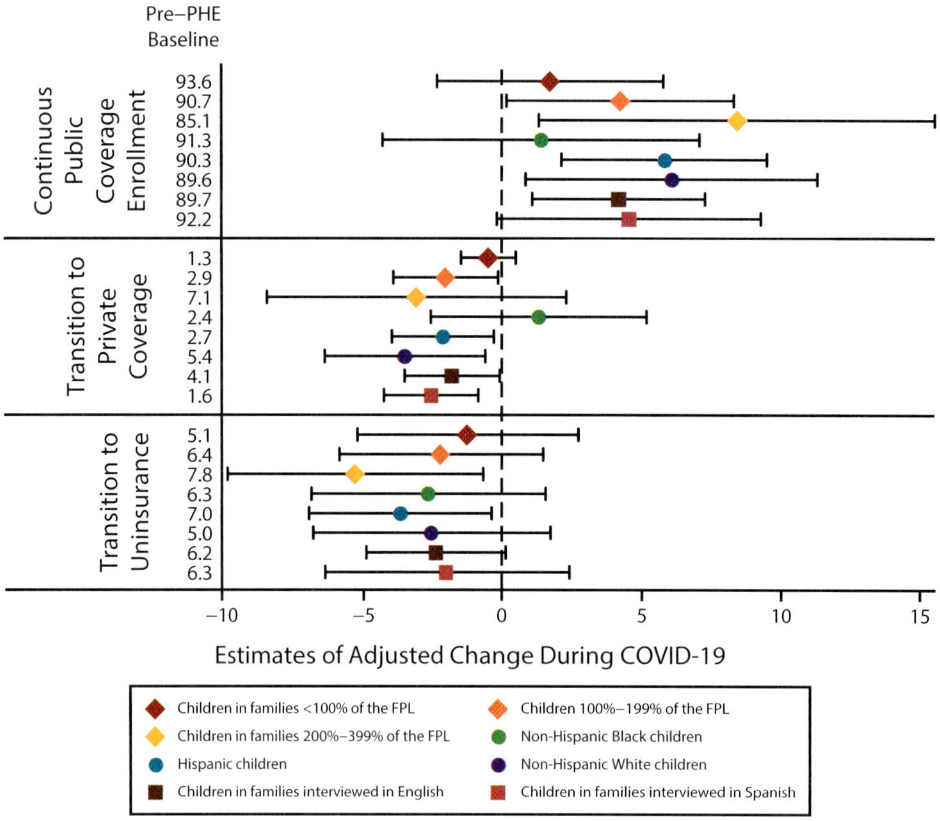

FIGURE 1— Stratified Estimates of Changes in Children's Public Coverage Continuity and Insurance Churning During the COVID-19 Public Health Emergency (PHE): United States, 2015–2021

Note. FPL = federal poverty *level (according to the US Department of Health and Human Services' Poverty Guidelines).* Data were derived from an analysis of 2015–2021 Medical Expenditure Panel Survey full-year consolidated files. Families interviewed in Spanish include interviews conducted in Spanish only and interviews conducted in a combination of Spanish and English. The model was adjusted for child's age and sex, family income, race/ethnicity, interview language, nativity, family size, and year fixed effects. The pre-PHE baseline represents the proportion of children with that coverage pattern type in the period 2015–2019, before the March 2020 PHE. Whiskers indicate 95% confidence intervals; those that do not cross the dashed line at 0 are statistically significant.

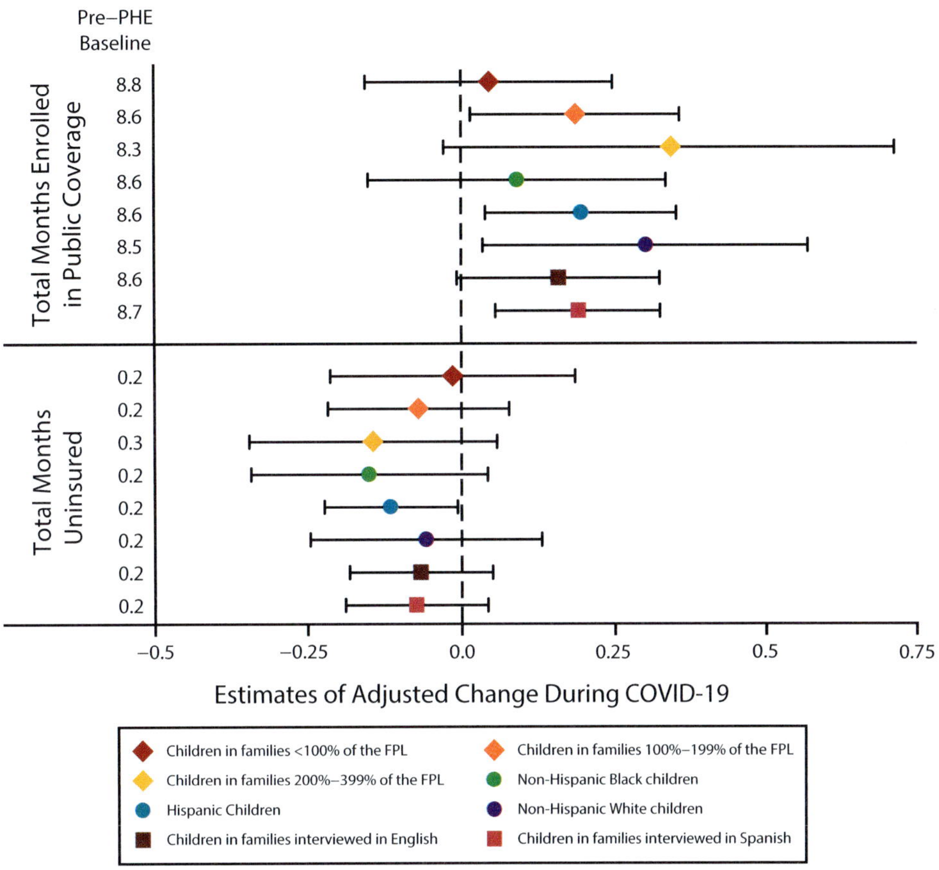

FIGURE 2— **Stratified Estimates of Changes in Children's Total Months of Public Coverage and No Insurance During the COVID-19 Public Health Emergency (PHE): United States, 2015–2021**

Note. FPL = federal poverty *level (according to the US Department of Health and Human Services' Poverty Guidelines).* Data were derived from an analysis of 2015–2021 Medical Expenditure Panel Survey full-year consolidated files. Families interviewed in Spanish include interviews conducted in Spanish only and interviews conducted in a combination of Spanish and English. The model was adjusted for child's age and sex, family income, race/ethnicity, interview language, nativity, family size, and year fixed effects. The pre-PHE baseline represents the number of months with that coverage pattern type among children in the period 2015–2019, before the March 2020 PHE. Whiskers indicate 95% confidence intervals; those that do not cross the dashed line at 0 are statistically significant.

FFCRA coverage provisions was associated with modest improvements in children's consistent public coverage enrollment and declines in transitions to private coverage and no insurance. Even prior to the FFCRA coverage provisions, children had largely stable public coverage and typically experienced only short periods of no insurance after losing public coverage. As a result, improvements in continuous public coverage enrollment during the PHE translated to only small increases in the total number of months of public coverage—less than 1 month—and no changes in the total number of months of no insurance.

Overall, 2.2% of Medicaid-enrolled children continued to transition to no insurance during the PHE disenrollment freeze. There are a number of reasons why respondents may have reported having no insurance despite the FFCRA continuous coverage provisions. First, our estimates could reflect Medicaid coverage loss for legitimate reasons such as moves between states or voluntary disenrollment. Second, states may not have complied immediately with continuous coverage requirements, leading to coverage loss before the coverage provisions were fully implemented.[17] Third, lack of insurance may have been misreported among respondents who were actually enrolled in Medicaid but were unaware of their ongoing enrollment during the continuous coverage provision (referred to as "Medicaid undercount").[18] Some states continued to send renewal forms and requests for documentation to Medicaid enrollees during the PHE, which could have contributed to confusion regarding Medicaid enrollment status.[19]

Increases in public coverage continuity were split between reductions in transitions to no insurance and transitions to private coverage. Overall, in our adjusted models, we found reductions in transitions from public coverage to private insurance of 2.3 percentage points during the PHE from transitions to private coverage among 6.2% of children before the PHE. Our estimates reflect reductions in children's public–private coverage churn rather than reductions in dual Medicaid and private coverage enrollment.

There are varying benefits of public and private coverage and implications for transitions from public to private coverage for children. Transitions in insurance coverage type, even from public to private without coverage gaps, can be disruptive to children's access to care in comparison with continuous Medicaid enrollment.[20] Private coverage typically offers higher physician payment rates, which can increase appointment availability relative to Medicaid,[21,22] but it also involves higher out-of-pocket costs for children's health care than Medicaid and CHIP.[23] When families are eligible for both Medicaid and private coverage, Medicaid can function as a secondary payer for private coverage for additional "wraparound" services, covering children's health care costs or services not otherwise covered.[24]

Children enrolled in CHIP available through expanded Medicaid eligibility in a state ("Medicaid expansion CHIP") can also use CHIP as a secondary payer for private coverage.[25] However, CHIP that is structured as insurance separate from Medicaid eligibility ("separate CHIP") cannot serve in this secondary coverage role, as children must be uninsured to be eligible in states with separate CHIP structures.[25]

An examination regarding the implications of the FFCRA continuous coverage policies for coverage inequities showed that the lowest-income children in families with incomes below 100% of the FPL, who had the highest pre-PHE baseline rates of stable public coverage before the FFCRA continuous coverage provisions, did not experience any significant coverage changes during the PHE. We found that children in families with incomes between 200% and 399% of the FPL experienced the largest increases in public coverage continuity and the largest decreases in no insurance during the PHE. The reason for this change could be that these children were closer to the Medicaid and CHIP income eligibility cutoffs and were therefore more likely to fluctuate in and out of eligibility before the PHE.[26] The FFCRA continuous coverage provisions froze disenrollment because of these income fluctuations, which might explain the larger coverage changes observed among children near the eligibility thresholds.

There were no significant coverage changes among non-Hispanic Black children during the PHE, whereas Hispanic children and non-Hispanic White children exhibited increases in public coverage continuity. There were notable reductions in transitions to no insurance among Hispanic children, who were the only group in our stratified models to show reductions in total months of no insurance during the FFCRA continuous coverage provisions.

Our results are consistent with previous research revealing reductions in inconsistent insurance among publicly insured children during the PHE, with higher predicted probabilities of inconsistent public coverage among Hispanic children and children in families who had incomes between 200% and 299% and 300% and 399% of the FPL during the period 2016 to 2021.[12] One previous study that also involved monthly MEPS data showed no evidence of significant changes in transitions from Medicaid or transitions to no insurance among children during the PHE in 2020 overall or stratified by children's race/ethnicity.[13]

Notably, the latter study incorporated a monthly measure of churning—rather than combining events over months—which would yield comparatively lower power to detect a policy effect.[13] The study authors suggested that the lower risks of insurance churning among children that predated the PHE continuous coverage policies may have been partly attributable to state continuous eligibility policies that were in place for Medicaid and CHIP in nearly half of all states, which may have dampened coverage gains for children from the FFCRA.[13] In studies comparing children's coverage changes during the PHE by whether states had 12-month continuous eligibility policies for children's Medicaid and CHIP, larger gains in children's Medicaid and CHIP enrollment during the PHE were observed in states that did not previously have such policies.[10,11]

The mandatory freeze on disenrollment under the FFCRA ended in April 2023, allowing states to begin "unwinding" the continuous coverage provisions and resume Medicaid disenrollment procedures over a 12- to 14-month period.[27,28] Our study revealed reductions in lack of insurance during the FFCRA among children in families with incomes between 200% and 399% of the FPL and Hispanic children, who had the highest rates of no insurance before the FFCRA policy changes. As a result, our findings might suggest that these children are at the highest risk for not having insurance and experiencing coverage loss as disenrollment is resumed under the FFCRA unwinding. Given that approximately half of all children are covered through Medicaid and CHIP, the unwinding is projected to have far-reaching effects on children's coverage stability, potentially resulting in coverage loss among upwards of 6.7 million children.[29]

Given that previous research showed that continuous eligibility policies reduce insurance churning and lack of insurance among children,[8] state adoption of 12-month continuous eligibility policies for children's Medicaid and CHIP may be protective against some coverage loss during the policy unwinding.[30,31] Children's 12-month continuous eligibility in Medicaid and CHIP became mandatory in all states starting in January 2024 under the Consolidated Appropriations Act of 2023.[32] Our results suggest that national continuous eligibility policies for children could increase continuous public coverage enrollments and reduce transitions to private coverage and no insurance. Our findings also suggest that children in families with incomes between 200% and 399% of the FPL, Hispanic children, and non-Hispanic White children may see the largest increases in public coverage under national continuous eligibility policies.

To further improve children's continuity of coverage, states could also consider pursuing multiyear continuous eligibility policies for children. Multiyear continuous eligibility policies are currently being implemented or under consideration in a growing number of states, following Oregon's lead in extending continuous Medicaid eligibility for children from birth to 6 years of age.[33,34] This approach may more closely follow the multiyear continuous eligibility that was in place under the FFCRA, resulting in increased public coverage continuity and reduced coverage inequities.

Limitations

Our study had several limitations. First, our analyses compared insurance stability and churning among publicly enrolled children before and during the PHE, and we could not employ a quasi-experimental design to evaluate a causal relationship between the FFCRA continuous coverage provisions and insurance coverage changes during the PHE. Second, our sample size was insufficient to be powered for further stratified analyses, including analyses by nativity, which we would have wanted to examine because of differences in public coverage eligibility by immigration status.[35] In addition, we were limited in stratified analyses of further racial/ethnic subgroups. Although we include stratified results for non-Hispanic Asian or Pacific Islander children and non-Hispanic Indigenous or other children in the supplement, these analyses should be considered exploratory as a result of the limited sample size.

Third, we examined coverage changes occurring within calendar years, during which there were already high levels of stable coverage among children, potentially owing to 12-month continuous eligibility policies that were already in place in approximately half of the states before the PHE. As a result, children's gains in coverage stability under the FFCRA might be greater over periods spanning multiple years rather than within the same year. Finally, survey results can be subject to reporting and recall bias, which can affect data reliability and validity. The risk of bias and less precise estimates in MEPS data may have been higher for the COVID-19 survey years because of lower response rates, although there has been no evidence of resulting systematic biases, including nonresponse bias, in MEPS data during the COVID-19 pandemic.[36]

Public Health Implications

We found that public coverage continuity among children increased during the FFCRA continuous coverage provisions, with reductions in insurance churning and lack of insurance. Children who had the highest baseline rates of no insurance—children in families with incomes between 200% and 399% of the FPL and Hispanic children—exhibited the largest declines in transitions to no insurance during the PHE. These results shed light on the potential effects of unwinding the FFCRA continuous coverage provisions on coverage inequities and offer evidence in support of continuous Medicaid and CHIP eligibility policies for promoting children's coverage stability. AJPH

ABOUT THE AUTHORS

At the time of conceptualization, Erica L. Eliason was with the Department of Health Services, Policy, & Practice, Brown University School of Public Health, Providence, RI. Aditi Vasan is with the Department of Pediatrics, University of Pennsylvania Perelman School of Medicine and PolicyLab, Children's Hospital of Philadelphia, Philadelphia. At the time of conceptualization, Daniel B. Nelson was with the Department of Population Medicine, Harvard Medical School, Boston, MA.

CORRESPONDENCE

Correspondence should be sent to Erica L. Eliason, PhD, MPH, Rutgers Center for State Health Policy, 112 Paterson St, 5th Floor, New Brunswick, NJ 08901 (e-mail: erica.eliason@rutgers.edu). Reprints can be ordered at https://www.ajph.org by clicking the "Reprints" link.

PUBLICATION INFORMATION

Full Citation: Eliason EL, Vasan A, Nelson DB. Children's insurance stability and coverage inequities during the COVID-19 continuous coverage provisions. *Am J Public Health*. 2025; 115(11):1848–1857.

Acceptance Date: October 7, 2024.

DOI: https://doi.org/10.2105/AJPH.2024.307900

ORCID iDs:

Erica L. Eliason https://orcid.org/0000-0002-5246-3176

Aditi Vasan https://orcid.org/0000-0001-8992-5672

Daniel B. Nelson https://orcid.org/0000-0001-9249-4439

CONTRIBUTORS

All of the authors contributed to research question conceptualization and design, interpretation of data and results, and the drafting of the article.

ACKNOWLEDGMENTS

Erica L. Eliason was supported by the National Institute of Child Health and Human Development under grant K99 HD111622.

This research was presented at the 2024 Association for Public Policy Analysis and Management Annual Fall Research Conference.

Note. The funders had no role in the design and conduct of the study; collection, management, analysis, and interpretation of the data; preparation, review, or approval of the article; or the decision to submit the article for publication.

CONFLICTS OF INTEREST

The authors have no conflicts of interest to disclose.

HUMAN PARTICIPANT PROTECTION

This study was considered exempt by the Rutgers University institutional review board because publicly available data were used.

REFERENCES

1. Cummings JR, Lavarreda SA, Rice T, Brown ER. The effects of varying periods of uninsurance on children's access to health care. *Pediatrics.* 2009;123(3):e411–e418. https://doi.org/10.1542/peds.2008-1874
2. Flores G, Lin H, Walker C, et al. The health and healthcare impact of providing insurance coverage to uninsured children: a prospective observational study. *BMC Public Health.* 2017;17(1):553. https://doi.org/10.1186/s12889-017-4363-z
3. Wherry LR, Miller S, Kaestner R, Meyer BD. Childhood Medicaid coverage and later-life health care utilization. *Rev Econ Stat.* 2018;100(2): 287–302. https://doi.org/10.1162/REST_a_00677
4. Goodman-Bacon A. The long-run effects of childhood insurance coverage: Medicaid implementation, adult health, and labor market outcomes. *Am Econ Rev.* 2021;111(8):2550–2593. https://doi.org/10.1257/aer.20171671
5. Satchell M, Pati S. Insurance gaps among vulnerable children in the United States, 1999–2001. *Pediatrics.* 2005;116(5):1155–1161. https://doi.org/10.1542/peds.2004-2403
6. Shen Y, Turner CB, Perkins RK, Moore A. Children's health insurance coverage and adequacy from 2016 to 2018: racial/ethnic disparities under the ACA. *J Public Health Res.* 2022;11(3): 22799036221102492. https://doi.org/10.1177/22799036221102492
7. Centers for Medicare & Medicaid Services. Continuous eligibility for Medicaid and CHIP coverage: enrollment strategies. Available at: https://www.medicaid.gov/medicaid/enrollment-strategies/continuous-eligibility-medicaid-and-chip-coverage/index.html. Accessed February 16, 2023.
8. Brantley E, Ku L. Continuous eligibility for Medicaid associated with improved child health outcomes. *Med Care Res Rev.* 2022;79(3):404–413. https://doi.org/10.1177/10775587211021172
9. Rachel Dolan MM, Tolbert J, Rudowitz R. Medicaid maintenance of eligibility (MOE) requirements: issues to watch. Available at: https://www.kff.org/medicaid/issue-brief/medicaid-maintenance-of-eligibility-moe-requirements-issues-to-watch. Accessed February 16, 2023.
10. Vasan A, Kenyon CC, Fiks AG, Venkataramani AS. Continuous eligibility and coverage policies expanded children's Medicaid enrollment: study examines state continuous eligibility and coverage policies and children's Medicaid enrollment during COVID-19. *Health Aff (Millwood).* 2023; 42(6):753–758. https://doi.org/10.1377/hlthaff.2022.01465
11. Singer PM, Mandle J, Nelson DB. Child enrollment in states with and without continuous coverage in Medicaid and CHIP during COVID-19. *Am J Public Health.* 2021;111(12):2103–2104. https://doi.org/10.2105/AJPH.2021.306550
12. Daw JR, Yekta S, Jacobson-Davies FE, Patrick SW, Admon LK. Consistency and adequacy of public and commercial health insurance for US children, 2016 to 2021. *JAMA Health Forum.* 2023; 4(11):e234179. https://doi.org/10.1001/jamahealthforum.2023.4179
13. Nelson DB, Goldman AL, Zhang F, Yu H. Continuous Medicaid coverage during the COVID-19 public health emergency reduced churning, but did not eliminate it. *Health Aff Sch.* 2023;1(5): qxad055. https://doi.org/10.1093/haschl/qxad055
14. Agency for Healthcare Research and Quality. Medical Expenditure Panel Survey HC-224 2020 full year consolidated data file. Available at: https://meps.ahrq.gov/data_stats/download_data/pufs/h224/h224doc.shtml. Accessed February 16, 2023.
15. Agency for Healthcare Research and Quality. Replicate File for BRR variance estimation: Medical Expenditure Panel Survey. Available at: https://meps.ahrq.gov/data_stats/download_data/pufs/h036brr/h36brr19doc.shtml. Accessed February 16, 2023.
16. Machlin S, Yu W, Zodet M. Computing standard errors for Medical Expenditure Panel Survey estimates. Available at: https://meps.ahrq.gov/survey_comp/standard_errors.jsp. Accessed February 16, 2023.
17. Pradhan R. Idaho dropped thousands from Medicaid in the pandemic's first years. Available at: https://kffhealthnews.org/news/article/idaho-medicaid-disenrollment-first-two-years-of-pandemic. Accessed February 16, 2023.
18. Boudreaux MH, Call KT, Turner J, Fried B, O'Hara B. Measurement error in public health insurance reporting in the American Community Survey: evidence from record linkage. *Health Serv Res.* 2015;50(6):1973–1995. https://doi.org/10.1111/1475-6773.12308
19. Brooks T, Gardner A, Osorio A, et al. Medicaid and CHIP eligibility and enrollment policies as of January 2022: findings from a 50-state survey. Available at: https://files.kff.org/attachment/REPORT-Medicaid-and-CHIP-Eligibility-and-Enrollment-Policies-as-of-January-2022.pdf. Accessed February 16, 2023.
20. Tumin D, Miller R, Raman VT, Uffman JC, Tobias JD. Patterns of health insurance discontinuity and children's access to health care. *Matern Child Health J.* 2019;23(5):667–677. https://doi.org/10.1007/s10995-018-2681-0
21. Rudowitz R, Burns A, Hinton E, Mohamed M. 10 things to know about Medicaid. Available at: https://www.kff.org/medicaid/issue-brief/10-things-to-know-about-medicaid. Accessed February 16, 2023.
22. Hsiang WR, Lukasiewicz A, Gentry M, et al. Medicaid patients have greater difficulty scheduling health care appointments compared with private insurance patients: a meta-analysis. *Inquiry.* 2019;56:46958019838118. https://doi.org/10.1177/0046958019838118
23. Kreider AR, French B, Aysola J, Saloner B, Noonan KG, Rubin DM. Quality of health insurance coverage and access to care for children in low-income families. *JAMA Pediatr.* 2016;170(1):43. https://doi.org/10.1001/jamapediatrics.2015.3028
24. Medicaid and CHIP Payment Access Commission. How Medicaid interacts with other payers. Available at: https://www.macpac.gov/subtopic/how-medicaid-interacts-with-other-payers. Accessed February 16, 2023.
25. US Government Accountability Office. Children's Health Insurance Program: efforts to measure and address potential substitution for private health insurance. Available at: https://www.gao.gov/assets/gao-20-12.pdf. Accessed February 16, 2023.
26. Kaiser Family Foundation. Medicaid/CHIP upper income eligibility limits for children, 2000–2024: trends in income eligibility limits for children. Available at: https://www.kff.org/medicaid/state-indicator/medicaidchip-upper-income-eligibility-limits-for-children. Accessed February 16, 2023.
27. Centers for Medicare & Medicaid Services. Key dates related to the Medicaid continuous enrollment condition provisions in the Consolidated Appropriations Act, 2023. Available at: https://www.medicaid.gov/media/148471. Accessed February 16, 2023.
28. Tolbert J, Ammula M. 10 things to know about the unwinding of the Medicaid continuous enrollment provision. Available at: https://www.kff.org/medicaid/issue-brief/10-things-to-know-about-the-unwinding-of-the-medicaid-continuous-enrollment-provision. Accessed February 16, 2023.
29. Alker J, Brooks T. Millions of children may lose Medicaid: what can be done to help prevent them from becoming uninsured? Available at: https://ccf.georgetown.edu/2022/02/17/millions-of-children-may-lose-medicaid-what-can-be-done-to-help-prevent-them-from-becoming-uninsured. Accessed February 16, 2023.

30. Federman S, Coleman A. Protecting kids from coverage losses during Medicaid redeterminations and beyond: five strategies for states. Available at: https://www.commonwealthfund.org/blog/2023/protecting-kids-coverage-losses-during-medicaid-redeterminations-and-beyond-five. Accessed February 16, 2023.
31. Eliason E, Nelson D, Vasan A. Continuous eligibility policies and CHIP structure affected children's coverage loss during Medicaid unwinding: article examines children's coverage during Medicaid unwinding. *Health Aff (Millwood)*. 2025;44(3):288–295. https://doi.org/10.1377/hlthaff.2024.01099
32. Hogan C, Volkov E, Peters C, De Lew N, Buchmueller T. New federal 12-month continuous eligibility expansion: over 17 million children could gain new protections from coverage disruptions. Available at: https://aspe.hhs.gov/sites/default/files/documents/5b52fb410eb225 17d4fc1bc4cac834bd/aspe-childrens-continuous-eligibility.pdf. Accessed February 16, 2023.
33. Williams E, Corallo B, Tolbert J, Burns A, Rudowitz R. Implications of continuous eligibility policies for children's Medicaid enrollment churn. Available at: https://www.kff.org/medicaid/issue-brief/implications-of-continuous-eligibility-policies-for-childrens-medicaid-enrollment-churn. Accessed February 16, 2023.
34. Burak EW. North Carolina and Hawaii make 10: states advancing Medicaid/CHIP multi-year continuous eligibility for young children. Available at: https://ccf.georgetown.edu/2023/11/16/north-carolina-and-hawaii-make-10-states-advancing-medicaid-chip-multi-year-continuous-eligibility-for-young-children. Accessed February 16, 2023.
35. Pillai A, Pillai D, Artiga S. State health coverage for immigrants and implications for health coverage and care. Available at: https://www.kff.org/racial-equity-and-health-policy/issue-brief/state-health-coverage-for-immigrants-and-implications-for-health-coverage-and-care. Accessed February 16, 2023.
36. Zuvekas SH, Kashihara D. The impacts of the COVID-19 pandemic on the Medical Expenditure Panel Survey. *Am J Public Health*. 2021;111(12):2157–2166. https://doi.org/10.2105/AJPH.2021.306534

Expansion of the Earned Income Tax Credit for Young Adults and Mental Health of US Home Renters, 2021–2023

Abdinasir K. Ali, PhD, MPH, and Wei Lyu, PhD

See also COVID-19 Benefits Cliff, pp. 1818–1857.

Objectives. To evaluate the impact of the temporary expansion of the Earned Income Tax Credit (EITC) for childless adults in 2021 on the mental health of home renters and homeowners.

Methods. We used US Behavioral Risk Factor Surveillance System data from 2021 through 2023. Mental health outcomes included the number of mentally unhealthy days in the past 30 days and an indicator for frequent mental distress (14 or more unhealthy days). We used a difference-in-differences design comparing outcome changes before and after the EITC expansion between young adults 18 to 24 years of age (treatment group) and adults 25 to 29 years of age (control group), separately for renters and homeowners.

Results. The EITC expansion was associated with statistically significant improvements in mental health among young renters but not homeowners. Specifically, after the expansion in 2022, renters 18 to 24 years of age experienced a mean of 2.21 fewer mentally unhealthy days and exhibited a 9.8 percentage point decrease in the probability of frequent mental distress relative to older renters.

Conclusions. Our findings suggest that antipoverty programs such as the EITC are associated with improvements in mental health among young adults who rent. (*Am J Public Health*. 2025;115(11): 1858–1867. https://doi.org/10.2105/AJPH.2025.308219)

AJPH November 2025, Vol. 115, No. 11

The number of renting households cost burdened during the COVID-19 pandemic had increased to more than 20 million as of 2022.[1] Also, nearly half of all renting households spend more than 30% of their incomes on rent.[2] Young adults who rent face more severe housing hardships as a result of worse socioeconomic conditions such as high poverty rates and widening gaps in income and education between young and older adults.[3,4] These housing hardships, coupled with low socioeconomic status, have been associated with depressive symptoms and declining mental health, especially among young adults.[5–7] Stress resulting from job losses caused by business closures and the general economic uncertainty during the COVID-19 pandemic further exacerbated mental health issues for renters.[8]

In response to the economic hardships during the COVID-19 pandemic, the government enacted the American Rescue Plan Act in March 2021, which included several income policies designed to support economically vulnerable populations. One key policy was the 1-year temporary expansion of the Earned Income Tax Credit (EITC) for childless adults. The EITC expansion increased the credit amount from $500 to $1500 and raised the adjusted gross income limit for claiming the credit from $16 000 to $21 000. It also expanded the age range of eligible workers by including younger adults 19 to 24 years of age, allowing them to qualify for the EITC for the first time.

The EITC was implemented in 1975 to encourage nonworking poor individuals with children to participate in the labor force and to reduce their tax burden upon entering the workforce.[9] Over the past several decades, the EITC has evolved into one of the largest antipoverty programs in the United States, and it had alleviated nearly 5.6 million people from poverty by 2018.[9,10] Many studies have demonstrated that the EITC reduces homelessness and evictions, improves housing affordability, decreases the number of mentally unhealthy days among married mothers, and improves infant health outcomes.[11–14]

Our aim in this study was to evaluate the impact of the temporary expansion of the childless EITC on the mental health of young adults according to housing tenure status. Many studies have evaluated the effects of the EITC on families with children and revealed improvements in mental health, nutrition, and child well-being.[15–17] However, to date, only a single study to our knowledge has evaluated the impact of the childless EITC expansion in 2021 on material well-being (e.g., food insufficiency, housing hardship, and difficulty meeting household expenses).[18] That study showed that the 2021 temporary EITC expansion was associated with a decline in housing hardship of 3.2 percentage points.[18] The temporary EITC expansion may offer crucial economic and mental health benefits for young renters, who face high poverty levels relative to all other age groups.[19] Upon receiving such a large cash payment as a lump sum, young adults could use the extra cash for household expenditures or other health improvement expenses and, in turn, improve their mental health outcomes.[20,21]

METHODS

We used 2021 to 2023 Behavioral Risk Factor Surveillance System (BRFSS) data for our study. The BRFSS is a nationally representative cross-sectional telephone survey conducted every month in all 50 states and the District of Columbia. The survey collects data on individuals' demographic and socioeconomic characteristics, health status, and behaviors by using random-digit dialing for both landlines and cell phones. The BRFSS was surveyed each month throughout the year with an overall response rate that ranged from 44% to 45% during the study period.[22,23]

We restricted our sample to childless adults 29 years or younger who were employed at the time of the survey and earned below $35 000 given that these individuals were likely to be affected by the EITC expansion. Information on individuals' employment status, parental status, and rental status was collected directly in the BRFSS questionnaires.[24] Income information was also obtained via a survey question that asked respondents to provide their annual household income from all sources.

Outcomes

Our study outcomes included a measure of mental health status captured by the number of days not in good mental health during the previous 30 days, indicating respondents' overall mental health status.[25] In addition, we evaluated a binary measure to indicate frequent mental distress, determined by whether individuals had bad mental health days for 14 or more days; this is considered a valid measure of mental health status because it is associated with mental health disorders.[25]

Research Design and Statistical Analysis

We used a difference-in-differences design to compare changes in mental health outcomes before and after the temporary EITC expansion between individuals 18 to 24 years old (eligible for the EITC for the first time) and those 25 to 29 years old, separately for renters and homeowners. Young adults 18 to 24 years of age who became temporarily eligible for the credit during the 2021 tax year were considered the treatment group given that they would receive the EITC for the first time if they filed their taxes in calendar year 2022. We selected individuals 25 to 29 years of age as the control group, as they were closest in age to the treatment group but were not affected by the temporary EITC expansion. We conducted our analysis around the actual timing of credit receipt by respondents. We included only data from February to June in each year because the EITC is typically claimed during the tax season of the following calendar year. For example, the first treatment period was February through June 2022, when individuals usually receive the EITC.[26,27] We excluded data from July to December of each year because people were unlikely to receive any credits during that period.

To better understand the effects of the temporary EITC expansion over time, we estimated an event-study difference-in-differences model to explore year-by-year changes in outcomes for 2022 and 2023 relative to 2021 (the reference year). Although the temporarily expanded EITC was available for receipt only in 2022 during filing for 2021 taxes, it is likely that some individuals who missed the deadline would claim the credit in the following years. Estimates suggest that 20% of qualified filers did not claim the EITC for tax year 2021.[28] Because the Internal Revenue Service (IRS) allows filers to claim the EITC retroactively for up to 3 years, some individuals may still receive their credits for tax year 2021 in 2023 or later. Thus, we included 2023 data in our analysis to account for this possibility and to assess whether the effects were different in 2023.

Specifically, we estimated the following equation:

$$Y_{ist} = \alpha + \beta_1 D_i \times Y2022_t + \beta_2 D_i \times Y2023_t + \pi \times D_i + X_{ist}\Phi + \theta_s + \omega_t + \epsilon_{ist}. \quad (1)$$

Y_{ist} represents the mental health outcome for individual i interviewed in state s at time t. D_i is a binary indicator equal to 1 for young adults 18 to 24 years old and 0 for adults 25 to 29 years old. $Y2022$ and $Y2023$ are binary indicators for calendar year 2022 and 2023, respectively, with 2021 as the reference year. X_{ist} includes individual characteristics such as race/ethnicity, income, sex, and insurance status. θ_s represents state fixed effects accounting for time-invariant differences across states, and ω_t represents time fixed effects to account for national trends shared across all individuals. The coefficient β_1 captures the effects of the 2021 EITC expansion on mental health among young renters 18 to 24 years old, and β_2 captures any prolonged effects that are present.

To examine the validity of the difference-in-differences design, we evaluated whether there were differential pretrends (i.e., parallel trend assumption) in outcomes during 2017 to 2019 between individuals 18 to 24 years old and those 25 to 29 years old, separately for renters and homeowners. We excluded 2020 to avoid any substantial changes related to the COVID-19 pandemic that might make the data not comparable between periods before and after the pandemic. The following model was estimated to evaluate the outcome pretrends:

$$Y_{ist} = \alpha + \delta_1 D_i \times Y2018_t + \delta_2 D_i \times Y2019_t + \pi \times D_i + X_{ist}\Phi + \theta_s + \omega_t + \epsilon_{ist}. \quad (2)$$

In Equation 2, $Y2018$ and $Y2019$ are binary indicators for 2018 and 2019, with 2017 as the reference year. All other parameters are defined the same as in Equation 1. The outcome pretrends between the treatment and control groups are captured by δ_1 and δ_2. The insignificance of δ_1 and δ_2 indicates that there were no outcome pretrends.

We further assessed the validity of our difference-in-differences design by conducting several falsification tests. First, we reestimated the model specified in Equation 1 using a sample of renters with incomes above \$50 000, who should be ineligible for any EITC benefits. Second, we reestimated the model with adults 25 to 29 years old as the treatment group and adults 30 to 34 years old as the control group. In this way, we hypothetically assumed that adults 25 to 29 years old were affected by the EITC expansion. Third, we used data from July to December in each year from 2021 to 2023, a period when most individuals would not receive any tax returns including the EITC from the IRS. Across all of these falsification tests, we expected to find null effects (i.e., the coefficients $\beta 1$ and $\beta 2$ would be statistically insignificant).

In addition, we performed several sensitivity checks to assess the robustness of our analysis. First, we reestimated the model using different month periods in each year based on the interview month (February–September, February–December, and January–July). Then we reestimated the model using alternative income samples in addition to our main sample, including a sample with incomes below \$25 000 and another with incomes below \$50 000. Moreover, we estimated an alternative model specification by adding year-by-state-specific trends (i.e., interaction terms between state and year) to account for state-specific trends in outcomes before and after the EITC expansion. We further added time trends for each sociodemographic subgroup (i.e., interaction terms between year and each sociodemographic covariate) in an additional specification to account for any time-varying confounding linked to differences in subgroup distributions between the treatment and control groups.

Finally, we estimated a model in which covariates were added for chronic conditions such as heart attack, coronary heart disease, stroke, asthma, skin cancer, melanoma, chronic obstructive pulmonary disease, depressive disorder, kidney disease, arthritis, and diabetes. These variables help further account for potential confounding related to respondents' underlying health status.

We estimated all regressions using ordinary least squares to provide directly interpretable estimates. All models were estimated separately for renters and homeowners. To further assess potential heterogeneity in the effects by sociodemographic subgroups, we also stratified the models by sex (male vs female) and race/ethnicity (non-Hispanic White vs non-White). We were unable to include other racial/ethnic groups as a result of the small sample sizes. The main estimates are reported from models that did not apply BRFSS sampling weights, as these models yielded more precise results (with lower standard errors). However, we also present results from weighted models as a sensitivity check. All estimates were considered statistically significant at the .05 level. We conducted all of our analyses using StataNow/SE version 18.5 (StataCorp LP, College Station, TX).

RESULTS

Table 1 reports summary descriptive statistics for treatment group (18–24 years old) and control group (25–29 years old) renters by year from 2021 to 2023 (i.e., tax years 2020, 2021, and 2022). Among young renters 18 to 24 years of age, the number of mentally unhealthy days fluctuated slightly, decreasing from a mean of 9.17 in 2021 to 8.88 in 2022 after the EITC expansion and then increasing to 9.37 in 2023 after the end of the expansion. Frequent mental distress followed a similar pattern. Mentally unhealthy days increased from 7.23 in 2021 to 9.06 in 2022 and 8.19 in 2023 for renters 25 to 29 years of age, whereas frequent mental distress rose from 23% in 2021 to more than 31% in 2022. Relative to older renters (the control group), younger renters (the treatment group) tended to include a higher proportion of women, to be less educated, to have lower incomes, and to include slightly more non-Hispanic Whites.

Similar descriptive statistics for homeowners are reported in Table A (available as a supplement to the online version of this article at http://www.ajph.org). Among young adult homeowners 18 to 24 years of age, the number of mentally unhealthy days increased from 6.81 in 2021 to 9.25 in 2022 after the EITC expansion and then decreased to 7.94 in 2023. In contrast, the number of mentally unhealthy days among homeowners 25 to 29 years of age declined from 8.19 in 2021 to 7.44 in 2022 and then rose to 11.19 in 2023.

Main Estimates

Table 2 presents the difference-in-differences estimates of the effects of the temporary childless EITC expansion on mental health outcomes, separately for renters and homeowners. Among renters, the estimates indicate that the EITC expansion in tax year 2021 for childless young workers 18 to 24 years old was associated with a statistically significant decline in number of mentally unhealthy days of 2.21 ($P < .01$) in 2022. On average, this represents approximately a 26% decrease in the number of mentally unhealthy days relative to the 2021 mean. In addition, the reduction in mentally unhealthy days corresponded to a statistically significant decrease of 9.8 percentage points in the probability of experiencing frequent mental distress in 2022, representing a reduction of 35% relative to the mean in 2021. We did not observe any statistically significant changes in either mental health outcome in 2023. However, these improvements in mental health outcomes were not observed among homeowners. Table 3 presents estimates of outcome pretrends from 2017 to 2019 BRFSS data. The estimates indicate no significant pretrends in outcomes, supporting the validity of our design.

Subgroup Analysis

Table 4 presents subgroup results by sex and race/ethnicity. Among renters with incomes below $35 000 who were employed and 18 to 24 years of age, both men and women and non-Hispanic White individuals saw significant reductions in mentally unhealthy days and frequency of mental distress. Specifically, men had 2.13 ($P < .05$) fewer mentally unhealthy days in 2022 and a 13 percentage point ($P < .01$) decrease in the probability of experiencing frequent mental distress. Women experienced 2.59 fewer mentally unhealthy days with no statistically significant changes in the probability of experiencing frequent mental distress. Non-Hispanic Whites experienced a reduction of 2.5 mentally unhealthy days and a 9.6 percentage point decrease in the probability of experiencing frequent mental distress in 2022. However, these effects were smaller and nonsignificant in 2023 across the subgroups we examined, consistent with the findings from the full sample.

Falsification Tests

Table B (available as a supplement to the online version of this article at http://www.ajph.org) reports the estimates for the falsification tests. We did not find any evidence that the temporary EITC expansion had effects on groups other than poor young childless workers 19 to 24 years old who had become eligible for the EITC for the first time. Specifically, the estimates for the sample of individuals with incomes above $50 000, hypothetically assuming adults 25 to 29 years old as the treatment group and limiting the months to July through December, were all statistically insignificant and small.

Sensitivity Checks

Table C (available as a supplement to the online version of this article at http://www.ajph.org) reports the results of the sensitivity checks in different month periods. The results were robust overall to using different month periods, including extending the month to September and adding back January. When extending the month to December, the estimates became much smaller and statistically insignificant, which was within our expectations because the credits were more likely to be used

TABLE 1— Descriptive Statistics Among Renters: Behavioral Risk Factor Surveillance System, United States, 2021–2023

	Childless Adults 18–24 Years of Age (Treatment Group)			Childless Adults 25–29 Years of Age (Control Group)		
	2021 (February–June)	2022 (February–June)	2023 (February–June)	2021 (February–June)	2022 (February–June)	2023 (February–June)
No. of observations	828	724	644	564	481	433
Outcomes						
Mean no. of mentally unhealthy days	9.17	8.88	9.37	7.23	9.06	8.19
Frequent mental distress, %	32.13	31.35	31.83	23.05	31.39	25.17
Covariates						
Female, %	47.71	44.48	44.72	44.68	42.00	35.10
Race/ethnicity, %						
Non-Hispanic White	66.79	61.74	54.04	62.94	58.42	53.58
Non-Hispanic Black	6.40	8.43	7.61	9.57	9.77	10.39
Non-Hispanic other	10.63	10.64	12.42	10.64	12.27	10.85
Hispanic	16.18	19.20	25.93	16.84	19.54	25.17
Married, %	6.52	6.22	7.61	9.75	7.90	9.01
Education, %						
Less than high school	4.95	5.25	6.99	5.32	5.20	8.78
High school	38.53	43.78	43.17	31.91	28.69	33.26
Some college	32.37	32.18	29.81	27.30	27.86	25.87
College or higher	24.15	18.78	20.03	35.46	38.25	32.10
Income, $, %						
<10 000	5.80	3.73	5.90	4.79	2.29	4.85
10 000–14 999	6.16	6.08	6.06	3.72	3.95	6.47
15 000–19 999	12.56	11.60	11.96	11.52	8.52	10.62
20 000–24 999	22.10	20.72	18.94	18.26	20.17	19.40
25 000–34 999	53.38	57.87	57.14	61.70	65.07	58.66
Insurance, %	83.45	84.53	81.83	81.56	77.13	73.21
Metropolitan area residence, %	73.91	75.69	78.88	76.42	78.38	81.29

Note. Descriptive statistics are derived from the analytical sample, which included childless adults 18–29 years old who were employed at the time of survey and had annual household incomes below $35 000. All of the variables shown are binary (0/1) indicators except for number of days in the past 30 days not in good mental health.

TABLE 2— Effects of the 2021 Expanded Childless Earned Income Tax Credit on Mental Health Among Renters and Homeowners: Behavioral Risk Factor Surveillance System, United States, 2021–2023

	Difference-in-Differences Estimate (SE)	
	Mentally Unhealthy Days	Frequent Mental Distress
Renters		
Year 2021 × age 18–24 (ref)	0	0
Year 2022 × age 18–24	−2.21** (0.80)	−0.098** (0.036)
Year 2023 × age 18–24	−0.76 (0.81)	−0.024 (0.037)
Outcome mean in 2021	8.39	0.28
No.	3674	3674
Homeowners		
Year 2021 × age 18–24 (ref)	0	0
Year 2022 × age 18–24	3.71 (2.07)	0.15 (0.091)
Year 2023 × age 18–24	−1.78 (2.25)	−0.026 (0.098)
Outcome mean in 2021	7.52	0.26
No.	553	553

Note. Standard errors are heteroskedasticity robust standard errors. The sample included childless adults aged 18–29 years who were employed at the time of the survey and had annual household incomes below $35 000. Effects were estimated from an event-study difference-in-differences model (Equation 1) and represent changes in the number of mentally unhealthy days and likelihood of experiencing frequent mental distress over the preceding 30 days upon receiving the Earned Income Tax Credit in 2022 and 2023. Models were estimated separately for renters and homeowners and controlled for sex, race/ethnicity, education, metropolitan/nonmetropolitan residence, and insurance status.
*$P < .05$; **$P < .01$.

TABLE 3— Outcome Pretrends Test of the Effects of the 2021 Expanded Childless Earned Income Tax Credit on Mental Health Among Renters and Homeowners: Behavioral Risk Factor Surveillance System, United States, 2021–2023

	Difference-in-Differences Estimate (SE)	
	Mentally Unhealthy Days	Frequent Mental Distress
Renters		
Year 2017 × age 18–24 (ref)	0	0
Year 2018 × age 18–24	−0.17 (0.61)	−0.030 (0.026)
Year 2019 × age 18–24	−0.58 (0.63)	−0.053 (0.028)
No.	5228	5228
Homeowners		
Year 2017 × age 18–24 (ref)	0	0
Year 2018 × age 18–24	1.12 (1.41)	0.065 (0.060)
Year 2019 × age 18–24	0.58 (1.51)	0.038 (0.064)
No.	970	970

Note. Standard errors are heteroskedasticity robust standard errors. The sample included childless adults aged 18–29 years who were employed at the time of the survey and had annual household incomes below $35 000. Effects were estimated from an event-study difference-in-differences model (Equation 2) and represent changes in the number of mentally unhealthy days and likelihood of experiencing frequent mental distress over the preceding 30 days upon receiving the Earned Income Tax Credit in 2022 and 2023. Models were estimated separately for renters and homeowners and controlled for sex, race/ethnicity, education, metropolitan/nonmetropolitan residence, and insurance status.

AJPH November 2025, Vol. 115, No. 11

TABLE 4— Effects of the 2021 Expanded Childless Earned Income Tax Credit on Mental Health Among Renters and Homeowners by Demographic Characteristics: Behavioral Risk Factor Surveillance System, United States, 2021–2023

	Male Sex		Female Sex		Non-Hispanic White Race/ Ethnicity		Non-White Race/Ethnicity	
	Mentally Unhealthy Days	Frequent Mental Distress	Mentally Unhealthy Days	Frequent Mental Distress	Mentally Unhealthy Days	Frequent Mental Distress	Mentally Unhealthy Days	Frequent Mental Distress
Renters								
Year 2021 × age 18–24 (ref)	0	0	0	0	0	0	0	0
Year 2022 × age 18–24	−2.13* (1.04)	−0.13** (0.046)	−2.59* (1.26)	−0.078 (0.059)	−2.50* (1.04)	−0.096* (0.048)	−1.79 (1.27)	−0.10 (0.057)
Year 2023 × age 18–24	−1.05 (1.04)	−0.037 (0.045)	−0.74 (1.32)	−0.024 (0.063)	−1.89 (1.09)	−0.057 (0.051)	0.80 (1.23)	0.024 (0.055)
Outcome mean in 2021	6.98	0.22	10.00	0.35	9.10	0.31	7.04	0.23
No.	2063	2063	1611	1611	2216	2216	1458	1458
Homeowners								
Year 2021 × age 18–24 (ref)	0	0	0	0	0	0	0	0
Year 2022 × age 18–24	6.38* (2.80)	0.30** (0.11)	−2.95 (3.74)	−0.13 (0.18)	6.37* (2.66)	0.31** (0.12)	−2.35 (4.04)	−0.20 (0.17)
Year 2023 × age 18–24	−2.05 (2.98)	−0.0056 (0.12)	−3.43 (3.91)	−0.14 (0.19)	−2.02 (3.04)	0.017 (0.13)	−0.20 (3.79)	−0.063 (0.17)
Outcome mean in 2021	5.71	0.19	10.3	0.36	8.28	0.28	5.56	0.18
No.	333	333	220	220	362	362	191	191

Note. Standard errors are heteroskedasticity robust standard errors. The sample included childless adults aged 18–29 years who were employed at the time of the survey and had annual household incomes below $35 000. Effects were estimated from an event-study difference-in-differences model (Equation 1) and represent changes in the number of mentally unhealthy days and likelihood of experiencing frequent mental distress over the preceding 30 days upon receiving the Earned Income Tax Credit in 2022 and 2023. Models were estimated separately for renters and homeowners and controlled for sex, race/ethnicity, education, metropolitan/nonmetropolitan residence, and insurance status.

*$P<.05$; **$P<.01$.

during the earlier months of the year. The results with alternative income samples are reported in Table D (available as a supplement to the online version of this article at http://www.ajph.org), and overall these results were similar to our main estimates.

Table E (available as a supplement to the online version of this article at http://www.ajph.org) reports the estimates for alternative model specifications, including adding year-by-state-specific trends, adding both year-by-demographics and year-by-state-specific trends, adding covariates for chronic conditions, and applying the BRFSS sampling weights. Overall, the results from these alternative specifications remained similar to our main findings. The only notable difference was that models incorporating BRFSS sampling weights had smaller effect sizes and were statistically insignificant. Because our analysis focused on a specific and relatively small sample, it is likely that certain observations that involved large sampling weights but were not overly affected by the EITC expansion (e.g., those from racial/ethnic minority groups) drove the weighted estimates toward the null.

DISCUSSION

Our study is the first to our knowledge to examine the impact of the temporary childless EITC expansion in 2021 on low-income childless young workers' mental health according to housing tenure. We found evidence that the temporary childless EITC expansion in 2021 was associated with improvements in mental health among renters but not homeowners. Specifically, our results suggest that the EITC expansion prevented a worsening trend in mental health that might otherwise have occurred. Young renters reported fewer days of poor mental health and had a lower likelihood of experiencing frequent mental distress, especially in 2022, the year they were eligible for the credit for the first time. We also found more pronounced improvements in mental health outcomes among men and non-Hispanic Whites.

Our findings indicate that the temporary EITC expansion in 2021 provided financial alleviation for young renters, who are disproportionately burdened by increasing housing costs in recent years. Between 2019 and 2023, median gross rental prices increased by 7.2%, from $1312 to $1406, marking the highest increase since 2011.[29] In addition, over the past 2 decades, inflation-adjusted median rents have increased by 21% while median annual incomes rose by only 2%.[30] Housing instability has been associated with worse mental health outcomes, including depression and anxiety,[31,32] and residents displaced from their neighborhoods because of the high cost of housing have experienced adverse mental health outcomes and exhibited increased use of health care services.[33] Therefore, the financial support offered by the EITC credit may have helped reduce the stress associated with meeting rising rents, contributing to improved mental health. Our findings are consistent with a recent study showing that cash transfers from the expanded American Rescue Plan Act Child Tax Credit improved the mental health of low-income parents who rented their homes.[34]

Our results are also consistent with the broader literature indicating sizable improvements in mental health associated with EITC payments.[35] For example, Evans and Garthwaite examined the effects of the 1993 EITC expansion and found that a $500 increase in EITC payments was associated with a "treatment on treated" effect of a 19% decrease in the number of mentally unhealthy days.[13] By comparison, our estimates indicate an "intent to treat" effect of a 25% decrease after the temporary EITC expansion for young adults, an effect associated with a payment of roughly $1500. However, this is still a lower bound estimate given that only about 80% of adults claimed the EITC; if we adjust for this figure, the effect size (as a "treatment on treated" effect) could be as large as 31%. Homeowners—who generally have greater economic stability—did not experience similar mental health benefits from the EITC expansion, suggesting that the policy's effects are more pronounced among those facing greater financial vulnerability.

The EITC is one of the major income support policies implemented as an antipoverty measure, and it was designed to encourage labor force participation; previous research indicates that the policy has had the desired effects of improving health and well-being.[9,14,20] For many young renters, the extra cash support provided by the EITC through the temporary expansion during the pandemic may have helped offset the rising cost of housing and other household expenditures, thus improving their mental health. These findings are important and provide further evidence of the impact of the EITC on the mental health of renters. We posit that the EITC provided supplemental income to vulnerable young adult renters, who were more likely than others to be adversely affected by the COVID-19 pandemic, thereby enhancing their income security and improving their mental health.

Limitations

This study has several limitations. First, the age groupings in the data are reported in 5-year intervals, and we were unable to select an accurate treatment group. The EITC expansion specifically affected individuals 19 to 24 years of age, but the closest group in the BRFSS is the 18- to 24-year group. Inclusion of individuals 18 years of age may have led to an underestimation of the effects. Second, the mental health outcomes in this study were based on self-reported data, which can be subject to reporting bias and inaccuracies. Moreover, the BRFSS data lack information on individual-level controls such as access to and use of mental health services, neighborhood characteristics, and family stressors. However, our model included education and whether the survey respondents had insurance coverage, variables that may have been highly affected by the pandemic among the individuals included in our study sample. We leave it to future research to address these gaps in data sources.

Another limitation is the potential for unobserved confounding factors that were not accounted for in our analysis. Although we used a difference-in-differences approach to mitigate such concerns, other policy changes or external economic factors coinciding with the EITC expansion could have influenced the observed mental health outcomes if they posed a different impact on young renters.

Public Health Implications

In 2022, about 80% of low-income renters spent more than 30% of their income on rent.[1] Housing affordability has become a major concern for renters, primarily because of stagnant wages and record rental prices over the past few decades. This has rendered many areas unlivable for low-income populations and the working poor. As a result, renters struggle to balance housing expenditures and other household expenditures, leaving them with fewer resources for health-improving needs. The implication of this study is that a well-targeted policy such as the EITC aimed at reducing poverty among young adults has the added benefit of helping to support vulnerable renters and therefore improving their mental health. AJPH

ABOUT THE AUTHORS

Abdinasir K. Ali is with the Department of Social and Behavioral Sciences, Harvard T. H. Chan School of Public Health, Boston, MA. Wei Lyu is with the Department of Health Services Administration, School of Health Professions, University of Alabama at Birmingham.

CORRESPONDENCE

Correspondence should be sent to Abdinasir K. Ali, PhD, MPH, Department of Social and Behavioral Sciences, Harvard T. H. Chan School of Public Health, Harvard University, Landmark West Wing, 4th Floor, Room 437 Quad, 401 Park Dr., Boston, MA 02215 (e-mail: aali@hsph.harvard.edu). Reprints can be ordered at http://www.ajph.org by clicking the "Reprints" link.

PUBLICATION INFORMATION

Full Citation: Ali AK, Lyu W. Expansion of the Earned Income Tax Credit for young adults and mental health of US home renters, 2021–2023. *Am J Public Health*. 2025;115(11):1858–1867.

Acceptance Date: June 13, 2025.

DOI: https://doi.org/10.2105/AJPH.2025.308219

ORCID iD:
Abdinasir K. Ali https://orcid.org/0000-0003-2191-2925

CONTRIBUTORS

Both of the authors substantially and equally contributed to the conception, design, analysis, and interpretation of the study. A. K. Ali wrote and revised the initial draft, with W. Lyu providing comments.

CONFLICTS OF INTEREST

The authors have no conflicts of interest to declare.

HUMAN PARTICIPANT PROTECTION

No protocol approval was needed for this study because publicly available data were used.

REFERENCES

1. Hermann A, Airgood-Obrycki W, Cahill N, Whitney P. Subsidizing the middle: policies, tradeoffs, and cost of addressing middle-income affordability challenges. Available at: https://www.jchs.harvard.edu/sites/default/files/research/files/harvard_jchs_middle_income_housing_hermann_etal_2024_updated.pdf. Accessed December 20, 2024.
2. Airgood-Obrycki W, Hermann A, Wedeen S. "The rent eats first": rental housing unaffordability in the United States. *Housing Policy Debate*. 2023;33(6):1272–1292. https://doi.org/10.1080/10511482.2021.2020866
3. Bialik K, Fry R. Millennial life: How young adulthood today compares with prior generations. Available at: https://www.pewresearch.org/social-trends/2019/02/14/millennial-life-how-young-adulthood-today-compares-with-prior-generations-2. Accessed December 20, 2024.
4. Sum A, Khatiwada I, McLaughlin J, Palma S. No country for young men: deteriorating labor market prospects for low-skilled men in the United States. *Ann Am Acad Polit Soc Sci*. 2011;635(1):24–55. https://doi.org/10.1177/0002716210393694
5. Mossakowski KN. The influence of past unemployment duration on symptoms of depression among young women and men in the United States. *Am J Public Health*. 2009;99(10):1826–1832. https://doi.org/10.2105/AJPH.2008.152561
6. Elliott S, West SM, Castro AB. Rent burden and depression among mothers: an analysis of primary caregiver outcomes. *J Policy Pract Res*. 2021;2(4):285–300. https://doi.org/10.1007/s42972-021-00040-3
7. Kim H, Burgard SA. Housing instability and mental health among renters in the Michigan Recession and Recovery Study. *Public Health*. 2022;209:30–35. https://doi.org/10.1016/j.puhe.2022.05.015
8. Ali AK, Wehby GL. State eviction moratoriums during the COVID-19 pandemic were associated with improved mental health among people who rent. *Health Aff (Millwood)*. 2022;41(11):1583–1589. https://doi.org/10.1377/hlthaff.2022.00750
9. Crandall-Hollick ML, Hughes JS. *The Earned Income Tax Credit (EITC): An Economic Analysis*. Washington, DC: Congressional Research Service; 2018.
10. Internal Revenue Service. States and local governments with Earned Income Tax Credit. Available at: https://www.irs.gov/credits-deductions/individuals/earned-income-tax-credit/states-and-local-governments-with-earned-income-tax-credit. Accessed December 20, 2024.
11. Hoynes H, Miller D, Simon D. Income, the Earned Income Tax Credit, and infant health. *Am Econ J*. 2015;7(1):172–211. https://doi.org/10.1257/pol.20120179
12. Pilkauskas N, Michelmore K. The effect of the Earned Income Tax Credit on housing and living arrangements. *Demography*. 2019;56(4):1303–1326. https://doi.org/10.1007/s13524-019-00791-5

13. Evans WN, Garthwaite CL. Giving mom a break: the impact of higher EITC payments on maternal health. *Am Econ J.* 2014;6(2):258–290. https://doi.org/10.1257/pol.6.2.258

14. Boyd-Swan C, Herbst CM, Ifcher J, Zarghamee H. The Earned Income Tax Credit, mental health, and happiness. *J Econ Behav Organ.* 2016;126:18–38. https://doi.org/10.1016/j.jebo.2015.11.004

15. Averett S, Wang Y. Effects of higher EITC payments on children's health, quality of home environment, and noncognitive skills. *Public Finance Rev.* 2018;46(4):519–557. https://doi.org/10.1177/1091142116654965

16. Hamad R, Collin DF, Rehkopf DH. Estimating the short-term effects of the Earned Income Tax Credit on child health. *Am J Epidemiol.* 2018;187(12):2633–2641. https://doi.org/10.1093/aje/kwy179

17. Batra A, Hamad R. Short-term effects of the Earned Income Tax Credit on children's physical and mental health. *Ann Epidemiol.* 2021;58:15–21. https://doi.org/10.1016/j.annepidem.2021.02.008

18. Lee J, Michelmore K, Pilkauskas N, Wimer C. *Effects of the Expansion of the Earned Income Tax Credit for Childless Young Adults on Material Wellbeing*. Cambridge, MA: National Bureau of Economic Research; 2024.

19. Wimer C, Nam J, Garfinkel I, Kaushal N, Waldfogel J, Fox L. Young adult poverty in historical perspective: the role of policy supports and early labor market experiences. *Soc Sci Res.* 2020;86:102390. https://doi.org/10.1016/j.ssresearch.2019.102390

20. Shields-Zeeman L, Collin DF, Batra A, Hamad R. How does income affect mental health and health behaviours? A quasi-experimental study of the Earned Income Tax Credit. *J Epidemiol Community Health.* 2021;75(10):929–935. https://doi.org/10.1136/jech-2020-214841

21. Golberstein E. The effects of income on mental health: evidence from the social security notch. *J Ment Health Policy Econ.* 2015;18(1):27–37.

22. Centers for Disease Control and Prevention. 2021 summary data quality report. Available at: https://www.cdc.gov/brfss/annual_data/2021/pdf/2021-DQR-508.pdf. Accessed December 20, 2024.

23. Centers for Disease Control and Prevention. 2023 summary data quality report. Available at: https://www.cdc.gov/brfss/annual_data/2023/pdf/2023-DQR-508.pdf. Accessed December 20, 2024.

24. Centers for Disease Control and Prevention. BRFSS questionnaires. Available at: https://www.cdc.gov/brfss/questionnaires/index.htm. Accessed December 20, 2024.

25. Cree RA, Okoro CA, Zack MM, Carbone E. Frequent mental distress among adults, by disability status, disability type, and selected characteristics—United States, 2018. *MMWR Morb Mortal Wkly Rep.* 2020;69(36):1238–1243. https://doi.org/10.15585/mmwr.mm6936a2

26. LaLumia S. The EITC, tax refunds, and unemployment spells. *Am Econ J.* 2013;5(2):188–221. https://doi.org/10.1257/pol.5.2.188

27. Rehkopf DH, Strully KW, Dow WH. The short-term impacts of Earned Income Tax Credit disbursement on health. *Int J Epidemiol.* 2014;43(6):1884–1894. https://doi.org/10.1093/ije/dyu172

28. Internal Revenue Service. EITC participation rate by states: tax years 2014 through 2021. Available at: https://www.eitc.irs.gov/eitc-central/participation-rate-by-state/eitc-participation-rate-by-states. Accessed December 20, 2024.

29. Fabina J. Largest annual real increase in gross rental costs since 2011: cost of rent and utilities rose faster than home values in 2023. Available at: https://www.census.gov/library/stories/2024/09/acs-rent-burden.html. Accessed December 20, 2024.

30. Joint Center for Housing Studies of Harvard University. America's rental housing. Available at: https://www.jchs.harvard.edu/sites/default/files/reports/files/Harvard_JCHS_Americas_Rental_Housing_2024.pdf. Accessed December 20, 2024.

31. Burgard SA, Seefeldt KS, Zelner S. Housing instability and health: findings from the Michigan Recession and Recovery Study. *Soc Sci Med.* 2012;75(12):2215–2224. https://doi.org/10.1016/j.socscimed.2012.08.020

32. Desmond M, Kimbro RT. Eviction's fallout: housing, hardship, and health. *Soc Forces.* 2015;94(1):295–324. https://doi.org/10.1093/sf/sov044

33. Lim S, Singh TP, Hall G, Walters S, Gould LH. Impact of a New York City supportive housing program on housing stability and preventable health care among homeless families. *Health Serv Res.* 2018;53(5):3437–3454. https://doi.org/10.1111/1475-6773.12849

34. Ali AK, Lyu W, Wehby GL. The effects of the expanded child tax credit on mental health of home renters and homeowners. *Ment Health Prev.* 2024;34:200341. https://doi.org/10.1016/j.mhp.2024.200341

35. Gangopadhyaya A, Blavin F, Braga B, Gates J. Credit where it is due: investigating pathways from Earned Income Tax Credit expansion to maternal mental health. *Health Econ.* 2020;29(9):975–991. https://doi.org/10.1002/hec.4034

Dialectical Processes of Health Framework as an Alternative to Social Determinants of Health Framework

Samuel R. Friedman, PhD, Suzan M. Walters, PhD, Ashly E. Jordan, PhD, MPH, David C. Perlman, MD, Georgios K. Nikolopoulos, PhD, Pedro Mateu-Gelabert, PhD, Diana Rossi, DSW, and Jerzy Eisenberg-Guyot, PhD, MPH

The social determinants of health (SDOH) framework has proven useful for research and practice in addressing the social causes of many health outcomes. However, its limitations may restrict its value as the world undergoes rapid ecological and social change.

We argue that SDOH does not adequately incorporate rapidly changing or "far upstream" social processes (particularly social movements), the dialectics of social conflict and creative social innovation, or bidirectional causation.

Ecosocial theory addresses some of these issues, yet dialectical frameworks offer additional insights during periods of rapid social change and disruption. The implications for research methods and practice are discussed. (*Am J Public Health*. 2025;115(11):1868–1876. https://doi.org/10.2105/AJPH.2025.308239)

AJPH November 2025, Vol. 115, No. 11

Changing times sometimes require us to reframe how we think about the world. This essay suggests that the ongoing changes in the world mean that we need to go beyond the social determinants of health approach to consider dialectical models that take macrosocial processes, events, and hard-to-predict popular mobilizations as circumstances that shape population health.

We are in a period of rapid climate change and other environmental transformations that threaten the health of billions of people.[1–3] Initial changes are already here, manifesting as heatwaves, massive fires on most continents, disastrous flooding, changes in land use and biodiversity that may drive emerging infections, and the like.[4] These disasters set in motion many ensuing problems, as when the hurricanes in the fall of 2024 that devastated Asheville, North Carolina, produced serious shortages of medical intravenous and peritoneal dialysis fluid supplies for patients throughout the East Coast of the United States.[5] A combination of harmful global climate change, warfare, economic stagnation, and governments that will not or cannot protect the people who live under them has led to widespread mass migration—which will likely greatly increase as environmental conditions worsen.[1,6,7] Political developments have included the Trump administration's abrupt termination of many domestic and international aid programs and much federally funded public health research,[8] as well as the growth of large fascist movements, which have produced ultranationalist and authoritarian governments like those in India (under Narendra Modi) and Hungary (under Viktor Orban), and which have intensified racial/ethnic and gender intersecting oppressions and injustices. Meanwhile, struggles for control over people, land, and resources underwrite humanitarian crises in places like Gaza,[9] Sudan,[10] Xinjiang,[11] and Yemen,[12] and escalating conflict among major powers threatens world war.[13,14] All of this exacerbates, and is stimulated by, ongoing climate change and by intermittent economic instability in a context of general economic stagnation, growing economic inequality, and rapid change in the geographic distributions of economic activities.[15–17] These processes may drive a range of adverse, unevenly distributed, and inequitable health outcomes, including pandemics.[18,19]

To understand these processes, and perhaps on that basis to intervene more effectively, requires intellectual frameworks that facilitate our understanding of rapidly changing sociopolitical and environmental processes, the social conflicts that emerge from them, and how these processes affect public health, belief systems, and people's varying capacities to act. In this essay, we suggest that these frameworks need to incorporate the insights of the social sciences regarding what some call "upstream" processes, with a special emphasis on social conflicts, power relationships, mass movements from below, and the organizational aspects of all sides to social conflicts. Studies of how social and environmental change affect health must address an important methodological challenge—how to understand and respond to unpredictable developments. Social movements and other reactions to sudden-onset, high-impact processes like wars, economic crises, mass migrations, pandemics, and social upheavals—referred to as Big Events[20–22]—sometimes can create largely unpredictable innovative ideas and organizations that affect sociopolitical struggles. In turn, such unexpected innovations can reshape societies and may transform the course of pandemics, wars, and public health and medicine more generally.

DIALECTICAL FRAMEWORKS

This essay proposes that a dialectical framework will be more useful in understanding our changing times than various social determinants of health (SDOH) or even ecosocial theories have been. Dialectics is a form of thinking and analysis that does not assume that relationships are linear or even continuous functions. It views entities and relationships as changing over time, which can include sudden qualitative reversals in their natures. As Bertell Ollman described it, "Dialectics is a way of thinking that brings into focus the full range of changes [processes] and interactions that occur in the world."[23(p19)]

Dialectical thinking sees wholes as consisting of multilevel, bidirectional, and often contradictory relationships (Figure 1). For example, societies are not static wholes but dynamic entities consisting of conflicting social groups, like the owning class and the working class. Moreover, dialectical thinking rejects the assumption that wholes are defined by the sum of their parts. Instead, wholes have emergent properties that their components lack (e.g., income inequality and degree of racial conflict are features of societies, not individuals). Of course, dialectical thinking recognizes that it is impossible at any moment to focus on entire wholes. As ecologist Richard Levins highlighted, models or frameworks that endeavor to look at everything at once would require infinite inputs that would take lifetimes to measure, or inputs that cannot readily be measured, and that would be too complex for the human mind (or for so-called "artificial intelligence") to comprehend.[24] Furthermore, wholes themselves are constantly

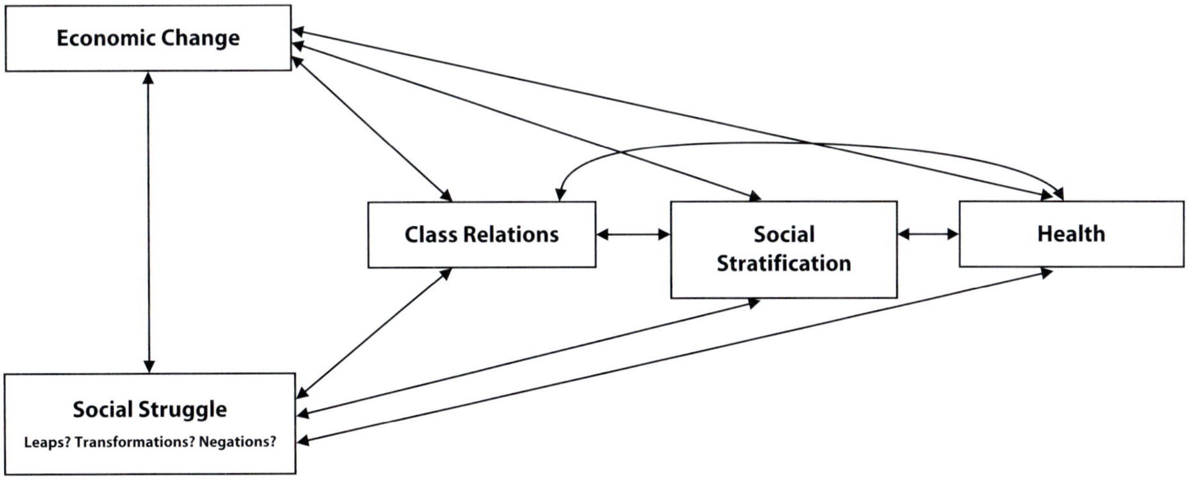

FIGURE 1— Patterns of Causation as Seen Through Dialectical Thinking

Note. Dialectical thinking sees patterns of causation as consisting of multilevel, bidirectional, and often contradictory relationships. Dialectical approaches will (usually) include a more complete set of supra-individual causes of health outcomes than social determinants of health approaches. They also typically consider causation to be bidirectional. Finally, as discussed in the text (section on Dialectical Frameworks), dialectical approaches often take account of the possibility of hard- or impossible-to-predict leaps in consciousness or organization and sudden transformations in relationships such as when organizations like labor unions or political parties change sides in a major conflict.

changing (and are doing so at paces that vary—as an example, consider the dynamics of global climate change). Changes in rates of change both reflect and are analogous to the processes of evolutionary change that, although sometimes gradual for long periods, may at other times be quite rapid, as in evolutionary punctuated equilibria.[25,26]

Sometimes change involves major reversals in the nature of organisms or organizations in a process of "negation," which results from contradictory processes within the organism or organizations, and which may arise unexpectedly.[27] A classic historical example is the transformation of the revolutionary European social democratic parties into supporters of the status quo at the beginning of World War I.[28–31] A biological example is that the introduction of HIV into a CD4 cell transforms it from a defender of the human body into a "factory of death" that churns out large numbers of additional HIV viruses.[32]

Dialectics pays close attention to transformations in social organization and in the consciousness and "definitions of the situations" held by ruling groups and by various population subgroups. These are subject to rapid transformations and even reversals in times of massive change, which is a major reason that dialectical frameworks are needed in such eras.

Methodologically, dialectical thinking makes explicit use of the power of abstraction by looking for internal conflicts within apparently unified organisms or processes, by analyzing processes from different viewpoints, and by identifying contradictions by asking "where is the rest of the world?"[33] Each such abstraction or combination of abstractions sacrifices concreteness to varying degrees, but dialectics provides a key way of thinking that may initially sacrifice precision but does so to maximize generality and realism.[23,24,33] There are extensive and somewhat divergent discussions and interpretations of dialectics; for further readings, see Engels,[34] Engels and Vujović,[35] Hegel and Wallace,[36] Friedman and Rossi,[37] Dietzgen,[38] Lukács,[39,40] and Levy et al.[41]

LIMITATIONS OF THE SOCIAL DETERMINANTS OF HEALTH FRAMEWORK

The SDOH framework has been useful both scientifically and pragmatically in its focus on supra-individual causes of health outcomes and their distributions across populations. However, this framework is much more applicable to situations and processes of relative stability than it is for analyzing and understanding processes undergoing rapid social, political, and environmental upheaval. Even for periods of relative stability, we would contend, SDOH has fundamental flaws that can be misleading. Its multilevel character is its chief strength, but the way that this is handled as an analytic and often overly deterministic (as opposed to dialectical[23,42]) model is a major flaw. The SDOH framework posits that social structures, including structural racism, patriarchy, private property, neoliberalism, imperialism, underdevelopment, income or wealth inequality, and political constitutional structures, drive the relative health of population groups. Politically, studies using the SDOH framework tend to support the arguments of human rights and social democratic models of social reform. Many astute practitioners of SDOH argue for changes in tax structures, welfare laws, labor laws, and laws and customs around gender roles and racial/ethnic domination that might reduce the health inequities and disparities that these structures produce. These can be useful. However, although the proposals may ameliorate the consequences of superordination–subordination relationships, or lead to modifications of their form (as in the change from Jim Crow segregation to current forms in the United States), they typically do not eradicate the subordinating processes themselves—which then continually produce and reproduce intergroup health inequities, eventually negating the enacted partial reforms.

The traditional SDOH framework uses standard statistical methods to study associations of health with individual-level or geographic-level measures of inequality, inequity, disempowerment, or injustice. Its strength as a framework is that it does promote the inclusion and consideration of some factors above the level of the individual in analyses, and does so in ways that allow for fairly straightforward statistical analysis.

SDOH approaches have produced important ecological and multilevel studies. These include studies demonstrating that people living in areas with higher levels of income or wealth generally have better health and, conversely, that people living in areas with lower levels of income or wealth generally have worse health (including infant mortality and adult all-cause and cause-specific mortality).[43–47] SDOH studies have also identified relationships between health care systems and a variety of health outcomes,[48–51] as well as between racial/ethnic and gender inequality and such outcomes, among many other areas.[52–57] As an example on a more specific level, the analyses of metropolitan areas conducted by Friedman et al. of health-related outcomes for people who inject drugs during the HIV/AIDS epidemic have shown that areas with more income inequality and higher arrest rates for "hard drug" use also have higher HIV prevalence, AIDS rates, and AIDS mortality, but that arrest rates do not have any effect on population rates of injection drug use.[58]

Why do we say that the SDOH framework is flawed? A key flaw is that it does not go far enough "upstream" in considering potent forces and processes that impact health—such as social conflicts, power relationships, and mass movements from below—and the organizational aspects of all sides to social conflicts and changes in these over time (Figure 1). That is, it often utilizes too narrow a level of abstraction,[23,59,60] considering more proximal components of social systems but not their macrosocial causes. For example, although SDOH frameworks often consider which individuals experience homelessness or are unstably housed, or study the extent of homelessness in a group or area, they rarely explore why there is such a high degree of homelessness or why homelessness exists in the first place. That is, they rarely look at the far "upstream" macrosocial causes of homelessness. Limiting how far upstream a framework "looks" is often rationalized as privileging a focus on "modifiable forces," but such limits often reflect what is seen as "politically feasible"[61] to modify, or as what one is willing to or can conceive of as being modified, and hence can constitute blinders. In contrast, frameworks more attuned to social conflict, including Marxist Political Economy of Health frameworks,[62,63] may draw attention to the balance of power between renters and landlords or workers and employers, or more fundamentally, the private or bureaucratic-class ownership of housing and productive property.

Furthermore, SDOH tends to consider "upstream factors" as static, and as unconnected to each other. A key example is the failure to consider economic systems, such as capitalism,[64,65] as wholes that link together "upstream" social determinants, including environmental conditions, war, housing, income, wealth, segregation, racism, sexism, and others. Here, some recent work on "commercial determinants of health," which has been suggested as a "subset" of SDOH, is a helpful start,[61] as are discussions of structural racism[54] and racial capitalism.[66,67]

SDOH also tends to consider only unidirectional forces (upstream to downstream) and often elides the fact that "downstream" factors and processes can impact those more "upstream" (e.g., that tenant organizing in a single building might spark citywide or even national tenants' movements, with broad societal repercussions).[68] This consideration is closely related to our final critique:

SDOH focuses on deterministic relationships between and within levels rather than incorporating a framework in which historical, time-varying and dialectic relationships between and within levels are reflected, limiting its ability to understand phenomena in rapid flux. We say that SDOH tends toward determinism despite recognizing that statistical error always appears in analyses. However, SDOH does not incorporate nondeterministic processes, like struggle, revolt, popularly based revolutions, or agency as constitutive parts of its framework, nor does it consider the extensive scholarship on the causes and processes involved in social movements of these types, which can have sudden onsets and changing intensities. (Sometimes this is described as free will, which we understand as existing within limits that Karl Marx described as follows: "[Humans] make their own history, but they do not make it as they please; they do not make it under self-selected circumstances, but under circumstances . . . transmitted from the past. The tradition of all dead generations weighs like a nightmare on the brains of the living."[69]) Philosophically, it uses a positivist framework to study health rather than a dialectical one. As such, it fails to incorporate the insights of Hegel, Marx, and other dialecticians, including ones who have applied dialectics to health issues, such as Richard Levins and Jaime Breilh.[70–74] (See also the Appendix, available as a supplement to the online version of this article at http://www.ajph.org.) In terms of sociopolitical analysis, social determinants of health approaches (as opposed to ecosocial, political economic, or dialectical ones) often fail to incorporate the insights of analysts who emphasize that systems of domination, oppression, exploitation, and inequality call forth opposition that can change processes and outcomes, often sustainably.[75–78]

DIALECTICAL APPROACHES TO SOCIAL STRUGGLE AND HEALTH

It may be—and on this, we are not sure, and call on the field for further discussion and research—that dialectical rigor might be incorporated into statistical models of the SDOH framework if they explicitly include measures and considerations of social movement formation, and their time-varying changes in strength, success, and failure. Such efforts should build on those that have been developed by social movement researchers such as

Charles Tilly or Doug McAdam.[79,80] (Friedman and his colleagues have incorporated social movement dynamics in their work on how Big Events can sometimes lead to HIV or other infectious outbreaks.[21]) The point is that along with the various upstream processes such as climate change or imperial invasions, or the extent and distribution of favelas and poverty, "movements from below" also have an impact on the various intermediate (and "far upstream") processes as well as on the hopes, beliefs, behaviors, and networks that affect infection transmission, exposures to occupational hazards, hypertension, and other risk factors and health outcomes. For example, Friedman et al. attempted to model this more specifically in an article on the Stigma System[42] that discusses the dialectics of struggle, the role of stigma, and specific organizational and community structures and conflicts that shape stigmas and their effects.

There are many examples of social movement processes of varying paces that have affected the trajectories of health outcomes. One example of a specific struggle from below in the United States that had important consequences for health was the wildcat strike wave that began in 1969 among West Virginia miners and other workers and that helped establish Black Lung compensation programs and the Occupational Safety and Health Administration, both of which beneficially affected workers and their health.[81,82] Structural characteristics that affect worker movements and their health have also been studied.[83,84] For example, structural and political sources of gay liberation movements include the growth of urban gay "ghettoes" and the ideological and organizational impacts of the civil rights movement, and gay and lesbian liberation movements formed the basis for many AIDS and women's health projects.[85,86] Tempalski et al. showed that the presence of local ACT UP chapters affected the likelihood that syringe exchanges would develop in US metropolitan areas (which in turn affected HIV/AIDS incidence).[87] The development of the Treatment Action Campaign (TAC) in South Africa strongly affected the politics and subsequent spread and uptake of antiretroviral therapy among South Africans.[88] There were upstream causes of the formation and actions of TAC, including the South African gay movement and the prior growth and strength of the struggle against apartheid—which itself can be analyzed in terms of social movement theory. Importantly, the politics of South African responses to AIDS were influenced by ideological factors. These include the subsumption of the politics of the South African Communist Party within those of the African National Congress (ANC), which tended to dampen struggles against the AIDS denialism of the ANC in power, and the presence of Trotskyists who took part in the freedom struggle, including working with elements of the Congress of South African Trade Unions, who formed an important part of the leadership of the TAC.

It is our expectation that these upstream forces and processes underlying social movements, together with variables reflecting transformations in their ideologies, leadership, and organization over time, will enable useful post hoc statistical analyses in an extended SDOH framework. This, however, leaves an important set of questions that require a fuller dialectical approach to address. To understand the issue requires a brief consideration of human agency at both the individual and collective levels.

We argue that there is an important aspect of human social struggle and social movement development that involves an unpredictable-in-advance element of human creativity and invention—in particular, the bottom-up creative agency of workers and oppressed people.[89] When confronting social crises and unknown situations, participants in social movements sometimes exhibit altruism and discover new forms of social organization, or new tactics, that can transform the outcomes of struggles—although it is unpredictable in advance whether they will (1) make such inventions or whether these innovations (2) enter the consciousness of, and engage the imaginations of, large numbers of people in ways that then affect subsequent history. Examples of successful innovations (each of which had precursors that did not "take off" in different situations) include the formation of soviets among workers and peasants in Russia in 1905,[90] the reinvention of the sit-down strike by Italian workers in 1920, and the Black student sit-ins in North Carolina in February 1960.[91–93] Each of these innovations, in turn, affected the outcomes of those and subsequent struggles that helped shape the social determinants of health and, in turn, the health of millions of people. Even at the social network level, human agency can lead members of stigmatized groups to support one another. For example, we have documented how people who use drugs develop normative and supportive mechanisms to promote each other's health, including the development of syringe exchange as an HIV prevention intervention.[94] We and other scholars have found that people who use drugs frequently engage in health-related actions to support their peers and embed safety within their networks.[95–97] We refer to these actions as "intraventions."[98,99] Such innovations cannot be predicted in advance, and thus may disrupt predictions from standard statistical models about how population health will unfold in the future. The implications of this for studying the social determination of health raise difficult theoretical and analytical issues. Some of these have, in turn, been considered by scholars and activists who have studied how social movement scholarship and Marxist frameworks might usefully be synthesized.[20]

These differences between the SDOH framework and dialectical approaches (including those that James Breilh and others call the Social Determination of Health framework) have both methodological and action implications.[73] SDOH usually focuses on positivistic and statistical methods, and on proposals for policy changes, whereas dialectical frameworks, while also taking into account the kinds of ideas and research results that SDOH frameworks generate, focus on the activities and strategies of the subordinated, and how they fare in the context of the structures, processes, and counterstrategies of the powerful. Methodologically, dialectical research might focus on case studies of effective popular organizations and their impacts on health, which might be thought of as a qualitative-historical positive deviance research design.[100,101]

Dialectical research could also incorporate statistical methods to analyze the historical or contemporary public health impact of social movements, which are often ignored in quantitative research.[77,84,102] For example, research could examine how social movements and ideologies have affected health behaviors and outcomes over time.

ECOSOCIAL THEORY AND DIALECTICAL MODELS

Much as Krieger's Ecosocial Theory built upon Political Economy of Health theories to more rigorously address the biological pathways linking social relations of power to population health,[103] we believe Ecosocial Theory can be enhanced by incorporating insights from dialectical approaches. Krieger's ecosocial model is presented in graphics (Figure 1.1, Table 2, and Table 2.3) included in her book *Ecosocial Theory, Embodied Truths, and the People's Health*.[104] This model depicts structures of oppression, exploitation, and injustice as relatively stable, although situated within historical context. It does not fully incorporate measures of struggle that go beyond resistance to include or lead to the development of beneficial responses or, more importantly, attempt to incorporate the different dimensions, organizations, and dialectics of struggle as constituent parts of its framework. The index of this valuable book,[104] like that of Krieger's earlier one,[103] includes no mention of social movement, war, rebellion, revolution, or migration—all of which are likely to be key shapers of population health over the next century.

Such an ecosocial framework suffices to study relatively stable structures or periods of relative equilibrium characterized by slowly changing processes, but it would benefit from the insights of dialectical approaches when analyzing rapidly and significantly changing processes and situations. At a time-invariant level of abstraction, it allows useful analyses by positing a form of oppression as static and conceptually holding it constant, reflecting neither gradual changes nor the sudden changes that resemble the punctuated equilibria in evolution.[26,105] However, the challenges of our time require new tools and analyses. Models that assume a slowly changing equilibrium can obscure the impacts of struggle, and perhaps reinforce dominant ideologies regarding the futility of such struggle. But as discussed at the beginning of this essay, we are in a period of rapid climate change and other environmental transformations in which planetary boundaries capable of sustaining life are being breached,[4] of mass migrations, of reactionary movements and of movements for human liberation, of intensifying imperial conflict and genocidal wars, of intermittent economic instability, and of consequent worsening and increasingly inequitable health outcomes.[1]

Krieger[106] issues a stirring wakeup call to take these threats seriously and to take the political determinants of health more seriously. To do so, we believe we will have to extend Ecosocial Theory to incorporate understandings of "factors" not as variables but as processes and relationships embedded in multilevel wholes that cause and themselves undergo change, and that do so in response to struggle and resistance. At a very macro but important level, the consequences of anthropogenic climate change (including global warming, ocean acidification, and others)[4] create an overarching situation of planetary health emergency that requires a fully dialectical perspective on social domination, social conflict, social transformation, and disease emergence and development to understand and address.

And as a fundamental characteristic of the dynamically but difficult-to-predict changing present and evolving future, won't mass social conflicts of the sort discussed continue to be major forces that can transform population health?

If so, we need models that can more richly and informatively incorporate them. *AJPH*

ABOUT THE AUTHORS

Samuel R. Friedman, Suzan M. Walters, and Jerzy Eisenberg-Guyot are with the Center for Opioid Epidemiology and Policy and Department of Population Health, NYU Grossman School of Medicine, New York, NY. Ashly E. Jordan, David C. Perlman, and Pedro Mateu-Gelabert are with the Center for Drug Use and HIV/HCV Research, New York, NY. Georgios K. Nikolopoulos is with the Medical School, University of Cyprus, Nicosia, Cyprus. Diana Rossi is a retired professor and researcher, and a founding member and consultant of Intercambios Civil Association, Buenos Aires, Argentina.

CORRESPONDENCE

Correspondence should be sent to Samuel R. Friedman, 250 Lawrence Ave, Highland Park, NJ 08904 (e-mail: Samuel.Friedman@NYULangone.org). Reprints can be ordered at http://www.ajph.org by clicking the "Reprints" link.

PUBLICATION INFORMATION

Full Citation: Friedman SR, Walters SM, Jordan AE, et al. Dialectical processes of health framework as an alternative to social determinants of health framework. *Am J Public Health*. 2025;115(11):1868–1876.

Acceptance Date: June 29, 2025.

DOI: https://doi.org/10.2105/AJPH.2025.308239

ORCID iDs:

Samuel R. Friedman https://orcid.org/0000-0003-2083-1226

David C. Perlman https://orcid.org/0000-0001-5674-025X

Georgios K. Nikolopoulos https://orcid.org/0000-0002-3307-0246

Jerzy Eisenberg-Guyot https://orcid.org/0000-0003-3851-267X

CONTRIBUTORS

All authors contributed equally to the conceptualization, writing, and review of this analytic essay.

ACKNOWLEDGMENTS

This work was funded by the US National Institute on Drug Abuse (grant nos. P30 DA011041, R01 DA058991, and K01DA053159).

Note. The contents are solely the responsibility of the authors and do not necessarily represent the official views of the National Institutes of Health.

CONFLICTS OF INTEREST

The authors have no potential or actual conflicts of interest.

HUMAN PARTICIPANT PROTECTION

This essay does not use data from human participants. The projects that paid for our efforts in writing this were approved by the institutional review boards of NYU Grossman School of Medicine and other relevant institutions.

REFERENCES

1. Deivanayagam TA, English S, Hickel J, et al. Envisioning environmental equity: climate change, health, and racial justice. *Lancet*. 2023;402(10395):64–78. https://doi.org/10.1016/S0140-6736(23)00919-4
2. Matlin SA, Depoux A, Schütte S, et al. Migrants' and refugees' health: towards an agenda of solutions. *Public Health Rev*. 2018;39(1):1–55. https://doi.org/10.1186/s40985-018-0104-9
3. Faber D. American oil-igarchy: how the corporate assault on liberal democracy and the climate are connected. *Capitalism Nature Socialism*. 2023;34(3):1–21. https://doi.org/10.1080/10455752.2023.2242653
4. Richardson K, Steffen W, Lucht W, et al. Earth beyond six of nine planetary boundaries. *Sci Adv*. 2023;9(37):eadh2458. https://doi.org/10.1126/sciadv.adh2458
5. Chicago Healthcare System Coalition for Preparedness and Response. Hurricane Helene: Baxter's manufacturing recovery in North Carolina. November 4, 2024. Available at: https://www.baxter.com/baxter-newsroom/hurricane-helene-updates. Accessed September 3, 2025.
6. Faber D, Schlegel C. Give me shelter from the storm: framing the climate refugee crisis in the context of neoliberal capitalism. *Capitalism Nature Socialism*. 2017;28:1–17. https://doi.org/10.1080/10455752.2017.1356494
7. Reyna S. Big pictures: capitalism, imperialism, climate change, war, and migration. 2024. Available at: https://www.google.com/url?sa=t&rct=j&q=&esrc=s&source=web&cd=&ved=2ahUKEwj7uJ7Z36iPAxVOv4kEHVlVMqYQFnoECBUQAQ&url=https%3A%2F%2Fwww.torontomu.ca%2Fcontent%2Fdam%2Fcentre-for-immigration-and-settlement%2Ftmcis%2Fpublications%2Fworkingpapers%2Fwp-2024-05-reyna.pdf&usg=AOvVaw0AKq_nQ1aZ8xHBZnmX0wM8&opi=89978449. Accessed August 26, 2025.
8. *Science News* Staff. Trump's proposed budget details drastic cuts to biomedical research and global health. June 2, 2025. *Science News*. Available at: https://www.science.org/content/article/trump-s-proposed-budget-details-dramatic-cuts-biomedical-research-and-global-health. Accessed September 4, 2025.
9. Farhat T, Ibrahim S, Abdul-Sater Z, Abu-Sittah G. Responding to the humanitarian crisis in Gaza: damned if you do . . . damned if you don't! *Ann Glob Health*. 2023;89(1):53. https://doi.org/10.5334/aogh.3975
10. Olu OO, Freeman AYS, Waya JLL, et al. Bridging the humanitarian-development divide in a protracted crisis: a case study of the use of a central plant to supply oxygen for COVID-19 case management in South Sudan. *Front Public Health*. 2023;11:1272328. https://doi.org/10.3389/fpubh.2023.1272328
11. Horton R. Offline: the health of the Uyghur people is all of our concern. *Lancet*. 2022;400(10355):798. https://doi.org/10.1016/S0140-6736(22)01737-8
12. Hashim HT, Miranda AV, Babar MS, et al. Yemen's triple emergency: food crisis amid a civil war and COVID-19 pandemic. *Public Health Pract (Oxf)*. 2021;2:100082. https://doi.org/10.1016/j.puhip.2021.100082
13. Achcar G. *The New Cold War*. Chicago, IL: Haymarket; 2023.
14. Wintour P. Are we heading for another world war—or has it already started? *The Guardian*. May 10, 2025. Available at: https://www.theguardian.com/news/ng-interactive/2025/may/10/are-we-heading-for-another-world-war-or-has-it-already-started. Accessed September 10, 2025.
15. Intergovernmental Panel on Climate Change. AR6 Synthesis Report: Climate Change 2023. 2023. Available at: https://www.ipcc.ch/report/sixth-assessment-report-cycle. Accessed March 25, 2024.
16. Roberts M. *The Long Depression: Marxism and the Global Crisis of Capitalism*. Chicago, IL: Haymarket; 2016.
17. Friedman SR, Perlman DC, Paraskevis D, Feldman J. Sociopolitical diagnostic tools to understand national and local response capabilities and vulnerabilities to epidemics and guide research into how to improve the global response to pathogens. *Pathogens*. 2023;12(8):1023. https://doi.org/10.3390/pathogens12081023
18. Friedman SR, Jordan AE, Perlman DC, Nikolopoulos GK, Mateu-Gelabert P. Emerging zoonotic infections, social processes and their measurement and enhanced surveillance to improve zoonotic epidemic responses: a "big events" perspective. *Int J Environ Res Public Health*. 2022;19(2):995. https://doi.org/10.3390/ijerph19020995
19. Wallace R. *Dead Epidemiologists*. New York, NY: Monthly Review Press. 2020.
20. Barker C, Krinsky J, Cox L, Nilsen AG. *Marxism and Social Movements*. Chicago, IL: Haymarket; 2014:473–473.
21. Friedman SR, Mateu-Gelabert P, Nikolopoulos GK, et al. Big Events theory and measures may help explain emerging long-term effects of current crises. *Glob Public Health*. 2021;16(8-9):1167–1186. https://doi.org/10.1080/17441692.2021.1903528
22. Friedman SR, Rossi D, Perlman DC. Historical and theoretical roots of the big events framework. *Int J Drug Policy*. 2024;133:104606. https://doi.org/10.1016/j.drugpo.2024.104606
23. Ollman B. *Dialectical Investigations*. New York, NY: Routledge; 1993:ix, 191.
24. Levins R. The strategy of model building in population biology. *Am Sci*. 1966;54(4):421–431.
25. Eldredge N, Gould SJ. Punctuated equilibria: an alternative to phyletic gradualism. In: Schopf TJM, ed. *Models in Paleobiology*. San Francisco, CA: Freeman Cooper; 1972:82–115.
26. Gould SJ. *The Structure of Evolutionary Theory*. Cambridge, MA: Harvard University Press; 2002.
27. Dunayevskaya R. *Philosophy and Revolution*. New York, NY: Lexington Books, 2003.
28. Anderson K. *Lenin, Hegel, and Western Marxism: A Critical Study*. Urbana: University of Illinois Press; 1995:311–311.

29. Friedman SR. Hegel's Absolutes and revolution: an expanded review of Eugene Gogol's *Toward a Dialectic of Philosophy and Organization*. *Crit Sociol (Eugene)*. 2015;41(6):929–934. https://doi.org/10.1177/0896920513518949
30. Gogol E. *Toward a Dialectic of Philosophy and Organization*. Boston, MA: Brill; 2012.
31. Schorske CE. *German Social Democracy, 1905–1917: The Development of the Great Schism*. Cambridge, MA: Harvard University Press; 1955.
32. The HIV Life Cycle. Updated April 9, 2025. Available at: https://hivinfo.nih.gov/understanding-hiv/fact-sheets/hiv-life-cycle#:~:text=Replication%3A%20Once%20integrated%20into%20the,(non%2Dinfectious)%20HIV. Accessed June 26, 2025.
33. Lewontin R, Levins R. *Biology Under the Influence: Dialectical Essays on Ecology, Agriculture, and Health*. New York, NY: Monthly Review Press; 2007.
34. Engels F. *Dialectics of Nature*. New York, NY: International Publishers; 1940.
35. Engels F, Vujović R. *Anti-Dühring*. New York, NY: International Publishers; 1939.
36. Hegel GWF, Wallace W. *Hegel's Logic*. Oxford, UK: Oxford University Press; 1975.
37. Friedman SR, Rossi D. Dialectical theory and the study of HIV/AIDS and other epidemics. *Dialect Anthropol*. 2011;35(4):403–427. https://doi.org/10.1007/s10624-011-9222-1
38. Dietzgen J. *Nature of Human Brain Work: An Introduction to Dialectics*. Binghamton, NY: PM Press; 2010.
39. Lukács G. *History and Class Consciousness: Studies in Marxist Dialectics*. Cambridge, MA: MIT Press; 1971:356–356.
40. Lukács G. *A Defence of History and Class Consciousness: Tailism and the Dialectic*. New York, NY: Verso; 2000.
41. Levy H, Macmurray J, Fox R, Arnot RP, Bernal JD, Carritt EF. *Aspects of Dialectical Materialism*. London, UK: Watts & Co; 1934.
42. Friedman SR, Williams LD, Guarino H, et al. The stigma system: how sociopolitical domination, scapegoating, and stigma shape public health. *J Community Psychol*. 2022;50(1):385–408. https://doi.org/10.1002/jcop.22581
43. Macinko JA, Shi L, Starfield B. Wage inequality, the health system, and infant mortality in wealthy industrialized countries, 1970-1996. *Soc Sci Med*. 2004;58(2):279–292. https://doi.org/10.1016/s0277-9536(03)00200-4
44. Kawachi I, Kennedy BP. Income inequality and health: pathways and mechanisms. *Health Serv Res*. 1999;34(1 pt 2):215–227.
45. Kuo CT, Kawachi I. County-level income inequality, social mobility, and deaths of despair in the US, 2000-2019. *JAMA Netw Open*. 2023;6(7):e2323030. https://doi.org/10.1001/jamanetworkopen.2023.23030
46. Krieger N, Rehkopf DH, Chen JT, Waterman PD, Marcelli E, Kennedy M. The fall and rise of US inequities in premature mortality: 1960-2002. *PLoS Med*. 2008;5(2):e46. https://doi.org/10.1371/journal.pmed.0050046
47. Khatana SAM, Venkataramani AS, Nathan AS, et al. association between county-level change in economic prosperity and change in cardiovascular mortality among middle aged US adults. *JAMA*. 2021;325(5):445–453. https://doi.org/10.1001/jama.2020.26141
48. Wilper AP, Woolhandler S, Lasser KE, McCormick D, Bor DH, Himmelstein DU. Health insurance and mortality in US adults. *Am J Public Health*. 2009;99(12):2289–2295. https://doi.org/10.2105/AJPH.2008.157685
49. Cooper H, Beane S, Yarbrough C, et al. Association of Medicaid expansion with health insurance, unmet need for medical care and substance use disorder treatment among people who inject drugs in 13 US states. *Addiction (Abingdon)*. 2023;119(3):582–592. https://doi.org/10.1111/add.16383
50. Gaffney AW, Himmelstein DU, Christiani DC, Woolhandler S. Socioeconomic inequality in respiratory health in the US from 1959 to 2018. *JAMA Intern Med*. 2021;181(7):968–976. https://doi.org/10.1001/jamainternmed.2021.2441
51. Cooper HL, Des Jarlais DC, Ross Z, Tempalski B, Bossak B, Friedman SR. Spatial access to syringe exchange programs and pharmacies selling over-the-counter syringes as predictors of drug injectors' use of sterile syringes. *Am J Public Health*. 2011;101(6):1118–1125. https://doi.org/10.2105/AJPH.2009.184580
52. Bailey ZD, Krieger N, Agénor M, Graves J, Linos N, Bassett MT. Structural racism and health inequities in the USA: evidence and interventions. *Lancet*. 2017;389(10077):1453–1463. https://doi.org/10.1016/S0140-6736(17)30569-X
53. Krieger N. Measures of racism, sexism, heterosexism, and gender binarism for health equity research: from structural injustice to embodied harm-an ecosocial analysis. *Annu Rev Public Health*. 2020;41:37–62. https://doi.org/10.1146/annurev-publhealth-040119-094017
54. Gee GC, Ford CL. Structural racism and health inequities: old issues, new directions. *Du Bois Rev*. 2011;8(1):115–132. https://doi.org/10.1017/S1742058X11000130
55. Hailu EM, Maddali SR, Snowden JM, Carmichael SL, Mujahid MS. Structural racism and adverse maternal health outcomes: a systematic review. *Health Place*. 2022;78:102923. https://doi.org/10.1016/j.healthplace.2022.102923
56. Brinda EM, Rajkumar AP, Enemark U. Association between gender inequality index and child mortality rates: a cross-national study of 138 countries. *BMC Public Health*. 2015;15:97. https://doi.org/10.1186/s12889-015-1449-3
57. Veas C, Crispi F, Cuadrado C. Association between gender inequality and population-level health outcomes: panel data analysis of Organization for Economic Co-operation and Development (OECD) countries. *EClinicalMedicine*. 2021;39:101051. https://doi.org/10.1016/j.eclinm.2021.101051
58. Friedman SR, Tempalski B, Brady JE, et al. Income inequality, drug-related arrests, and the health of people who inject drugs: reflections on seventeen years of research. *Int J Drug Policy*. 2016;32:11–16. https://doi.org/10.1016/j.drugpo.2016.03.003
59. Levins R. Strategies of Abstraction. In: Levins R, Lewontin R, eds. *Biology Under the Influence*. New York, NY: MR Press; 2007.
60. Muntaner C, Chung H. Commentary: macrosocial determinants, epidemiology, and health policy: should politics and economics be banned from social determinants of health research? *J Public Health Policy*. 2008;29(3):299–306. https://doi.org/10.1057/jphp.2008.23
61. Schwartz S, Prins SJ, Campbell UB, Gatto NM. Is the "well-defined intervention assumption" politically conservative? *Soc Sci Med*. 2016;166:254–257. https://doi.org/10.1016/j.socscimed.2015.10.054
62. Harvey M. The Political Economy of Health: revisiting its Marxian origins to address 21st-century health inequalities. *Am J Public Health*. 2021;111(2):293–300. https://doi.org/10.2105/AJPH.2020.305996
63. Krieger N. Social epidemiologic alternatives: sociopolitical and psychosocial frameworks. In: *Epidemiology and the People's Health: Theory and Context*. New York, NY: Oxford University Press; 2011:163–201.
64. Eisenberg-Guyot J, Prins SJ. The impact of capitalism on mental health. In: Bhugra D, Moussaoui D, Craig TJ, eds. *Oxford Textbook of Social Psychiatry*. New York, NY: Oxford University Press; 2022:195–205.
65. Friedman SR, Krawczyk N, Perlman DC, et al. The opioid/overdose crisis as a dialectics of pain, despair, and one-sided struggle. *Front Public Health*. 2020;8:540423. https://doi.org/10.3389/fpubh.2020.540423
66. Laster Pirtle WN. Racial capitalism: a fundamental cause of novel coronavirus (COVID-19) pandemic inequities in the United States. *Health Educ Behav*. 2020;47(4):504–508. https://doi.org/10.1177/1090198120922942
67. Cooper HLF, Fullilove MT. *From Enforcers to Guardians: A Public Health Primer on Ending Police Violence*. Baltimore, MD: Johns Hopkins University Press; 2020:281.
68. Krieger N. Proximal, distal, and the politics of causation: what's level got to do with it? *Am J Public Health*. 2008;98(2):221–230. https://doi.org/10.2105/AJPH.2007.111278
69. Marx K. *The Eighteenth Brumaire of Louis Bonaparte*. New York, NY: International Publishers, 1967.
70. Levins R. *The Dialectical Biologist*. Cambridge, MA: Harvard University Press; 1985.
71. Levins R. Dialectics and systems theory. *Sci Soc*. 1998;7(4):557–582. https://doi.org/10.1080/09505439809526525
72. Levins R. The internal and external in explanatory theories. *Sci Cult (Lond)*. 2009:7(4):557–582. https://doi.org/10.1080/09505439809526525
73. Breilh J. *Critical Epidemiology and the People's Health*. New York, NY: Oxford University Press; 2021.
74. Breilh J. The social determination of health and the transformation of rights and ethics. *Glob Public Health*. 2023;18(1):2193830. https://doi.org/10.1080/17441692.2023.2193830
75. Borrell C, Espelt A, Rodríguez-Sanz M, Navarro V. Politics and health. *J Epidemiol Community Health*. 2007;61(8), 658–659. https://doi.org/10.1136/jech.2006.059063
76. Navarro V. A critique of the ideological and political positions of the Willy Brandt Report and the WHO Alma Ata Declaration. *Soc Sci Med*. 1984;18(6):467–474. https://doi.org/10.1016/0277-9536(84)90002-9
77. Gamson WA. *The Strategy of Social Protest*. Homewood, IL: Wadsworth Pub; 1990:357–357.
78. Beissinger MR. *The Revolutionary City: Urbanization and the Global Transformation of Rebellion*. Princeton, NJ: Princeton University Press; 2022.

79. McAdam D, Snow DA. *Social Movements: Readings on Their Emergence, Mobilization, and Dynamics.* Los Angeles, CA: Roxbury Pub Co; 1997.

80. Tilly C. *From Mobilization to Revolution*. Reading, MA: Addison-Wesley; 1978.

81. Hopkins GW. *The Miners for Democracy: Insurgency in the United Mine Workers of America, 1970-1972*. Chapel Hill, NC: University of North Carolina Press; 1976.

82. Hume B. *Death and the Mines.* New York, NY: Grossman Publishers; 1971.

83. DeFina R, Hannon L. De-unionization and drug death rates. *Soc Curr.* 2019;6(1):4–13. https://doi.org/10.1177/2329496518804555

84. Wallace M. Dying for coal: the struggle for health and safety conditions in American coal mining, 1930-82. *Social Forces.* 1987;66(2):336–364.

85. Drucker P. *Warped: Gay Normality and Queer Anticapitalism.* Chicago, IL: Haymarket Press; 2015.

86. Adam B. *The Rise of a Gay and Lesbian Movement.* Revised Edition. New York, NY: Twayne Publishers; 1995:221–221.

87. Tempalski B, Flom PL, Friedman SR, et al. Social and political factors predicting the presence of syringe exchange programs in 96 US metropolitan areas. *Am J Public Health.* 2007;97(3):437–447. https://doi.org/10.2105/AJPH.2005.065961

88. Decoteau CL. *Ancestors and Antiretrovirals: The Biopolitics of HIV/AIDS in Post-Apartheid South Africa.* Chicago, IL: University of Chicago Press; 2013:324–324.

89. Conner CD. *A People's History of Science: Miners, Midwives, and Low Mechanicks.* London, UK: Hachette UK; 2009.

90. Trotsky L. *1905*. Chicago, IL: Haymarket Books; 2017.

91. Torigian M. The occupation of the factories: Paris 1936, Flint 1937. *Comp Stud Soc Hist.* 1999;41(2):324–347. https://doi.org/10.1017/S0010417599002108

92. White AA. The Depression Era sit-down strikes and the limits of liberal labor law. *Seton Hall L Rev.* 2010;40:1.

93. Zinn H. *SNCC: The New Abolitionists.* Vol 1. Boston, MA: South End Press; 2002.

94. Friedman SR, Des Jarlais DC, Sotheran JL, Garber J, Cohen H, Smith D. AIDS and self-organization among intravenous drug users. *Int J Addict.* 1987;22(3):201–219. https://doi.org/10.3109/10826088709027425

95. Moore LD, Wenger LD. The social context of needle exchange and user self-organization in San Francisco: possibilities and pitfalls. *J Drug Issues.* 1995;25(3):583–598. https://doi.org/10.1177/002204269502500305

96. Palamar JJ, Acosta P, Sutherland R, Shedlin MG, Barratt MJ. Adulterants and altruism: a qualitative investigation of "drug checkers" in North America. *Int J Drug Policy.* 2019;74:160–169. https://doi.org/10.1016/j.drugpo.2019.09.017

97. Bathje GJ, Pillersdorf D, Kacere L, Bigg D. Helping behaviour among people who use drugs: altruism and mutual aid in a harm reduction program. *J Community Appl Soc Psychol.* 2020;30(2):119–131. https://doi.org/10.1002/casp.2432

98. Friedman SR, Maslow C, Bolyard M, Sandoval M, Mateu-Gelabert P, Neaigus A. Urging others to be healthy: "intravention" by injection drug users as a community prevention goal. *AIDS Educ Prev.* 2004;16(3):250–263. https://doi.org/10.1521/aeap.16.3.250.35439

99. Mateu-Gelabert P, Guarino H, Quinn K, et al. Young drug users: a vulnerable population and an underutilized resource in HIV/HCV prevention. *Curr HIV/AIDS Rep.* 2018;15(4):324–335. https://doi.org/10.1007/s11904-018-0406-z

100. Schulman S. *Let the Record Show: A Political History of ACT UP New York, 1987-1993.* New York, NY: Farrar, Straus, and Giroux; 2021.

101. Friedman SR, Casriel C. Drug users' organizations and AIDS policy. *AIDS Public Policy J.* 1988;3(2):30–36.

102. Dean A, McCallum J, Venkataramani AS, Michaels D. The effect of labor unions on nursing home compliance with OSHA's workplace injury and illness reporting requirement. *Health Aff (Millwood).* 2023;42(9):1260–1265. https://doi.org/10.1377/hlthaff.2023.00255

103. Krieger N. *Epidemiology and the People's Health: Theory and Context.* New York, NY: Oxford University Press; 2011:381.

104. Krieger N. *Ecosocial Theory, Embodied Truths, and the People's Health.* New York, NY: Oxford University Press; 2021.

105. Eldredge N, Gould SJ. Punctuated equilibria: an alternative to phyletic gradualism. In: Schopf TJM, ed. *Models in Paleobiology.* San Francisco, CA: Freeman, Cooper & Co; 1972:82–115.

106. Krieger N. Theorizing epidemiology, the stories bodies tell, and embodied truths: a status update on contending 21(st) c CE epidemiological theories of disease distribution. *Int J Soc Determinants Health Health Serv.* 2024;54(4):331–342. https://doi.org/10.1177/27551938241269188

How Anti-Immigrant Policies Impact Research Among Latinx and Undocumented People Who Use Drugs

Zena K. Coronado, BS, Sedona L. Koenders, MS, Kelly R. Knight, PhD, Julia Lechuga, PhD, Andrea M. López, PhD, and Carlos Martinez, PhD

See also Pinedo and Escobar, p. 1809.

Since January 2025, anti-immigrant policies, criminalization, and xenophobic rhetoric have rapidly intensified, threatening the health and well-being of Latinx communities. Under new executive orders, funding and research related to racial health disparities and equity is being scaled back or halted.

The negative effects of immigration enforcement on the health of Latinx communities have been well documented. Less is known about how the implementation of these policies and associated anti-immigrant rhetoric impacts researchers' ability to conduct health equity science among vulnerable Latinx communities. The current anti-immigrant political climate is likely to have detrimental effects on health equity research and lead to increases in morbidity and mortality among Latinx people who use drugs (PWUD).

This analytic essay draws on data from 4 case studies of research with Latinx PWUD residing in 3 US states. We discuss how anti-immigration policies and xenophobic rhetoric affect the ability to conduct research with Latinx PWUD. We offer strategies to support the continuation of health equity research in the context of an increasingly hostile sociopolitical landscape. (*Am J Public Health*. 2025;115(11):1877–1886. https://doi.org/10.2105/AJPH.2025.308234)

AJPH November 2025, Vol. 115, No. 11

We are in a rapidly escalating crisis regarding the health and well-being of Latinx communities targeted by US immigration enforcement. The federal government has promised to execute the largest mass deportation effort in US history[1] and has implemented immigration-related executive orders aimed at removing undocumented immigrants.[2,3] On January 21, 2025, several executive orders were signed, including the expansion of the "expedited removal" process by Immigration and Customs Enforcement (ICE) and 287(g) agreements, which authorize state and local law enforcement entities to enforce immigration laws to the fullest extent possible.[2] These recent actions represent an escalation of the policies implemented under previous federal administrations. Between 2016 and 2020, the 287(g) program underwent a historic expansion, with 135 agreements established between ICE and law enforcement agencies across 21 states.[2] The administration implemented law enforcement raids in homes and businesses targeting undocumented immigrants while blocking access to asylum at the US southern border.[4,5]

The negative effects of immigration enforcement on the health of Latinx communities have been well documented.[6–9] Intensified policing, immigration raids and detention, and fear of deportation create a distressing intersectional effect in Latinx communities, reducing mobility, creating mistrust of government entities, producing negative mental and physical health impacts, and decreasing health care utilization.[6–8,10–13] Fear of deportation leads to adverse mental health conditions such as trauma-related distress and negative physical health outcomes, including chronic stress and hypertension,[6,14] and reduces prevention behavior, such as HIV testing.[15,16] Furthermore, immigration detention is associated with depression and posttraumatic stress disorder (PTSD).[17–19] Although these policies affect Latinx immigrants directly, the structural vulnerability they exacerbate can have "spillover effects" on their families and the mental health of wider communities over time.[20–22] For example, witnessing immigration raids and experiencing the deportation of a parent during childhood are both associated with increased odds of psychological distress and receiving a PTSD diagnosis.[23,24] Knowing a person who has been deported is associated with positive screens for anxiety and depression.[20,21]

In the wake of the 2024 US presidential election, scientists and health care providers urgently alerted public health communities that the increased "hypercriminalization"[25] of immigrants would likely further negatively impact health and service access for Latinx people, including those with and without legal citizenship status.[26–28] Here, we argue that hypercriminalization of immigration also negatively affects health equity science, an already underexamined population health domain. Health equity science investigates patterns and underlying contributors to health inequities and builds an evidence base that can guide action in surveillance, policy, communication, and scientific inquiry toward eliminating inequities.[29] As researchers who work in a variety of settings across the United States, we understand that the current administration's policies will likely exacerbate health inequities impacting Latinx communities, particularly among the most vulnerable, including people who are homeless and use substances. What has been less examined is how the enactment of these policies, drastic cuts in funding for health equity research, and associated anti-immigrant rhetoric may severely jeopardize our ability as research scientists to conduct health equity science among these communities.

Latinx people experience significant health disparities in substance use disorders and are disproportionately impacted by opioid overdose mortality.[9,30–32] Between 2010 and 2021, the overdose rate rose by 287.5% among Latinx people, compared with a rise of 160% among non-Latinx people.[9] The rise in overdose-related deaths among Latinx people is being driven by co-use of fentanyl and stimulants: between 2007 and 2019, fatal overdoses from opioids and cocaine co-use rose 729%, and opioid and methamphetamine co-use increased by 4600%.[30] Existing barriers to access medications for opioid use disorder experienced by the general population are exacerbated among Latinx communities through limited access to insurance, fear of deportation, or difficulty navigating the health care system.[31,33–37] Although undocumented status increases risk of homelessness and may increase overdose mortality, little is known about how substance use patterns intersect with these risks and the service needs among undocumented Latinx people who use drugs (PWUD).[38,39]

Latinx immigrants are disproportionately affected by immigration enforcement policies and portrayed as the dominant adversary in the illicit drug market. Public vilification portrays Latinx immigrants as responsible for drug trade–related crime and public disorder, increasing their susceptibility to multiple forms of stigma (e.g., structural, enacted, and anticipated stigma), which is associated with increased risk of overdose.[40] The current targeting of immigrants is amplified by the racialized media rhetoric surrounding the sale of illicit drugs. For example, in San Francisco, California, there has been consistent media coverage focused on Honduran immigrants, alleging that they are the primary sellers of fentanyl and therefore to blame for public disorder in the city.[41–44] This has reinforced the xenophobic narratives of drug scares throughout US history, which depict immigrants as menacing foreigners seeking to threaten the health and safety of the country[45,46] and as direct threats to "deserving citizens." Pervasive media coverage vilifying immigrants has contributed to a series of legislative proposals, including the recently approved Laken Riley Act, aimed at increasing punishment for undocumented immigrants, especially those involved in the illicit drug market.[47] Racialized reporting on the seizure of illicit drugs by law enforcement, particularly along the US–Mexico border, is a consistent feature in the media that influences public opinion toward Latinx immigrant communities.[26]

Here, we present barriers that our research teams foresee or already experience conducting health equity research with Latinx PWUD to understand the causes of disproportionate overdose rates and to implement harm reduction interventions. Since January 2025, we have encountered barriers inhibiting the ability to continue engaging in health equity science efforts. We conclude by discussing strategies that may promote resilience to continue to conduct health equity research to reduce harms among Latinx PWUD during this time of heightened vulnerability.

CASE STUDIES

In this section, we illustrate the challenges we have faced that are likely to escalate under conditions of hypercriminalization of Latinx PWUD through 4 case studies in 3 states that include 1 needs assessment, 2 research studies, and the implementation of 1 intervention.

Harm Reduction: San Francisco

In 2019, San Francisco County was among the 3 counties in California with the highest opioid-related death rates among Latinx PWUD.[33] Alarmed by this trend, the San Francisco AIDS Foundation petitioned the San Francisco Department of Public Health (SFDPH) in 2021 to determine the barriers and gaps in harm reduction services experienced by Latinx PWUD. Harm reduction services have been shown to effectively reduce overdose mortality rates and disease transmission,[48–52] yet racial inequities permeate overdose prevention efforts, including syringe exchange programs,[53] naloxone distribution programs,[54,55] overdose response training,[56] and opioid treatment programs.[50,57,58]

In response, the SFDPH commissioned a team to conduct a needs assessment aimed at examining the conditions, challenges, and barriers impacting Latinx PWUD who are primarily Spanish or Mayan language speakers.[59] This was the first assessment of its kind in California to prioritize the challenges faced by Latinx PWUD in accessing harm reduction services. We found that several intersectional factors limited or prevented access to services, including a lack of familiarity or discomfort with approaching service providers and the language inaccessibility of programs. Nearly half of the participants (n = 105) were undocumented and 12% reported not seeking drug treatment services through fear of being intercepted by police or immigration authorities.

This was the case despite San Francisco's provision of public health insurance to undocumented individuals and its status as a sanctuary city, which limits cooperation between police officers and federal immigration authorities. The sense of insecurity experienced by some Latinx PWUD was described by a transgender Latina participant, who explained:

> I feel unprotected. Trans girls suffer discrimination. We are supposed to be in a sanctuary city that protects us but at the same time we feel unprotected. (43 years old, transgender woman)

Past experiences with police and immigration authorities may have affected our participants' current health-seeking behaviors. We found that 10% of our participants had been placed into custody by immigration authorities at least once. Additionally, 29% of participants reported that they had experienced mistreatment from police. The findings of this needs assessment are consistent with other work demonstrating that barriers to accessing harm reduction services and substance use treatment are experienced more acutely by immigrants, particularly those with vulnerable legal status.[10,34,60]

Binational Work: US–Mexico Border

The 2000-mile US–Mexico border region connects 4 US states with Mexico, forming interdependent sister cities like Ciudad Juarez (CJ), Mexico, and El Paso (EP), Texas.[61] The CJ–EP region is impacted by significant health disparities, including high rates of substance use, infectious diseases, and chronic conditions.[62] Binational coalitions leverage resources to deploy and evaluate health interventions, including harm reduction efforts, public health surveillance,[63] and program development and evaluation.[64] The US–Mexico border region is a focal point for drug and US immigration policy enforcement[65] and is often politicized as a key area of criminal activity in need of control.[66] Federal immigration enforcement policies like the Migrant Protection Protocols exacerbate stigma by exposing asylum seekers to discrimination, seclusion,[67] and substance use as a form of coping.[35] Immigrants who use drugs also face violence from the Mexican government's strategies to comply with US "War on Drugs" policies.

Between 2018 and 2022, we implemented a binational harm reduction intervention for PWUD in CJ–EP. The intervention was informed by a study consisting of 40 in-depth interviews with PWUD aimed at understanding how violence between drug trafficking organizations and drug market enforcement strategies by militarized police affected the substance use risk environment. Our results indicate that border militarization in response to US drug enforcement policies exposed PWUD to systemic violence on both sides of the border. The following illustrates the exposure to violence from multiple sources experienced by a woman who uses drugs amid cartel violence and border militarization in CJ.

> At the time that it [the violence] began, about four years, almost reaching five, they [militarized and federal law enforcement entities] arrived and there were deaths of working girls [women participating in the sex work trade] they killed them there in the room, it was two friends that I lost, the hooded people came in and beat us and forced us to use drugs and if you did not cooperate with them they themselves planted drugs on you for the police to take their turn, many things like that. (34 years old, woman)

This systemic violence paralyzed the outreach work of health and harm reduction organizations that were providing PWUD essential services to reduce substance use harms and collecting needed information for evaluation and surveillance. A man recounted the difficulty he encountered in accessing harm reduction supplies in CJ because of the reduced frequency with which staff working at a harm reduction organization conducted outreach to distribute supplies.

> During the violence I struggled more to get 'the cuetes' [needles] exchanged. In other words, during the violence they [refers to the staff at the harm reduction organization] would come out to our neighborhood occasionally. And before, well, they would come more often. In other words, there were more supplies available . . . I could even stop by with people I know and ask them for clean syringes. (39 years old, man)

Our research documents that US-driven drug enforcement policies result in militarization, human rights violations, and structural violence while destabilizing health and harm reduction efforts.[68]

Community-based organizations play an essential role in implementing harm reduction services to curb infectious disease transmission and substance use harm. We found that violence and distrust often disrupt these efforts.[68] Trust is critical to engaging immigrants in health services and scientific research and to ensuring the validity of the data that are generated.[69]

Recruitment Challenges in 5-County Study: Maryland

In 2019, our research team released a report based on a Rapid Ethnographic Assessment of PWUD (n = 72) and related stakeholders as part of the Statewide Assessment of Drug Use and Services Region 5 Report[70] commissioned by the Maryland Department of Health. Our research was focused on 5 counties in Maryland's Capital Region (counties bordering Washington, DC) and southern Maryland. Our research team has extensive experience engaging marginalized communities, including racialized populations who use drugs.[71] During the initial stages of data collection, it became clear that we were not recruiting Latinx PWUD proportionate to the county populations, nor was there much data about substance use and overdose from the perspective of Latinx people in the region. Because our broader ethnographic approach includes contextualizing substance use in relation to individual, community, and structural factors,[72] we designed a Latinx-focused substudy in Prince George's and Montgomery Counties, the counties with the largest Latinx populations in the region.

This substudy took place concurrently with the parent study in 2019, when the threat of immigration raids became commonplace in Maryland. We focused this substudy on providers that served Latinx people, because, consistent with Rapid Ethnographic Assessment methods, we first wanted to establish the landscape of services and risk for Latinx PWUD. We used a structurally oriented theoretical framework as the basis for data collection and analysis that considered legacies of racism, trauma, and social exclusion in producing drug-related risk. A participant in the substudy described the following:

> [T]he ongoing attacks, it just exacerbates everything else. If you're already dealing with the trauma of coming here and then dealing with the trauma of then living here under all this anti-immigrant rhetoric, I think it just exacerbates everything else. And it distracts from everything else, too. Like we were talking about people being fearful to leave their house and being out and about in the community. Then it makes everything else that much more secondary. So, yes, I may want to connect to these services or go into treatment. And I was already thinking twice about it, and now these raid threats are here. It just pushes everything back even more and potentially exacerbates all the needs in our community. (Service provider; age and gender are not provided to protect the service provider's privacy and anonymity.)

Substance use happened in the context of various immigration or enforcement-related concerns. People experienced prolonged and extensive trauma related to migration and family separation. Many people had fled their home countries under intense duress, including during childhood or adolescence. The political climate in Maryland was a critical mediator for whether people were willing to engage with treatment services, and this is compounded by concerns about stigma or criminalization for disclosing substance use. Participants experienced intense anguish, worry, and anxiety about the political climate and could not prioritize harm reduction or drug treatment. During eras of hypercriminalization, robust longitudinal research is impacted, and yet there is an urgent need to continue to fill the knowledge gap regarding how harm reduction efforts intersect with long-standing racial disparities in the provision of services.

Impacts of Political Rhetoric: San Francisco

In February 2024, we began data collection on a longitudinal qualitative and ethnographic study examining fentanyl-stimulant polysubstance use and overdose vulnerability among people experiencing homelessness in San Francisco, California (n = 66). We established a goal of including at least 25% Latinx-identifying individuals, intentionally oversampling to address the increased risk of overdose mortality among this group and to contribute to the limited existing research on this population. We anticipated and ultimately experienced difficulty finding eligible Latinx participants despite trying various recruitment strategies. We were able to enroll and interview 11 Latinx participants.

Current policies and the political climate may also affect our ability to find participants for follow-up. Stigmatizing narratives from public officials and media outlets about the purportedly disproportionate role of immigrants in San Francisco's drug trade may already be placing Latinx PWUD at greater risk.[73,74] In 2023, the *San Francisco Chronicle* published a controversial investigation into Honduran immigrants who were part of the drug market, including quotes from locals such as, "They're ruining the neighborhood in so many ways. They're poisoning people. . . . They're this cancer, this aggressive, metastasizing cancer on the Tenderloin—the dealers and the addicts."[41] Despite limited evidence that Hondurans play an outsized role in San Francisco's illicit drug market, public officials and media have centered blame on them for the city's overdose crisis.[42] This has sparked efforts to dismantle the city's sanctuary city policy and make it easier to deport individuals arrested with illicit drugs.[43,75]

Some participants have attributed shifts in the local drug market and supply to increased policing and criminalization targeting Honduran drug dealers. As a non-Honduran drug seller stated when interviewed by journalists, "The one good thing is they really cracked down on the Hondos [Hondurans]. Makes it easier for the rest of us."[44] These shifts have direct impacts on the substance use risk landscape, such as increased risk of overdose because of an unreliable drug supply, increased risk of police encounters and arrest, and unstable access to medications and services for avoiding withdrawal. One participant illustrated the effects of these shifts:

> Just that one change in daytime [police activity] made it hard to find [fentanyl], made prices go up. It's crazy. So, we were sick at daytime when we adjusted to it. And that really bad fentanyl that came out—even though we were still using, we would go two days being sick, because we couldn't find anything [strong] enough to keep us well. Or we couldn't find it. . . . Honestly, what I've seen, the cops are at a lot more spots. I know that plays a big part in it. . . . So, I think it's a big part of them being busted [for selling], or making it hard to sell. (35 years old, woman)

As research has demonstrated, the overdose crisis has coincided with highly stigmatizing media narratives.[76] Stigma toward PWUD acts as a barrier to implementing evidence-based programs and policies, such as expanding access to pharmacological treatment. The merging of harmful rhetoric about immigrants with negative portrayals of substance users is likely to exacerbate these risks.

DISCUSSION

The current anti-immigrant political climate is likely to have a detrimental effect on health equity research, with potential impacts on how we understand trends in morbidity and mortality among Latinx PWUD. The problematic history of exploitation and abuse in health care and research has already resulted in deep distrust among communities of color.[77] The anticipated 2025 to 2029 US administration's mass deportation and intensified "War on Drugs" policies will exacerbate distrust, fear, and violence, hindering health service delivery and research recruitment and participation. As substance use researchers, we find the interaction between drug and immigration policies to be of particular concern. However, we acknowledge that there are numerous additional mental and physical health impacts that take place at the intersection of immigration status, race, ethnicity, primary language, and other stigmatized statuses.

The conflation of antidrug and anti-immigrant sentiment has a long history in the United States. Immigrants and communities of color have been scapegoated and made targets of drug panics since the late 19th century.[45] These practices have had intergenerational effects on the health and well-being of immigrant communities.[20–22] Racialized portrayals have led to a simplistic, popularized view that the overdose crisis will be solved by doubling efforts to enforce draconian "War on Drugs" policies. In March 2025, the Alien Enemies Act of 1798 was invoked at the federal level to target undocumented immigrants, alleged migrant gang and cartel members, and drug dealers for arrest and deportation.[78] Latinx immigrants are not only targets of immigration enforcement policies but also compounded targets of "War on Drugs" enforcement policies.[79] Although the current administration's hypercriminalization efforts seek to target "dangerous" criminals, intense policing is ubiquitous among all people suspected of being undocumented, and this has been a historical trend in communities of color more generally.[25,80,81] Latinx communities, especially those who are undocumented, will avoid public spaces to prevent potential interactions with law enforcement or ICE to reduce their risk of deportation.[12]

An increasingly punitive immigration and drug policy enforcement environment may paralyze health equity research efforts and limit access to lifesaving tools and treatment of Latinx PWUD during a critical period of escalating overdose vulnerability among racialized communities.[79] Research remains fundamental for understanding the changing causes of overdose mortality in the fourth wave of the overdose crisis (the era primarily affecting communities of color who are also polysubstance users) to develop strategies to reduce mortality and mediate harms. These strategies include scaling up harm reduction efforts in most affected communities, engaging in rapid surveillance and response to crises, and conducting community-engaged research to develop evidence-based interventions that are responsive to localized needs. Service avoidance by vulnerable communities results in several public health consequences, including a rise in avoidable health care costs for conditions that worsen through lack of medical attention and greater risk of overdose.[6–10] This should be of particular concern for researchers and advocates in California and Texas, the 2 states found to have the highest count of US drug overdose deaths among Latinx people.[33,82]

Documenting the impacts of this era of hypercriminalization is an essential public health priority to understand the escalation of enforcement in the context of already compounded health disparities. We contend that diminished research in these arenas will have cascading negative public health impacts. We propose the following strategies to increase resilience and facilitate the conduct of health equity research in this political climate:

1. strengthen collaborations with trusted community-based organizations using participatory approaches to maintain the trust of Latinx PWUD;
2. strengthen trauma-informed practices for recruitment modalities and limit high-threshold or trauma-inducing interactions with research studies;
3. commit to research engagement with those most at risk for criminalization, despite ongoing barriers; and
4. advocate simultaneously for expansion of sanctuary city policies and protections from enforcement agencies in clinical settings (Box 1).

These practices will be vital to bridging gaps in scientific knowledge and fostering trust in a highly politicized and stigmatized environment. More broadly, researchers and academic institutions must collectively advocate against the current dismantling of health equity research and initiatives across federal agencies, including long-standing funding streams. Latinx PWUD are one example of a highly vulnerable community, but the patterns they experience are a window into broader trends in experiences of criminalization and violence that produce health inequities.

At this urgent moment, when the significance of critical health equity research is being cast in a negative light, we must deepen our cross-site and interdisciplinary engagements with each other and the communities in which we work. Methodologies that center trust and rapport building become especially important when people are already fearful of institutional engagement.[69] It is crucial that we consistently evaluate how we conduct research, ensuring that our methodologies remain sensitive to rapid changes and can adequately document the experiences of our participants, especially in the context of an increasingly hostile sociopolitical landscape.[69] Furthermore, the importance of retaining and expanding diversity among those conducting research cannot be overstated. When working with structurally marginalized communities, such as Latinx immigrants, having researchers with shared backgrounds and lived experiences facilitates all aspects of the research process.[99,100] As we await final decisions and outcomes related to the future of National Institutes of Health (NIH) funding resulting from the current administration's directives, it is already evident that the elimination of funding mechanisms, such as NIH Administrative and Research Supplements to Promote Diversity in Health-Related Research, will reduce opportunities for underrepresented public health and clinical researchers. Researchers who use intersectional approaches to examine health disparities within Latinx communities may experience compounded methodological barriers, such as participant recruitment challenges, an issue that is already constrained by structural barriers and the need to oversample marginalized populations.

As immigration-related presidential executive orders and other legislation continue to be implemented, Latinx PWUD will become increasingly

BOX 1— Strategies to Facilitate Health Equity Research Among Latinx People Who Use Drugs: United States, 2025

Key Strategies for Researchers	Examples of Actions
Strengthen collaborations with trusted community-based organizations (CBOs).	• Use participatory approaches to gain and maintain trust among criminalized communities (such as Latinx people who use drugs).[71] • Place an emphasis on collaborations that benefit both parties.[71] • Spend time observing and listening to safety concerns raised by impacted communities prior to, during, and after data collection.[71] • Codesign research projects with CBOs and engage CBOs in research dissemination.[83–85] • Build in expertise data collection efforts in research protocols that include perspectives of stakeholders from CBOs to understand policy landscape and community concerns.[83–85]
Strengthen trauma-informed practices.	• Limit high threshold or trauma-inducing interactions in research.[86] • Conduct trauma-informed training with research staff for recruitment and to reduce precipitating trauma responses.[87] • Provide referrals to participants who need mental health support.[87]
Commit to research engagement with those most at risk for criminalization.	• Implement extensive protections for participant privacy and confidentiality, including how data are stored.[88–90] • Nonfederal funders establish research funding opportunities focused specifically on criminalized communities.[91–93] • Emphasize your personal dedication to working in collaboration with impacted communities, not only in how you speak but also in the approaches you use.[71] • Collaborate and provide support to researchers who are also committed to the work.[94]
Advocate simultaneously for expansion of sanctuary city policies and protections from enforcement agencies in clinical settings.	• Ensure participants and staff know their rights and local policies.[88,89] • Connect clinical staff to trainings on legal protections (particularly in clinical settings—both physical and records).[91,95] • Researchers who have subject matter expertise may serve as expert witnesses in court cases.[96] • Provide research data to policymakers and legal representatives to have evidence to cite in their arguments for sanctuary city policies.[97,98]

vulnerable to targeted actions and be placed at risk for harsher legal consequences. The current political climate vilifies Latinx communities and threatens many with the risk of deportation. As anti-immigrant policies and xenophobic and racist rhetoric continue to increase, conducting research with Latinx people will likely become even more challenging, particularly with those who are undocumented. Given the rapid and comprehensive enforcement, it is now more important than ever to document their experiences using both qualitative and quantitative methodologies. The next wave of the overdose crisis will undoubtedly be shaped by the enforcement policies taking effect at present. Health equity research is a critical component to mitigating significant effects on morbidity and mortality. AJPH

ABOUT THE AUTHORS

Zena K. Coronado is with the Division of Health Equity and Society, Zuckerberg San Francisco General Hospital and Trauma Center, University of California, San Francisco. Sedona L. Koenders and Kelly R. Knight are with the Department of Humanities and Social Sciences, School of Medicine, University of California, San Francisco. Julia Lechuga is with the Department of Medicine and School of Medicine, University of California, San Francisco. Andrea M. López is with the Department of Anthropology, University of Maryland, College Park. Carlos Martinez is with the Department of Latin American and Latino Studies, University of California, Santa Cruz.

CORRESPONDENCE

Correspondence should be sent to Zena K. Coronado, UCSF Pride Hall, 2540 23rd St, 4th Floor, San Francisco, CA 94110 (e-mail: zdhatt@umd.edu). Reprints can be ordered at https://www.ajph.org by clicking the "Reprints" link.

PUBLICATION INFORMATION

Full Citation: Coronado ZK, Koenders SL, Knight KR, Lechuga J, López AM, Martinez C. How anti-immigrant policies impact research among Latinx and undocumented people who use drugs. *Am J Public Health*. 2025;115(11):1877–1886.

Acceptance Date: June 20, 2025.

DOI: https://doi.org/10.2105/AJPH.2025.308234

ORCID iDs:

Zena K. Coronado https://orcid.org/0009-0002-8828-6105

Kelly R. Knight https://orcid.org/0000-0002-5838-8592

Julia Lechuga https://orcid.org/0000-0002-3303-8692

Carlos Martinez https://orcid.org/0000-0001-6596-2807

CONTRIBUTORS

All authors contributed equally to the conceptualization of the manuscript, analysis and interpretation of data, drafting and revisions of the manuscript, and the approval of the final version.

ACKNOWLEDGMENTS

Research reported in this article was supported by the National Institute on Drug Abuse of the National Institutes of Health (award no. R01DA057672), the National Institutes of Health and National Institute on Minority Health and Health Disparities (award no. MD010657), and the Maryland Department of Health through the Centers for Disease Control and Prevention (award no. CDC-RFA-TP18-1802).

Note. The contents are solely the responsibility of the authors and do not necessarily represent the official views of the National Institutes of Health, Maryland Department of Health, or Centers for Disease Control and Prevention.

CONFLICTS OF INTEREST

The authors have no financial or nonfinancial conflicts of interests to disclose.

HUMAN PARTICIPANT PROTECTION

All research studies received institutional review board approval from the researchers' respective organizations.

REFERENCES

1. Inskeep S. Trump promised the "largest deportation" in US history. Here's how he might start. NPR. November 14, 2024. Available at: https://www.npr.org/2024/11/12/nx-s1-5181962/trump-promises-a-mass-deportation-on-day-1-what-might-that-look-like. Accessed February 6, 2025.
2. After day one: a high-level analysis of Trump's first executive actions. American Immigration Council. January 22, 2025. Available at: https://www.americanimmigrationcouncil.org/research/after-day-one-high-level-analysis-trumps-first-executive-actions. Accessed February 18, 2025.
3. NPR Staff. All the executive orders Trump has signed after 1 week in office. NPR. January 28, 2025. Available at: https://www.npr.org/2025/01/28/nx-s1-5276293/trump-executive-orders. Accessed February 6, 2025.
4. López WD. Immigration worksite raids are violent, militarized, and rooted in racial discrimination—and politicians love them for it. *Pract Anthropol.* 2022;44(1):31–35. https://doi.org/10.17730/0888-4552.44.1.31
5. Martinez C. Waiting in captivity: slow borders, predatory bureaucracies, and the necrotemporality of asylum deterrence. *Refuge.* 2023;39(2):1–17. https://doi.org/10.25071/1920-7336.41069
6. Cabral J, Cuevas AG. Health inequities among Latinos/Hispanics: documentation status as a determinant of health. *J Racial Ethn Health Disparities.* 2020;7(5):874–879. https://doi.org/10.1007/s40615-020-00710-0
7. Friedman AS, Venkataramani AS. Chilling effects: US immigration enforcement and health care seeking among Hispanic adults. *Health Aff (Millwood).* 2021;40(7):1056–1065. https://doi.org/10.1377/hlthaff.2020.02356
8. Kline N. Pathogenic policing: immigration enforcement and health in the US South. Rutgers University Press; 2019. Available at: https://www.rutgersuniversitypress.org/pathogenic-policing/9780813595320. Accessed February 6, 2025.
9. Romero R, Friedman JR, Goodman-Meza D, Shover CL. US drug overdose mortality rose faster among Hispanics than non-Hispanics from 2010 to 2021. *Drug Alcohol Depend.* 2023;246:109859. https://doi.org/10.1016/j.drugalcdep.2023.109859
10. Martinez O, Wu E, Sandfort T, et al. Evaluating the impact of immigration policies on health status among undocumented immigrants: a systematic review. *J Immigr Minor Health.* 2015;17(3):947–970. https://doi.org/10.1007/s10903-013-9968-4
11. Rhodes SD, Mann L, Simán FM, et al. The impact of local immigration enforcement policies on the health of immigrant Hispanics/Latinos in the United States. *Am J Public Health.* 2015;105(2):329–337. https://doi.org/10.2105/AJPH.2014.302218
12. Asad AL. On the radar: system embeddedness and Latin American immigrants' perceived risk of deportation. *Law Soc Rev.* 2020;54(1):133–167. https://doi.org/10.1111/lasr.12460
13. Maldonado CZ, Rodriguez RM, Torres JR, Flores YS, Lovato LM. Fear of discovery among Latino immigrants presenting to the emergency department. *Acad Emerg Med.* 2013;20(2):155–161. https://doi.org/10.1111/acem.12079
14. Garcini LM, Daly R, Chen N, et al. Undocumented immigrants and mental health: a systematic review of recent methodology and findings in the United States. *J Migr Health.* 2021;4:100058. https://doi.org/10.1016/j.jmh.2021.100058
15. Suro B, Lechuga J, Galletly CL, Glasman L. The influence of perceived immigration context and healthcare utilization immigration law concerns on Latinx immigrants' HIV testing. *J Lat Psychol.* 2022;10(2):156–167. https://doi.org/10.1037/lat0000171
16. Aborode AT, Lawal L, Agwuna FO, Adewunmi RO, Ubechu SC, Badri R. Health disparities among illegal immigrants and homeless people in the USA: a struggle within. *IJS Global Health.* 2023;6(6):e0362. https://doi.org/10.1097/GH9.0000000000000362
17. Zayas LH, Villatoro AP, Londoño T, Fuentes-Balderrama J. Emotional wellbeing of asylum-seeking children after release from immigration detention. *Hisp J Behav Sci.* 2024;46(4):206–222. https://doi.org/10.1177/07399863241304083
18. Minero LP, Domínguez S, Budge SL, Salcedo B. Latinx trans immigrants' survival of torture in US detention: a qualitative investigation of the psychological impact of abuse and mistreatment. *Int J Transgend Health.* 2022;23(1–2):36–59. https://doi.org/10.1080/26895269.2021.1938779
19. Priestley I, Cherian S, Paxton G, et al. The impact of immigration detention on children's mental health: systematic review. *Br J Psychiatry.* Published online April 10, 2025:1–10. https://doi.org/10.1192/bjp.2025.29
20. Dadras O, Hazratzai MS. The silent trauma: US immigration policies and mental health. *The Lancet Reg Health Am.* 2025;44:101048. https://doi.org/10.1016/j.lana.2025.101048
21. Pinedo M, Valdez CR. Immigration enforcement policies and the mental health of US citizens: findings from a comparative analysis. *Am J Community Psychol.* 2020;66(1–2):119–129. https://doi.org/10.1002/ajcp.12464
22. MacLean SA, Agyeman PO, Walther J, Singer EK, Baranowski KA, Katz CL. Characterization of the mental health of immigrant children separated from their mothers at the US-Mexico border. *Psychiatry Res.* 2020;286:112555. https://doi.org/10.1016/j.psychres.2019.112555
23. Pinedo M, Escobar C. Childhood parental deportations, immigration enforcement experiences, and posttraumatic stress disorder among US-born Latino adults, 2021. *Am J Public Health.* 2024;114(S6):S495–S504. https://doi.org/10.2105/AJPH.2024.307660
24. Rojas-Flores L, Clements ML, Hwang Koo J, London J. Trauma and psychological distress in Latino citizen children following parental detention and deportation. *Psychol Trauma.* 2017;9(3):352–361. https://doi.org/10.1037/tra0000177
25. Rios VM. The hypercriminalization of Black and Latino male youth in the era of mass incarceration. In: Marable M, Steinberg I, Middlemass K, eds. *Racializing Justice, Disenfranchising Lives: The Racism, Criminal Justice, and Law Reader.* New York, NY: Palgrave Macmillan US; 2007:17–33. https://doi.org/10.1057/9780230607347_2
26. López-Hinojosa I, Zhang J, López-Hinojosa K, Baig AA, Tung EL, Martinez-Cardoso A. "We have to lie low . . . that sort of poisons me more and more": a qualitative study of violent political rhetoric and health implications for Spanish and Chinese speaking immigrants. *Soc Sci Med.* 2024;341:116504. https://doi.org/10.1016/j.socscimed.2023.116504
27. Page KR, Spiegel PB, Cuneo CN. Detained at the doctor's office: US immigration policy endangers health. *BMJ.* 2025;388:r304. https://doi.org/10.1136/bmj.r304
28. Yang LH, Eger MA, Link BG. The human cost of politicizing immigration: migration stigma, US politics, and health. *JAMA.* 2024;332(8):619–620. https://doi.org/10.1001/jama.2024.11126
29. Burton DC, Kelly A, Cardo D, et al. Principles of health equity science for public health action. *Public Health Rep.* 2024;139(3):277–283. https://doi.org/10.1177/00333549231213162
30. Townsend T, Kline D, Rivera-Aguirre A, et al. Racial/ethnic and geographic trends in combined stimulant/opioid overdoses, 2007–2019. *Am J Epidemiol.* 2022;191(4):599–612. https://doi.org/10.1093/aje/kwab290
31. Cano M. Racial/ethnic differences in US drug overdose mortality, 2017–2018. *Addict Behav.* 2021;112:106625. https://doi.org/10.1016/j.addbeh.2020.106625
32. Pinedo M. The impact of deportation policies on the substance using behaviors of US-citizen Latinos. *Int J Drug Policy.* 2020;75:102605. https://doi.org/10.1016/j.drugpo.2019.11.013
33. Valdez A, Cepeda A, Frankeberger J, Nowotny KM. The opioid epidemic among the Latino population in California. *Drug Alcohol Depend Rep.* 2022;2:100029. https://doi.org/10.1016/j.dadr.2022.100029
34. Mancini MA, Salas-Wright CP, Vaughn MG. Drug use and service utilization among Hispanics in the United States. *Soc Psychiatry Psychiatr Epidemiol.* 2015;50(11):1679–1689. https://doi.org/10.1007/s00127-015-1111-5
35. Hernandez OLO. Migrant trajectories and health experiences: processes of health/illness/care for drug use among migrants in the Mexico–United States border region. Critical Medical Anthropology Perspectives in and from Latin America. January 1, 2020. Available at: https://www.academia.edu/42346533/Migrant_trajectories_and_health_experiences_Processes_of_health_illness_care_for_drug_use_among_migrants_in_the_Mexico_United_States_border_region. Accessed February 25, 2025.
36. Cano M, Gelpí-Acosta C. Variation in US drug overdose mortality within and between Hispanic/Latine subgroups: a disaggregation of national data. *SSM Ment Health.* 2022;2:100095. https://doi.org/10.1016/j.ssmmh.2022.100095

37. Spencer M, Garnett M, Miniño A. Drug overdose deaths in the United States, 2002–2022. National Center for Health Statistics. 2024. Available at: https://dx.doi.org/10.15620/cdc:135849. Accessed February 25, 2025.
38. Chinchilla M, Gabrielian S. Stemming the rise of Latinx homelessness: lessons from Los Angeles County. *J Soc Distress Homeless.* 2020;29(2):71–75. https://doi.org/10.1080/10530789.2019.1660049
39. Pierce K, Sun D, Feldmeyer B. Staying under the radar? Immigration effects on overdose deaths and the impact of sanctuary jurisdictions. *Societies.* 2023;13(6):135. https://doi.org/10.3390/soc13060135
40. Tsai AC, Kiang MV, Barnett ML, et al. Stigma as a fundamental hindrance to the United States opioid overdose crisis response. *PLoS Med.* 2019;16(11):e1002969. https://doi.org/10.1371/journal.pmed.1002969
41. Cassidy M, Lurie G. This is the hometown of San Francisco's drug dealers. *San Francisco Chronicle.* 2023. Available at: https://www.sfchronicle.com/projects/2023/san-francisco-drug-trade-honduras. Accessed February 25, 2025.
42. Valdez J. San Francisco mayor apologizes for saying "a lot of" drug dealers are Honduran. *Los Angeles Times.* October 21, 2022. Available at: https://www.latimes.com/california/story/2022-10-20/san-francisco-mayor-apologizes-honduran-drug-dealers-comments. Accessed February 6, 2025.
43. Thadani T. Undocumented fentanyl dealers in SF could be easier to deport under new proposal. *San Francisco Chronicle.* February 14, 2023. Available at: https://www.sfchronicle.com/sf/article/fentanyl-dealers-crime-sf-deport-immigration-17782315.php. Accessed February 6, 2025.
44. Cassidy M, Lurie G, Fagan K. SF's shifting drug trade. *San Francisco Chronicle.* December 31, 2023:A001.
45. Martinez C, Guzman L. *SF Chronicle*'s "Honduran Drug Dealers" series fuels xenophobia. Filter. July 21, 2023. Available at: https://filtermag.org/san-francisco-honduras-fentanyl-xenophobia. Accessed February 6, 2025.
46. Reinarman C. The social construction of drug scares. In: Adler PA, Adler P, eds. *Constructions of Deviance: Social Power, Context, Interaction.* 8th ed. Belmont, CA: Wadsworth Publishing Co; 2015:92–104.
47. Bustillo X. Trump signs first bill of his second presidency, the Laken Riley Act, into law. *NPR.* January 29, 2025. Available at: https://www.npr.org/2025/01/29/g-s1-45275/trump-laken-riley-act. Accessed February 25, 2025.
48. van Santen DK, Lodi S, Dietze P, et al. Comprehensive needle and syringe program and opioid agonist therapy reduce HIV and hepatitis C virus acquisition among people who inject drugs in different settings: a pooled analysis of emulated trials. *Addiction.* 2023;118(6):1116–1126. https://doi.org/10.1111/add.16147
49. Abdul-Quader AS, Feelemyer J, Modi S, et al. Effectiveness of structural-level needle/syringe programs to reduce HCV and HIV infection among people who inject drugs: a systematic review. *AIDS Behav.* 2013;17(9):2878–2892. https://doi.org/10.1007/s10461-013-0593-y
50. Lambdin BH, Bluthenthal RN, Wenger LD, et al. Overdose education and naloxone distribution within syringe service programs—United States, 2019. *MMWR Morb Mortal Wkly Rep.* 2020;69(33):1117–1121. https://doi.org/10.15585/mmwr.mm6933a2
51. *Harm Reduction Framework.* Rockville, MD: Center for Substance Abuse Prevention, Substance Abuse and Mental Health Services Administration; 2023.
52. Wheeler E, Jones S, Gilbert MK, Davidson PJ. Opioid overdose prevention programs providing naloxone to laypersons—United States, 2014. *MMWR Morb Mortal Wkly Rep.* 2015;64(23):631–635.
53. Kinnard EN, Bluthenthal RN, Kral AH, Wenger LD, Lambdin BH. The naloxone delivery cascade: identifying disparities in access to naloxone among people who inject drugs in Los Angeles and San Francisco, CA. *Drug Alcohol Depend.* 2021;225:108759. https://doi.org/10.1016/j.drugalcdep.2021.108759
54. Barboza GE, Angulski K. A descriptive study of racial and ethnic differences of drug overdoses and naloxone administration in Pennsylvania. *Int J Drug Policy.* 2020;78:102718. https://doi.org/10.1016/j.drugpo.2020.102718
55. Dayton L, Tobin K, Falade-Nwulia O, et al. Racial disparities in overdose prevention among people who inject drugs. *J Urban Health.* 2020;97(6):823–830. https://doi.org/10.1007/s11524-020-00439-5
56. Kim K, Oh H, Miller D, Veloso D, Lin J, McFarland W. Prevalence and disparities in opioid overdose response training among people who inject drugs, San Francisco: naloxone training among injectors in San Francisco. *Int J Drug Policy.* 2021;90:102778. https://doi.org/10.1016/j.drugpo.2020.102778
57. Goedel WC, Shapiro A, Cerdá M, Tsai JW, Hadland SE, Marshall BDL. Association of racial/ethnic segregation with treatment capacity for opioid use disorder in counties in the United States. *JAMA Netw Open.* 2020;3(4):e203711. https://doi.org/10.1001/jamanetworkopen.2020.3711
58. Lagisetty PA, Ross R, Bohnert A, Clay M, Maust DT. Buprenorphine treatment divide by race/ethnicity and payment. *JAMA Psychiatry.* 2019;76(9):979–981. https://doi.org/10.1001/jamapsychiatry.2019.0876
59. Martinez C, Altenberg N, Casas J, Parmenter I. Unido/Xs Contra La Sobredosis (United against Overdose): a needs assessment report from the San Francisco Harm Reduction for Spanish and Maya Speaking Communities Project (2021-2022). San Francisco AIDS Foundation. 2022:21. Available at: https://www.academia.edu/88206266/Unido_xs_Contra_la_Sobredosis_United_against_Overdose_A_Needs_Assessment_Report_from_the_San_Francisco_Harm_Reduction_for_Spanish_and_Maya_Speaking_Communities_Project. Accessed February 6, 2025.
60. Lough M, DeFries T, Brady K, Block A. Immigrants and substance use disorders: a legal and medical perspective—part II. Applying medical evidence and expertise on SUDs to immigration cases. Immigrant Legal Resource Center. 2023. Available at: https://www.ilrc.org/sites/default/files/2023-08/Immigrants%20and%20Substance%20and%20Alcohol%20Use%20Disorder-A%20Legal%20and%20Medical%20Perspective%20%28Part%20II%29.pdf. Accessed February 6, 2025.
61. Ganster P, Sweedler A, Scott J, Dieter-Eberwein W. On the road to interdependence? The United States-Mexico border region. In: *Borders and Border Regions in Europe and North America.* San Diego, CA: San Diego University Press; 1997:237–239.
62. Rosales CB, Carvajal S, de Zapien JEG. Editorial: emergent public health issues in the US–Mexico border region. *Front Public Health.* 2016;4:93. https://doi.org/10.3389/fpubh.2016.00093
63. Weinberg M, Waterman S, Lucas CA, et al. The US-Mexico Border Infectious Disease Surveillance Project: establishing binational border surveillance. *Emerg Infect Dis.* 2003;9(1):97–102. https://doi.org/10.3201/eid0901.020047
64. Rodríguez-Saldaña J. Challenges and opportunities in border health. *Prev Chronic Dis.* 2005;2(1):A03.
65. Heyman J. The US-Mexico border since 2014: overt migration contention and normalized violence. In: *Handbook on Human Security, Borders and Migration.* Edward Elgar Publishing; 2021:54–70. Available at: https://china.elgaronline.com/edcollchap/edcoll/9781839108891/9781839108891.00008.xml. Accessed February 25, 2025.
66. Burrow CL. Media framing of US-Mexico border immigration: a content analysis of national and border news articles. Dept of Criminal Justice. New Mexico State University. 2024. Available at: https://www.proquest.com/docview/3066739081/abstract/884852A41F624EF8PQ/1?sourcetype=Dissertations%20&%20Theses. Accessed February 25, 2025.
67. Mercado A, Garcini L, Venta A, Paris M. "Remain In Mexico": stories of trauma and abuse. *Health Aff (Millwood).* 2021;40(7):1170–1173. https://doi.org/10.1377/hlthaff.2020.02331
68. Lechuga J, Ramos R, Dickson-Gomez J, et al. Institutional violence from police militarization and drug cartel wars as a "big event" and its influence on drug use harms and HIV risk in people who inject drugs on the US–Mexico border. *Int J Drug Policy.* 2023;119:104125. https://doi.org/10.1016/j.drugpo.2023.104125
69. Huslage M, Rai A, Held ML. Building partnerships and trust: research with vulnerable immigrant communities. *Fam Soc.* 2022;103(2):235–246. https://doi.org/10.1177/10443894211034776
70. Lopez AM. Statewide Assessment of Drug Use and Services (SEADS) Region 5 Report 2019. Available at: https://drive.google.com/file/d/1S4xRU7EKFEONjAUhgOSh-a2aj4nv96F-/view?usp=drive_link. Accessed February 6, 2025.
71. Lopez AM, Thomann M, Dhatt Z, et al. Understanding racial inequities in the implementation of harm reduction initiatives. *Am J Public Health.* 2022;112(S2):S173–S181. https://doi.org/10.2105/AJPH.2022.306767
72. Sangaramoorthy T, Kroeger KA. *Rapid Ethnographic Assessments: A Practical Approach and Toolkit For Collaborative Community Research.* London, UK: Routledge; 2020. https://doi.org/10.4324/9780429286650
73. Pagones S. Honduran migrants working for Mexican cartels brazenly took over San Francisco's drug market thanks to lax policies. New York Post. July 10, 2023. Available at: https://nypost.com/2023/07/10/honduran-migrants-mexican-cartels-overtaking-san-francisco. Accessed February 6, 2025.
74. Woodhouse L. The criminal order beneath the "chaos" of San Francisco's Tenderloin. Real Clear

Investigations. June 16, 2022. Available at: https://www.realclearinvestigations.com/articles/2022/06/16/the_criminal_order_beneath_the_chaos_of_san_franciscos_tenderloin_836918.html. Accessed February 6, 2025.

75. Cassidy M, Lurie G, Barnerd-Smith J. New front in SF drug crackdown: 3 accused of dealing hauled back from Honduras. *San Francisco Chronicle*. February 24, 2024. Available at: https://www.sfchronicle.com/crime/article/sf-drugs-honduran-fugitives-18684729.php. Accessed February 6, 2025.

76. McGinty EE, Stone EM, Kennedy-Hendricks A, Barry CL. Stigmatizing language in news media coverage of the opioid epidemic: implications for public health. *Prev Med.* 2019;124:110–114. https://doi.org/10.1016/j.ypmed.2019.03.018

77. Hattery AJ, Smith E, Magnuson S, et al. Diversity, equity, and inclusion in research teams: the good, the bad, and the ugly. *Race Justice.* 2022; 12(3):505–530. https://doi.org/10.1177/21533687221087373

78. Treisman R. Trump is promising deportations under the Alien Enemies Act of 1798. What is it? *NPR*. October 19, 2024. Available at: https://www.npr.org/2024/10/19/nx-s1-5156027/alien-enemies-act-1798-trump-immigration. Accessed February 6, 2025.

79. Guilamo-Ramos V, Benzekri A, Wilson L, Abram MD. Avoiding a new US "war on drugs." *BMJ.* 2025;388:r225. https://doi.org/10.1136/bmj.r225

80. Brennan D. Undocumented people (en)counter border policing: near and far from the US border. *Migr Soc.* 2018;1(1):156–163. https://doi.org/10.3167/arms.2018.010114

81. Theodore N. *Insecure Communities: Latino Perceptions of Police Involvement in Immigration Enforcement*. Chicago, IL: Dept of Urban Planning and Policy, University of Illinois at Chicago; 2013:28.

82. Centers for Disease Control and Prevention, National Center for Health Statistics. National Vital Statistics System. Mortality 2018-2023 on CDC WONDER Online Database. Released in 2024. Available at: http://wonder.cdc.gov/ucd-icd10-expanded.html. Accessed February 6, 2025.

83. Young-Ponder K, Dones M, Coronado ZK, Perry E, Kushel M. *Latine Experiences of Homelessness in the California Statewide Study of People Experiencing Homelessness.* San Francisco, CA: UCSF Benioff Homelessness and Housing Initiative; 2025.

84. Kushel M, Moore T, Birkmeyer J, et al. *Toward a New Understanding: The California Statewide Study of People Experiencing Homelessness.* San Francisco, CA: UCSF Benioff Homelessness and Housing Initiative. 2023.

85. California Statewide Study of People Experiencing Homelessness. University of California San Francisco Benioff Homelessness and Housing Initiative. Available at: https://homelessness.ucsf.edu/our-impact/studies/california-statewide-study-people-experiencing-homelessness. Accessed February 6, 2025.

86. Simon C, Vincent L, Coulter A, et al. The Methadone Manifesto: treatment experiences and policy recommendations from methadone patient activists. *Am J Public Health.* 2022;112(S2):S117–S122. https://doi.org/10.2105/AJPH.2021.306665

87. Macias C, Barreira P, Hargreaves W, Bickman L, Fisher W, Aronson E. Impact of referral source and study applicants' preference for randomly assigned service on research enrollment, service engagement, and evaluative outcomes. *Am J Psychiatry.* 2005;162(4):781–787. https://doi.org/10.1176/appi.ajp.162.4.781

88. Kassis SB. Confidentiality protections in research involving people with substance use disorders. Alcohol, Other Drugs, and Health: Current Evidence. July 1, 2013. Available at: https://www.bu.edu/aodhealth/2013/07/01/confidentiality-protections-in-research-involving-people-with-substance-use-disorders. Accessed February 6, 2025.

89. Rudolph AE, Young AM, Havens JR. A rural/urban comparison of privacy and confidentiality concerns associated with providing sensitive location information in epidemiologic research involving persons who use drugs. *Addict Behav.* 2017;74:106–111. https://doi.org/10.1016/j.addbeh.2017.06.006

90. National Institute on Drug Abuse. Guidelines for developing a data and safety monitoring plan. October 11, 2018. Available at: https://nida.nih.gov/research/clinical-research/guidelines-developing-data-safety-monitoring. Accessed February 6, 2025.

91. Public Health Awakened. Public health actions for immigrant rights: a short guide to protecting undocumented residents and their families for the benefit of public health and all society. February 9, 2018. Available at: https://publichealthawakened.org/wp-content/uploads/2017/03/DPH-Actions-in-Support-of-Undocumented-Populations-UPDATED_2018.02.09.pdf. Accessed February 25, 2025.

92. Fazio L. When the government cancels your research grant, here's what you can do. *Nature.* 2025;641(8064):824. https://doi.org/10.1038/d41586-025-01547-5

93. Kozlov M, Mallapaty S. Exclusive: NIH to terminate hundreds of active research grants. *Nature.* 2025;639(8054):281–282. https://doi.org/10.1038/d41586-025-00703-1

94. Centers for Medicare & Medicaid Services. Health Equity Data Access Program Grant. October 1, 2024. Available at: https://www.cms.gov/priorities/health-equity/grants-awards/data-access-program. Accessed February 6, 2025.

95. Berlinger N, Zacharias RL. Resources for teaching and learning about immigrant health care in health professions education. *AMA J Ethics.* 2019;21(1):E50–57. https://doi.org/10.1001/amajethics.2019.50

96. Rubinfeld DL, Cecil JS. Scientists as experts serving the court. *Daedalus.* 2018;147 (4):152–163. https://doi.org/10.1162/daed_a_00526

97. Mohyeddin I. Data shows sanctuary policies make communities safer, healthier and more prosperous. National Immigration Law Center. March 5, 2025. Available at: https://www.nilc.org/articles/data-shows-sanctuary-policies-make-communities-safer-healthier-and-more-prosperous. Accessed June 14, 2025.

98. Kromm JN, Frattaroli S, Vernick JS, Teret SP. Public health advocacy in the courts: opportunities for public health professionals. *Public Health Rep.* 2009;124(6):889–894. https://doi.org/10.1177/003335490912400618

99. Salas J, Waxman E, Gupta P, Bernstein H, Echave P, Gallardo LH. When researchers build trust, "hard-to-reach" undocumented communities aren't so hard to reach. Urban Institute. 2022. Available at: https://www.urban.org/urban-wire/when-researchers-build-trust-hard-reach-undocumented-communities-arent-so-hard-reach. Accessed February 18, 2025.

100. Willig C, Rogers WS. *The SAGE Handbook of Qualitative Research in Psychology.* London, UK: SAGE Publications Ltd; 2017. https://doi.org/10.4135/9781526405555

Blood Transfusions for Pregnancy Loss in Texas Before and After Abortion Bans, 2017–2023

Amanda Nagle, MPH, Goleen Samari, PhD, MPH, MA, Lauren Thaxton, MD, MBA, MSBS, and Alison Gemmill, PhD, MPH

See also Horvath, p. 1812.

Objectives. To measure changes in blood transfusion related to pregnancy loss in Texas after the 2021 Senate Bill 8 (SB8), which banned abortion after the detection of fetal cardiac activity (6-week ban), and the ban that was enforced after the 2022 *Dobbs v Jackson* Supreme Court decision, which banned abortion at all gestational durations (total ban).

Methods. We used administrative data from all Texas hospital, emergency, and ambulatory surgical facilities from January 2017 through September 2023. Using time series analysis, we assessed if the number of pregnancy loss encounters that received blood transfusions, an indicator of severe morbidity, was different than expected after the 6-week and total bans.

Results. We identified 320 696 pregnancy loss encounters and 7408 related blood transfusions. During the 6-week ban, transfusion numbers were similar to expected. During the total ban, the quarterly mean number of pregnancy loss encounters that received blood transfusions was 385.8, which was 50.7 more transfusions (15.1%) than the 335.1 expected based on historical data (2-sample t test $P = .03$).

Conclusions. Texas's total abortion ban was associated with an increase in severe morbidity among people experiencing pregnancy loss. (*Am J Public Health*. 2025;115(11):1887–1894. https://doi.org/10.2105/AJPH.2025.308224)

AJPH November 2025, Vol. 115, No. 11

Pregnancy loss—encompassing ectopic pregnancies, miscarriages or early pregnancy losses, molar pregnancies, and stillbirths—is a common experience that affects an estimated 20% of recognized pregnancies in the United States.[1] Pregnancy loss can be a serious medical event requiring timely medical care,[2] as people experiencing loss can face severe complications, including hemorrhage,[3] shock, cardiac arrest, and death.[4]

There is qualitative evidence that abortion bans are impacting treatment and health outcomes for some people experiencing pregnancy loss[5–7] because management of pregnancy loss includes abortion care.[8–11] Following the Supreme Court's *Dobbs v Jackson Women's Health Organization* decision in June 2022, 14 states banned abortion at any gestational duration.[10] As of June 2025, 12 states ban abortion at all gestational durations with limited exceptions.[12] Since *Dobbs,* case studies have documented instances when people experiencing pregnancy loss were denied recommended medications and procedures from hospitals[6] because of providers' fear of legal repercussions for providing treatment, and obstetricians/gynecologists working in states with abortion bans report "clinically inappropriate delays" in pregnancy loss care attributed to abortion restrictions.[5] The abortion bans also pushed some patients to forgo care or seek care in other states, sometimes leading to more severe morbidity and need for invasive intervention.[6]

Before the *Dobbs* decision, Texas was the first state to ban abortion after the detection of fetal cardiac activity (around 6 weeks gestation) through Senate Bill 8 (SB8), which was implemented on September 1, 2021. The law's enforcement deputized citizens to sue anyone suspected of "aiding or abetting" a prohibited abortion for up to $10 000.[13] This resulted in a chilling effect on the provision of evidence-based, standard pregnancy loss care.[14] For example, some Texas hospitals shifted to exclusively offering expectant management (i.e., a "wait and see" approach) for patients experiencing the loss of a previable fetus.[7] Following the *Dobbs* decision in June 2022, Texas enacted a ban on abortion at any gestational duration (total ban) except when the life of the woman is threatened and made providing an abortion a felony punishable by life in prison and a \$100 000 fine.[13]

Few studies have quantitatively examined the health consequences for people experiencing pregnancy loss in states with abortion bans. One exception is a study of the 2 Texas hospitals that shifted to exclusively offering expectant management for previable fetuses with indications for delivery, rather than active management (i.e., induction of labor). They found that the change in practice was associated with increased morbidity among patients, but the study had a limited generalizability and sample size.[7] The current study builds on earlier work by using all-payer administrative data from the entire state of Texas to examine whether 1 type of severe morbidity—hemorrhage requiring blood transfusion—increased among patients diagnosed with pregnancy loss following abortion restrictions. Specifically, we studied the changes after SB8 (6-week ban) and the post-*Dobbs* ban (total ban). We focused on hemorrhage requiring transfusion because it is a life-threatening event that is sensitive to delays and denials of care, and is common enough to have statistical power to detect changes.

METHODS

Data came from public use data sets of inpatient and outpatient (including emergency department) data reported to the Texas Department of State Health Services (DSHS) for the period January 2017 through September 30, 2023. These data contain information from all Texas hospitals and ambulatory surgery centers for the entire period and freestanding emergency medical centers beginning in October 2020. The reporting of emergency department records began in 2016, and January 2017 is the earliest a consistent time series for this analysis can begin. In the DSHS-provided data, each record represents a single "encounter," which includes up to 25 diagnoses and 25 procedures for a patient during their stay, which may last many days.[15] In the outpatient data, diagnoses are coded using the *International Classification of Diseases, 10th Revision* (*ICD-10*; Geneva, Switzerland: World Health Organization; 1992), and procedures are coded with Current Procedural Terminology (CPT) codes (https://www.aapc.com/codes/cpt-codes/36430). In the inpatient data, both diagnoses and procedures were coded using *ICD-10*. For patient privacy, DSHS public use data contain the calendar quarter of admission and do not include exact admission dates. The data also include information on patient age, race and ethnicity, and the type of insurer, if any, that paid the medical bill.

Measures

Our primary outcome measures were the number of blood transfusions among pregnancy loss encounters in each quarter. We identified pregnancy loss encounters using the following diagnoses codes: missed and spontaneous abortion (O02.1xx, O03.xxx), blighted ovum (O02.0xx), hydatidiform molar pregnancy (O01.9xx), ectopic pregnancy (O08.xxx and O00.xxx), preterm premature rupture of membranes first and second trimester (O42.011, O42.012) with labor within 24 hours, intrauterine demise (O36.4xx), and stillbirth (Z37.1xx, Z37.2xx, Z37.3xx), where *x* represents any character.[16] Blood transfusions were identified using 64 *ICD-10* codes defined for severe maternal morbidity[17] and CPT code 36430.[18] To identify these codes, the first author undertook a detailed review of all potentially relevant *ICD-10* and CPT codes, in consultation with clinical and coding experts. All codes used in this study are described in Appendix A (available as a supplement to the online version of this article at https://ajph.org).

Our main exposure was the abortion policy context, which divided our quarterly data into 3 time periods: before the bans (January 2017 through September 2021, not including the COVID-19 period, April 2020 through March 2021), 6-week ban period (October 2021 through June 2022), and total ban period (July 2022 through September 2023). We excluded the COVID-19 period from this analysis as conceptions,[19] hospital usage, and maternal health[20] were impacted and not informative for estimating future expected trends.

We present distributions of patients by demographic characteristics and pregnancy loss type for the overall study period and for each policy context period. Demographic characteristics included age, race and ethnicity (Hispanic, non-Hispanic White, non-Hispanic Black, other, and more than 1 race), payer of the medical bill (private insurance or TRICARE, Medicaid, and charity, indigent or unknown other), and type of pregnancy loss.

Analysis

We evaluated changes in the number and rate of transfusions among pregnancy loss encounters after the 6-week ban and the total ban. To estimate expected trends in the absence of these policies, we fit a linear regression model using data from the prebans period (i.e., before October 2021 and excluding COVID-19 quarters), incorporating quarterly fixed effects to adjust for seasonality:

$$y_t = \beta_0 + \beta_1 X_t + \beta_2(Q2)_t + \beta_3(Q3)_t + \beta_4(Q4)_t + \varepsilon_t \quad (1)$$

In this model, y_t is the number of transfusions in quarter t. X_t is a continuous variable indicating the number of quarters since January 1, 2017, and $Q2$ through $Q4_t$ are binary indicators for calendar quarters 2 through 4, with quarter 1 as the reference. We include these quarterly indicators to account for well-documented seasonality in conceptions and pregnancy losses, which could confound observed changes over time.[21–23]

Using this model, we fit a linear equation to approximate the expected number of transfusions in each quarter. We extrapolated trends (i.e., expected trends) through 2023 based on the predictions from the model. We calculated residuals for each quarter by subtracting the expected number of transfusions from the observed values. To determine whether observed numbers of transfusions during the 6-week ban or total ban periods were significantly different from expected trends, we conducted a 2-sample t test on the residuals, comparing the mean residuals during these periods to the mean residual during the prebans period, which, by design, is zero. As a robustness check, we conducted a simulation-based prediction interval test using 1000 draws from the model's predictive distribution. Inference was consistent with the primary analysis, indicating that conclusions were not sensitive to modeling assumptions. We also repeated the analysis on the rate of transfusion per pregnancy loss visit in Appendix B (available as a supplement to the online version of this article at https://ajph.org).

We conducted the analysis in R version 4.4.1 (R Foundation for Statistical Computing, Vienna, Austria).

Sensitivity Analysis

Vaginal bleeding during pregnancy is seen in 15% to 25% of pregnancies and makes up 1.6% of emergency department visits in the United States.[24] This is commonly diagnosed as "threatened abortion," and the pregnancy may later end in spontaneous abortion. If the patient receives a diagnosis of spontaneous abortion in addition to the threatened abortion in the recorded encounter, the encounter is included in the primary analysis. However, some threatened abortion encounters are treated with pregnancy-ending care (e.g., procedural abortion or induction of labor) and do not receive a diagnosis of spontaneous abortion. These are the cases most likely to see a change in management practices after the implementation of abortion restrictions because there may still be fetal cardiac activity or another indicator that keeps the diagnosis as threatened rather than spontaneous abortion. Since the management of threatened abortion cases may change by withholding procedural care, we repeated the primary analysis considering pregnancy loss encounters and threatened abortion encounters as a sensitivity analysis. This approach is likely too broad and includes many encounters for pregnancies that continue to birth. Therefore, we conducted a second sensitivity analysis including all pregnancy loss cases and threatened abortion encounters that end in procedural abortion, induction of labor, hysterectomy, or extraction of products of conception. These cases of threatened abortion and pregnancy ending care are likely pregnancy losses. We cannot track medication management using misoprostol and mifepristone because the data contain only procedure codes.

Although complications from abortion (medically coded as induced terminations) are very rare, sometimes people seek care at hospitals after abortion, and 1 in 1000 abortion clients receives a blood transfusion.[25–27] Some encounters diagnosed as pregnancy losses could have been care needed after an induced abortion if the induction was not disclosed. This misclassification could be greater after restrictive policies because patients may be less likely to share that they had an abortion, and providers may be less likely to use the induced termination billing codes. Therefore, we conducted a third sensitivity analysis including codes for complications from induced termination (under O07: failed induced termination, and O04: complications following induced termination). See Appendix A for a complete list of codes used.

RESULTS

There were 320 696 pregnancy loss encounters in Texas facilities between January 1, 2017, and September 30, 2023. Table 1 presents the distribution of pregnancy loss encounters by patient age, patient race and ethnicity, payer, and type of pregnancy loss for each period. Most encounters were among patients aged 20 to 35 years

TABLE 1— Patient Characteristics of Pregnancy Loss Encounters: Texas Facilities, January 2017–September 2023

	Before Bans (n = 204 719), No. (%)	6-Week Ban (n = 42 739), No. (%)	Total Ban (n = 73 238), No. (%)	Overall (n = 320 696), No. (%)
Age group, y				
10–14	216 (0.1)	47 (0.1)	55 (0.1)	318 (0.1)
15–19	14 696 (7.2)	2 661 (6.2)	4 567 (6.2)	21 924 (6.8)
20–24	41 515 (20.3)	8 415 (19.7)	14 772 (20.2)	64 702 (20.2)
25–29	51 565 (25.2)	10 572 (24.7)	18 289 (25.0)	80 426 (25.1)
30–34	48 570 (23.7)	10 580 (24.8)	18 025 (24.6)	77 175 (24.1)
35–39	33 814 (16.5)	7 323 (17.1)	12 298 (16.8)	53 435 (16.7)
40–44	12 970 (6.3)	2 821 (6.6)	4 707 (6.4)	20 498 (6.4)
45–64	1 369 (0.7)	320 (0.7)	522 (0.7)	2 211 (0.7)
Missing	4 (0.0)	0 (0)	3 (0.0)	147 (0.0)
Race/ethnicity				
Hispanic	84 275 (41.2)	18 759 (43.9)	33 373 (45.6)	136 407 (42.5)
Non-Hispanic White	66 001 (32.2)	12 749 (29.8)	20 319 (27.7)	99 069 (30.9)
Non-Hispanic Black	32 032 (15.6)	7 118 (16.7)	12 597 (17.2)	51 747 (16.1)
Other and more than 1 race	15 753 (7.7)	2 609 (6.1)	4 370 (6.0)	22 732 (7.1)
Missing	6 658 (3.3)	1 504 (3.5)	2 579 (3.5)	10 741 (3.3)
Payer				
Private insurance or TRICARE	49 760 (24.3)	10 067 (23.6)	17 701 (24.3)	77 604 (24.2)
Medicaid	72 325 (35.3)	14 946 (35.0)	25 076 (34.2)	112 347 (35.0)
Charity, indigent, or unknown	39 407 (19.2)	7 996 (18.7)	13 202 (18.0)	60 605 (18.9)
Other	43 227 (21.1)	9 730 (22.8)	17 183 (23.5)	70 140 (21.9)
Type of pregnancy loss				
Spontaneous abortion	100 269 (49.0)	22 170 (51.9)	39 743 (54.3)	162 182 (50.6)
Missed abortion	55 919 (27.3)	10 455 (24.5)	15 837 (21.6)	82 211 (25.6)
Ectopic pregnancy	28 443 (13.9)	6 102 (14.3)	10 873 (14.8)	45 418 (14.2)
Intrauterine demise or stillbirth	12 910 (6.3)	2 745 (6.4)	4 609 (6.3)	20 264 (6.3)
Blighted ovum	5 695 (2.8)	1 029 (2.4)	1 635 (2.2)	8 359 (2.6)
PPROM first or second trimester	998 (0.5)	147 (0.3)	313 (0.4)	1 458 (0.4)
Hydatidiform molar pregnancy	485 (0.2)	91 (0.2)	228 (0.3)	804 (0.3)

Note. PPROM = preterm premature rupture of membranes. TRICARE is insurance provided by the military.

(69.4%). Medicaid was the most common payer (35.0%) and spontaneous and missed abortions were the most common diagnoses, making up 76.2% of encounters. In the entire period, 7408 pregnancy loss encounters received blood transfusions (or 2.31%).

Table 2 shows the observed and expected counts of transfusion in each period, and Figure 1 shows the quarterly number of transfusions among pregnancy loss encounters, along with expected values based on a model prediction. The model demonstrated a strong fit in the prebans period, with an R^2 of 0.86; this indicates that a high proportion of variance in transfusion counts in the prebans period is explained by the model. During this period, the number of transfusions among pregnancy loss encounters increased steadily, with an estimated slope of 2.3 additional transfusions per quarter. There was also evidence of seasonality, which was expected given that both pregnancy and spontaneous abortion exhibit seasonal patterns.[22,23]

The mean number of transfusions under the 6-week ban was not different from expected. Under the total ban, the mean number of blood transfusions was 385.8, which was 50.7 more transfusions (15.1%) than expected.

TABLE 2— Pregnancy Loss Visits and Blood Transfusions: Texas Facilities, January 2017–September 2023

Period[a]	Quarters	Pregnancy Loss Encounters	Blood Transfusions	Expected	Observed	Mean Residual	P[b]
Before bans	15	204 719	4 480	298.7	298.7	0.0	. . .
6-week ban	3	42 739	999	326.9	333.0	6.1	.79
Total ban	5	73 238	1 929	335.1	385.8	50.7	.03

[a]Before bans = January 2017 through September 2021, not including COVID-19 period, April 2020 through March 2021; 6-week ban = October 2021 through June 2022; total ban = July 2022 through September 2023.
[b]*P* value is with the 2-sample *t* test comparing the mean of period residuals to prebans residuals.

In a 2-sample *t* test comparing the residuals of the prebans and total ban periods, the mean residual of the total ban period was significantly greater (mean residuals = 0.0 vs 50.7; *P* = .03). Additional results on transfusion rates per 100 pregnancy loss encounters can be found in Appendix B. In brief, the mean rate of transfusions per encounter was also significantly greater than expected under the total ban (mean residuals = 0.00 vs 0.20; *P* = .03).

In the first sensitivity analysis, we included all threatened abortion visits. There were 299 589 encounters for threatened abortion in the study period, of which 212 received blood transfusions. Including these cases did not change the direction of the results or the significance of the findings (Table 3).

In the second sensitivity analysis, it was uncommon in Texas during the study period for encounters with a diagnosis of threatened abortion and no additional diagnosis of spontaneous abortion to receive an abortion procedure or induction of labor—only 137 cases in 5.75 years. Of these, 9 received blood transfusions during the encounter. This may reflect the practice of how cases are coded as well as medical care practices. The results including these cases are not different than the primary analysis.

In the third sensitivity analysis, 1096 visits for care following induced

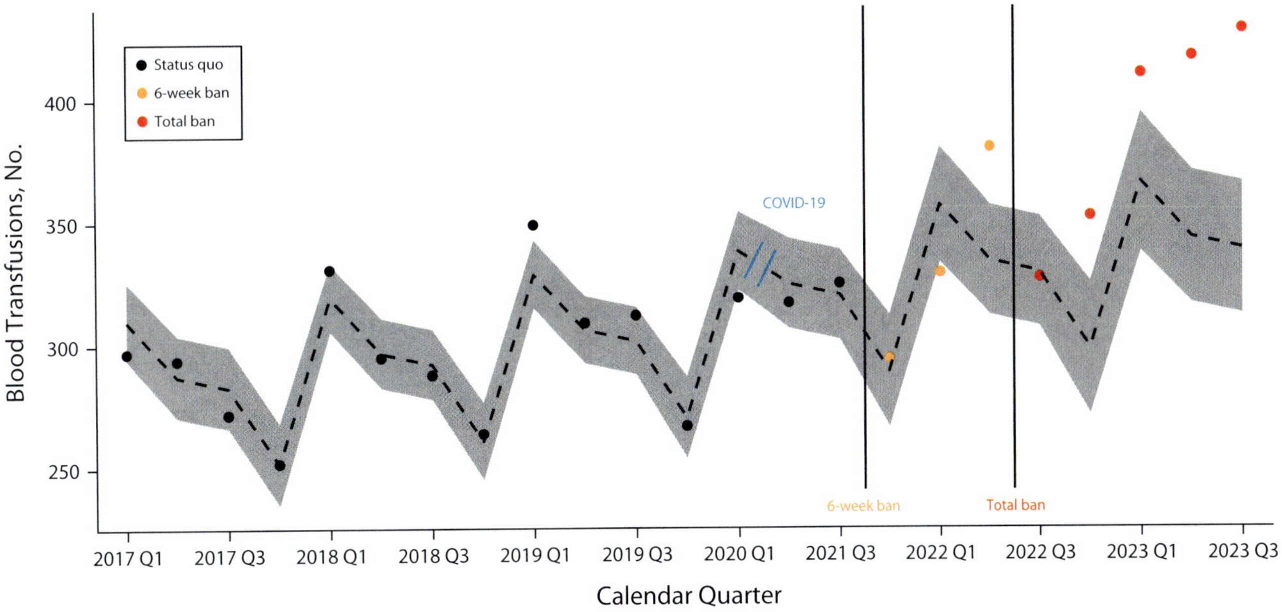

FIGURE 1— Number of Hospital and Facility Visits With Diagnosis of Pregnancy Loss and Blood Transfusion: Texas, January 2017–September 2023

Note. Q = quarter. Figure 1 illustrates the number of blood transfusions to eligible encounters and the expected number of transfusions in Texas over time. The dashed line, representing the expected number of transfusions, was estimated from a regression model using 2017 to September 2021 data, not including the COVID-19 period of April 2020 through March 2021. The shaded region represents the 95% confidence interval for the expected number of transfusions. Individual points represent observed quarterly transfusion counts.

TABLE 3— Sensitivity Analyses Including All and Some Threatened Abortion Encounters: Texas Facilities, January 2017–September 2023

Data Treatment	Encounters	Transfusions	Difference From Primary Analysis	Residual No. Transfusions *Dobbs* Period	P^a
Only encounters with pregnancy loss diagnosis	320 696	7 408	Primary analysis	50.7	.03
Primary analysis + encounters with threatened abortion cases	620 285	7 620	299 589 encounters 212 transfusions	61.7	.02
Primary analysis + encounters with threatened abortion code and procedure that would end a pregnancy	320 832	7 417	136 encounters 9 transfusions	50.9	.03
Primary analysis + encounters for complications following induced terminations	321 792	7 488	1 096 encounters 80 transfusions	47.8	.04

[a]*P* value derived from *t* test comparing number of transfusions.

terminations of pregnancy. Of these, 80 received blood transfusions. Including these cases did not change the results. This demonstrates that the primary results are not explained by differential coding of care following induced abortions.

DISCUSSION

Among patients presenting at Texas hospital, emergency, and ambulatory surgical facilities diagnosed with pregnancy loss, blood transfusions increased above expected trends during Texas's total abortion ban that followed the *Dobbs* decision, but not during the 6-week ban period. Delays in and denials of care may have contributed to this increased severe morbidity.[6,7]

We were not able to test mechanisms behind the greater than expected blood transfusions or identify why we saw changes after the total ban after *Dobbs* and not after the 6-week ban of SB8. However, the specifics of the policies point to 2 factors that may be responsible: difference in enforcement mechanisms and difference in diagnostic information required. The potential punishment for providing a restricted abortion under SB8 was a $10 000 fine in civil court initiated by a lawsuit.[28] This is less severe than the penalties under the total ban, which include criminal charges, significant jail time, and a $100 000 fine.[29]

Second, the abortion ban at all gestations (total ban) and the ban after detection of cardiac activity (6-week ban) require different amounts of diagnostic information before providers can provide pregnancy loss care. Under the 6-week ban, providers could legally intervene in pregnancy loss cases when no cardiac activity was detected. The total ban, by contrast, requires documentation of both gestational duration and absence of cardiac activity to determine that the pregnancy is not viable (e.g., a pregnancy with no cardiac activity at five weeks is typical, compared with a pregnancy with no cardiac activity at 11 weeks). This potentially introduces additional hurdles, especially in urgent or ambiguous clinical scenarios.[30]

Limitations and Strengths

Study limitations included the inability to capture pregnancy losses in other settings, such as private doctors' offices. However, most cases of severe morbidity related to pregnancy loss would receive treatment at an included facility. Another limitation is the use of a prepost design without comparison states; data availability and cost constraints make it challenging to use comparable data from other states. A challenge of this design is that other changes in the period could influence the outcome. However, we are not aware of coding or care changes related to blood transfusion in this period, and we have removed the quarters most impacted by COVID-19 to ensure they did not affect inferences. We were also unable to link encounters together for individuals who have more than 1 visit for a single pregnancy loss. Accordingly, we used pregnancy loss encounter as the unit of analysis and were not able to measure rates of blood transfusion per pregnancy loss. Sensitivity analyses showed that the findings were robust to inclusion of other codes related to pregnancy loss and codes for care after induced terminations. In addition, there was no evidence that abortion safety or efficacy changed during the study period[26,31] or that abortion counts among Texans changed greatly.[32] A limitation of the modeling is the quarterly nature of the data, which provides fewer data points to model the expected number of transfusions than monthly or weekly data would provide.

Finally, this analysis relied on coding generated for billing purposes and not primarily for research. There can be errors and subjectivity in billing codes. We relied on diagnoses of pregnancy loss to identify cases and may have missed cases that were provided procedural or medication management of pregnancy loss, but a diagnosis of pregnancy loss was not recorded (on purpose or in error). In this way, we took a conservative approach to sample identification because cases where pregnancy viability (loss status) was ambiguous were the cases most likely to be affected by abortion bans. An additional challenge posed by the billing codes was that coding of symptoms as related to pregnancy loss versus induced termination relied on disclosure from the patient. Although serious complications from abortion are rare,[25,26] it is likely that some patients who sought care after having an abortion did not disclose the abortion, and these visits were classified as pregnancy loss visits. Care for complications from induced abortion may also have been delayed or denied because of abortion restrictions or patient fear of abortion restrictions,[6] potentially resulting in higher morbidity. Changes in care for induced terminations may have contributed to the increase in transfusions measured here.

Strengths of this study included having data from all payers and hospital systems in a large state. The data also included many years, allowing us to use 15 observations before SB8 from which to model prebans trends. This also allowed us to avoid using the year directly before as a comparison group, as is common when researching change from policy shocks. In this case, comparison with the previous year would be a problem because the COVID-19 pandemic made the previous year unusual. This has obscured maternal morbidity changes in other studies.[33]

Public Health Implications

Overall, these findings suggest that Texas's abortion ban may contribute to increased severe morbidity among Texans experiencing pregnancy loss, resulting in additional short- and long-term health consequences for women and increased costs to families and health systems. Many women are at increased risk for severe morbidity, as 100 000 early pregnancy losses (miscarriages) occur annually in Texas,[34] in addition to ectopic pregnancies and stillbirths. Furthermore, these findings have national implications as more than 1 million pregnancy losses occur annually in the United States,[34] and the policy environment in Texas is not unique. As of June 2025, 11 other states banned abortion at any gestational duration.[12] Our findings also reinforce earlier studies showing that timely, evidence-based pregnancy loss care is essential to health and that denial or delays in care have serious health consequences. For example, a recent analysis of inpatient hospitalizations in Texas for second-trimester pregnancy losses found that sepsis rates rose 50% in 2022.[35]

This is one of the first peer-reviewed studies to quantitatively measure changes in pregnancy loss health after *Dobbs v Jackson Women's Health Organization*. Qualitative research has found that patient factors (e.g., waiting to present for care out of fear of criminalization or expectation of poor-quality care) and care provision factors (e.g., withholding care because of fetal cardiac tones or the perception that procedural care is never legal) are extant.[6] More qualitative and quantitative research is needed to determine how these factors may contribute to this increase in need for blood transfusion and other severe morbidities. AJPH

ABOUT THE AUTHORS

Amanda Nagle is with the Population Research Center at the University of Texas at Austin. Goleen Samari is with the Department of Population and Public Health Sciences in the Keck School of Medicine of the University of Southern California, Los Angeles. Lauren Thaxton is with the Department of Obstetrics and Gynecology at the University of Colorado Anschutz Medical Campus, Aurora. Alison Gemmill is with the Department of Population, Family and Reproductive Health at Johns Hopkins Bloomberg School of Public Health, Baltimore, MD.

CORRESPONDENCE

Correspondence should be sent to Amanda Nagle, 305 E 23rd St, Austin, TX 78712 (e-mail: anagle@utexas.edu). Reprints can be ordered at https://www.ajph.org by clicking the "Reprints" link.

PUBLICATION INFORMATION

Full Citation: Nagle A, Samari G, Thaxton L, Gemmill A. Blood transfusions for pregnancy loss in Texas before and after abortion bans, 2017–2023. *Am J Public Health*. 2025;115(11): 1887–1894.

Acceptance Date: June 16, 2025.

DOI: https://doi.org/10.2105/AJPH.2025.308224

ORCID iDs:

Amanda Nagle https://orcid.org/0000-0003-3646-9903

Goleen Samari https://orcid.org/0000-0002-9506-3586

Lauren Thaxton https://orcid.org/0000-0002-1368-0709

Alison Gemmill https://orcid.org/0000-0001-5879-9730

CONTRIBUTORS

A. Nagle conceptualized the research question, curated the data, conducted data analysis, and wrote the initial draft. G. Samari advised on statistical methodology and edited the article. L. Thaxton provided methodological expertise on medical coding, conditions, and treatment. A. Gemmill contributed to statistical analysis and interpretation and critically reviewed the article for substantive content.

ACKNOWLEDGMENTS

This research was supported by grants P2CHD042849 (Population Research Center at The University of Texas at Austin), T32HD007081

(Training Program in Population Studies awarded to the Population Research Center at The University of Texas at Austin), P2CHD042854 (Hopkins Population Center), and R01HD114292, all from the Eunice Kennedy Shriver National Institute of Child Health and Human Development.

The authors thank Diane Coffey, PhD, for providing feedback on drafts of this article.

CONFLICTS OF INTEREST

The authors have no conflicts of interest to disclose.

HUMAN PARTICIPANT PROTECTION

This secondary data analysis was designated as not human participant research by The University of Texas at Austin institutional review board.

REFERENCES

1. Rossen LM, Ahrens KA, Branum AM. Trends in risk of pregnancy loss among US women, 1990–2011. *Paediatr Perinat Epidemiol.* 2018; 32(1):19–29. https://doi.org/10.1111/ppe.12417
2. Freedman LR, Landy U, Steinauer J. When there's a heartbeat: miscarriage management in Catholic-owned hospitals. *Am J Public Health.* 2008;98(10):1774–1778. https://doi.org/10.2105/AJPH.2007.126730
3. Nanda K, Lopez LM, Grimes DA, Peloggia A, Nanda G. Expectant care versus surgical treatment for miscarriage. Cochrane Pregnancy and Childbirth Group. *Cochrane Database Syst Rev.* 2012;2012(3):CD003518. https://doi.org/10.1002/14651858.CD003518.pub3
4. Saraiya M, Green CA, Berg CJ, Hopkins FW, Koonin LM, Atrash HK. Spontaneous abortion–related deaths among women in the United States—1981–1991. *Obstet Gynecol.* 1999;94(2): 172–176. https://doi.org/10.1016/S0029-7844(99)00280-X
5. Sabbath EL, McKetchnie SM, Arora KS, Buchbinder M. US obstetrician-gynecologists' perceived impacts of post–*Dobbs v Jackson* state abortion bans. *JAMA Netw Open.* 2024;7(1):e2352109. https://doi.org/10.1001/jamanetworkopen.2023.52109
6. Grossman D, Joffe C, Kaller S, et al. Care post-*Roe*: documenting cases of poor-quality care since the *Dobbs* decision. September 2024. Advancing New Standards in Reproductive Health; Texas Policy Evaluation Project. Available at: https://www.ansirh.org/sites/default/files/2023-05/Care%20Post-Roe%20Preliminary%20Findings.pdf. Accessed December 10, 2024.
7. Nambiar A, Patel S, Santiago-Munoz P, Spong CY, Nelson DB. Maternal morbidity and fetal outcomes among pregnant women at 22 weeks' gestation or less with complications in 2 Texas hospitals after legislation on abortion. *Am J Obstet Gynecol.* 2022;227(4):648–650.e1. https://doi.org/10.1016/j.ajog.2022.06.060
8. American College of Obstetricians and Gynecologists. Early pregnancy loss. *Practice Bulletin.* 2018;(200). Available at: https://www.acog.org/clinical/clinical-guidance/practice-bulletin/articles/2018/11/early-pregnancy-loss. Accessed September 28, 2023.
9. Weigel G, Sobel L, Salganicoff A. Understanding pregnancy loss in the context of abortion restrictions and fetal harm laws. KFF. December 4, 2019. Available at: https://www.supremecourt.gov/opinions/URLs_Cited/OT2021/19-1392/19-1392-12.pdf. Accessed August 22, 2025.
10. Nandi P, Roncari DM, Werner EF, Gilbert AL, Ramos SZ. Navigating miscarriage management post-*Dobbs*: health risks and ethical dilemmas. *Womens Health Issues.* 2024;34(5):449–454. https://doi.org/10.1016/j.whi.2024.05.004
11. Upadhyay UD, Coplon L, Atrio JM, Villalonga M; on behalf of the Society of Family Planning Clinical Affairs Committee. Society of Family Planning Committee Statement: Abortion nomenclature. *Contraception.* 2023;126:110094. https://doi.org/10.1016/j.contraception.2023.110094
12. Guttmacher Institute. Interactive map: US abortion policies and access after *Roe*. September 3, 2025. Available at: https://states.guttmacher.org/policies. Accessed November 7, 2023.
13. Texas State Law Library. History of abortion laws. Available at: https://guides.sll.texas.gov/abortion-laws/history-of-abortion-laws. Accessed August 7, 2024.
14. Arey W, Lerma K, Carpenter E, et al. Abortion access and medically complex pregnancies before and after Texas Senate Bill 8. *Obstet Gynecol.* 2023;141(5):995–1003. https://doi.org/10.1097/AOG.0000000000005153
15. Texas Department of State Health Services. Health data researcher information. Available at: https://www.dshs.texas.gov/center-health-statistics/texas-health-care-information-collection. Accessed August 22, 2025.
16. Reproductive Health Access Project. Coding for miscarriage care (early pregnancy loss). 2024. Available at: https://www.reproductiveaccess.org/resource/coding-epl. Accessed August 23, 2024.
17. Alliance for Innovation on Maternal Health. Severe maternal morbidity. Severe maternal morbidity code list. April 2023. Available at: https://saferbirth.org/severe-maternal-morbidity. Accessed April 22, 2025.
18. Codify by AAPC. CPT 36430, under venipucture and transfusion procedures. Available at: https://www.aapc.com/codes/cpt-codes/36430?srsltid=AfmBOopqapGLDQJjf63CmzGX-Eg3Tqnc-mAyxhI1zyt0bg2Euo0Zumqs. Accessed December 10, 2024.
19. Stout MJ, Van De Ven CJM, Parekh VI, et al. Use of electronic medical records to estimate changes in pregnancy and birth rates during the COVID-19 pandemic. *JAMA Netw Open.* 2021;4(6): e2111621. https://doi.org/10.1001/jamanetworkopen.2021.11621
20. Kotlar B, Gerson EM, Petrillo S, Langer A, Tiemeier H. The impact of the COVID-19 pandemic on maternal and perinatal health: a scoping review. *Reprod Health.* 2021;18(1):10–39. https://doi.org/10.1186/s12978-021-01070-6
21. Gemmill A, Casey JA, Margerison CE, Zeitlin J, Catalano R, Bruckner TA. Patterned outcomes, unpatterned counterfactuals, and spurious results: perinatal health outcomes following COVID-19. *Am J Epidemiol.* 2022;191(11): 1837–1841. https://doi.org/10.1093/aje/kwac110
22. Wesselink AK, Wise LA, Hatch EE, et al. A prospective cohort study of seasonal variation in spontaneous abortion. *Epidemiology.* 2022; 33(3):441–448. https://doi.org/10.1097/EDE.0000000000001474
23. Wesselink AK, Wise LA, Hatch EE, et al. Seasonal patterns in fecundability in North America and Denmark: a preconception cohort study. *Hum Reprod.* 2020;35(3):565–572. https://doi.org/10.1093/humrep/dez265
24. Wittels KA, Pelletier AJ, Brown DFM, Camargo CA. United States emergency department visits for vaginal bleeding during early pregnancy, 1993-2003. *Am J Obstet Gynecol.* 2008;198(5): 523.e1–523.e6. https://doi.org/10.1016/j.ajog.2007.11.011
25. Upadhyay UD, Desai S, Zlidar V, et al. Incidence of emergency department visits and complications after abortion. *Obstet Gynecol.* 2015;125(1): 175–183. https://doi.org/10.1097/AOG.0000000000000603
26. Upadhyay UD, Koenig LR, Meckstroth K, Ko J, Valladares ES, Biggs MA. Effectiveness and safety of telehealth medication abortion in the USA. *Nat Med.* 2024;30(4):1191–1198. https://doi.org/10.1038/s41591-024-02834-w
27. Schummers L, Darling EK, Dunn S, et al. Abortion safety and use with normally prescribed mifepristone in Canada. *N Engl J Med.* 2022;386(1): 57–67. https://doi.org/10.1056/NEJMsa2109779
28. Bohra N. Texas law banning abortion as early as six weeks goes into effect as the US Supreme Court takes no action. *The Texas Tribune.* August 31, 2021. Available at: https://www.texastribune.org/2021/08/31/texas-abortion-law-supreme-court. Accessed November 8, 2023.
29. Klibanoff E. Texans who perform abortions now face up to life in prison, $100,000 fine. *The Texas Tribune.* August 25, 2022. Available at: https://www.texastribune.org/2022/08/25/texas-trigger-law-abortion. Accessed November 8, 2023.
30. Presser L, Surana K. A third woman has died under Texas' abortion ban as doctors reach for riskier miscarriage treatments. *The Texas Tribune.* November 27, 2024. Available at: https://www.texastribune.org/2024/11/27/texas-abortion-death-porsha-ngumezi. Accessed March 25, 2025.
31. Aiken ARA, Romanova EP, Morber JR, Gomperts R. Safety and effectiveness of self-managed medication abortion provided using online telemedicine in the United States: a population based study. *Lancet Reg Health Am.* 2022;10:100200. https://doi.org/10.1016/j.lana.2022.100200
32. Society of Family Planning. #WeCount Report April 2022 through June 2024. October 22, 2024. https://doi.org/10.46621/728122kflzwf. Accessed December 10, 2024.
33. Stevenson AJ. The pregnancy-related mortality impact of a total abortion ban in the United States: a research note on increased deaths due to remaining pregnant. *Demography.* 2021;58(6): 2019–2028. https://doi.org/10.1215/00703370-9585908
34. Nobles J, Hwang S, Bennett E, Jacques L. Abortion restrictions threaten miscarriage management in the United States. *Health Aff (Millwood).* 2024; 43(9):1219–1224. https://doi.org/10.1377/hlthaff.2023.00982
35. Presser L, Suozzo A, Chou S, Surana K. Texas banned abortion. Then sepsis rates soared. ProPublica. February 20, 2025. Available at: https://www.propublica.org/article/texas-abortion-ban-sepsis-maternal-mortality-analysis. Accessed April 22, 2025.

Abortion Restrictions and Infant Mortality in the United States, 2018–2023

Michaela R. Anderson, MD, Gordon Burtch, PhD, and Brad N. Greenwood, PhD

Objectives. To evaluate the impact of state-level abortion restrictions enacted between 2018 and 2023 on infant mortality in the United States, comparing mortality trends across restricting and nonrestricting states.

Methods. Using a difference-in-differences approach, we drew infant mortality data from the Centers for Disease Control and Prevention's WONDER (Wide-ranging Online Data for Epidemiologic Research) database and categorized deaths by age and cause, incorporating information on abortion restrictions and legal exceptions from the Center for Reproductive Rights and the Kaiser Family Foundation. We calculated estimates at the state-year level.

Results. Infant mortality increased by 7.2% in restricting states. The increase is predominantly attributable to early (aged < 1 day) and late (aged 1 month to 1 year) infant deaths. Effects were largest for perinatal and noncongenital causes of death. Health exceptions did not significantly moderate the effects.

Conclusions. Curtailing abortion access increases infant deaths. Fetal and maternal health exceptions do not moderate this effect. Excess deaths are not exclusively attributable to congenital abnormalities. Further work is needed to understand how restrictions contribute to late deaths and the long-term effects of infant deaths on families and communities. (*Am J Public Health*. 2025;115(11):1895–1902. https://doi.org/10.2105/AJPH.2025.308228)

AJPH November 2025, Vol. 115, No. 11

In June 2022, the US Supreme Court's holding in *Dobbs v Jackson Women's Health Organization* (hereafter *Dobbs*)[1] foundationally changed abortion access in the United States by returning control of abortion to state legislatures. As of November 2024, 21 states have introduced new restrictions on abortion, including more stringent gestational limitations and outright bans.[2,3] Such restrictions have subsequently been linked to reduced trust in clinicians,[4] increased mental distress,[5,6] increased cost and distance of travel to obtain an abortion,[7] and increased foster care placements.[8]

Before *Dobbs* was decided, researchers documented an increase in Texas's infant mortality rate following the passage of Senate Bill 8 (SB-8), also known as the Texas Heartbeat Act.[9] Based on a study of nearly 100 000 infant deaths and 28 comparison states, Gemmill et al.[9] found an approximately 12% increase in rates of infant and neonatal mortality. Yet, our understanding of whether similar effects manifest in states that enacted abortion restrictions after *Dobbs* was decided[1] is still emerging,[10] and the degree to which such effects vary with states' incorporation of legal exceptions (e.g., for maternal health or fetal abnormality) is unknown. We addressed these gaps, investigating whether restrictions on abortion access have yielded a national increase in infant mortality and whether such effects are attenuated by legal exceptions.

It is plausible that these effects will extend beyond Texas. If the newly implemented restrictions create barriers to abortion access, through either increased travel costs or lost wages,[7] then infant mortality could reasonably be expected to increase. This could stem from either (1) the continuation of pregnancies with congenital issues because those children are less likely to survive outside the womb, or (2) the restriction compelling women without the resources or ability to care for a child to carry a fetus to term.[11] However, SB-8 differs from the legislation enacted in other states in material ways. Specifically, SB-8 contains both limited exceptions for maternal health and life-limiting fetal anomalies and creates penalties for anyone aiding a woman in securing an abortion (e.g., physicians, cab drivers),[12] raising the possibility that SB-8 may have a unique impact on infant mortality. Thus, it is possible that the observed effects might not generalize to other states, a notion consistent with recent research finding that abortion rates have increased since *Dobbs* was decided.[13]

METHODS

We designed a population-based observational study to evaluate the impact of newly implemented abortion restrictions on infant mortality across US states.

Data

Consistent with previous work, we measured the effect of abortion restrictions on infant mortality using data from the Centers for Disease Control and Prevention's WONDER (Wide-ranging Online Data for Epidemiologic Research) database.[9] The Centers for Disease Control and Prevention (CDC) compiles data on every death in the United States based on death certificates. For our analyses, we collected annual data on infant deaths (children aged < 1 year) for all 50 states and the District of Columbia. The sample spans 2018 to 2023. We began the sample in 2018 to avoid integration challenges associated with administrative updates to WONDER. The resulting panel contained a balanced window of observations (i.e., each location was observed the same number of times) around the newly instituted abortion restrictions, the bulk of which occurred between June and September 2022.

We also collected state-year counts of death from WONDER among 4 mutually exclusive groups based on age at time of death: infants younger than 1 day, infants aged 1 to 7 days, infants aged 7 to 28 days, and infants aged 28 days to 1 year.[14] Furthermore, we collected data on deaths among older children (aged 1 or 2 years), and state-year counts of infant deaths by cause of death, focusing in particular on the distinction between deaths from perinatal (*International Classification of Diseases, 10th Revision*, Geneva, Switzerland: World Health Organization; 1992; [*ICD-10*] codes P00–P96), congenital (*ICD-10* codes Q00–Q99), and all other causes.

Importantly, our analysis focused on a state-year panel because the CDC suppresses counts in geographies and time periods when between 1 and 9 deaths occurred. Total infant deaths per year always exceeds this threshold, but this is not the case for monthly counts in some states, particularly deaths among infants in narrower age ranges or deaths from specific causes. To ensure robustness, we examined monthly panels as well, in which we observed consistent effects. We also collected data on annual state births from the CDC's National Vital Statistics System to enable birth-adjusted estimations, for which we set the number of births as exposure, which is empirically equivalent to including the number of births as an offset. The CDC records data on all US births based on birth certificates.

We combined these panels with information on the timing of new abortion restrictions based on data from the Center for Reproductive Rights.[2] We focused on a joint indicator of bans or gestational limits not permitted under *Roe v Wade*.[15] A treatment schedule is provided in Appendix Figure A (available as a supplement to the online version of this article at http://www.ajph.org). Summary statistics are in Appendix Table A. Note that our analysis does not consider restrictions enjoined by courts at the time of our analysis.

Statistical Analysis

To identify the effect of abortion restrictions on infant deaths, we used a difference-in-differences approach, exploiting the staggered implementation of restrictions across states over time.[16] We cast states that instituted a new abortion restriction as treated as of the period when the restriction was introduced. Using this treatment, as seen in Equation 1, we report a series of estimations leveraging various outcomes. To ensure robustness, we used a variety of estimators (both linear and Poisson regression). All estimations included state and year fixed effects.

$$Deaths^{\rho}_{s,t} \sim Abortion\ Ban_{s,t} + \delta_s + \tau_t \quad (1)$$

Here, *Deaths* refers to the outcomes of interest, indexed by ρ (i.e., deaths in general, deaths among certain age groups, or deaths from certain causes). We repeated the estimations for each outcome. The subscripts s and t index states and years. *Abortion Ban* is a binary indicator of treatment, reflecting the implementation of either an outright ban or a gestational limit; δ indexes the state fixed effects; and τ indexes the year fixed effects. In all estimations, we clustered SEs by state.[17] It should be noted that alternative model specifications (e.g., state-specific linear trends) consistently achieved lower scores on both the Akaike and Bayesian information criteria.

We also assessed any heterogeneity in the effect that may arise from legal exceptions to new restrictions, specifically health exceptions for the mother (health exception) and those involving lethal fetal abnormality (fetal exception), as compiled by the Kaiser Family Foundation. We introduced binary indicators, which indicate an exception in a state's law. We incorporated the moderating effect of these exceptions by interacting them with the treatment indicator (i.e., abortion ban).

As noted, we employed multiple estimators. Consistent with previous work, our primary regressions were based on a Poisson pseudomaximum likelihood estimator (i.e., a nonlinear difference-in-differences estimation), wherein we modeled the death outcomes as an exponential function of treatment.[18] Recent work indicates that a Poisson estimator is preferable to a linear regression that accounts for the exponential relationship via a log transformation of the dependent variable, particularly when confronted with many zeros, because the log-linear approach can result in estimation bias and yields estimates that depend on the scale of the outcome.[19]

Additionally, in deference to recent work documenting biases that can occur when treatments are staggered in time and space,[20] we repeated our estimations using the Gardner[21] 2-stage difference-in-differences estimator. We also used the extended form Poisson difference-in-differences estimator proposed by Wooldridge,[22] which also permits a robust estimation in the presence of staggered treatments. These estimates are presented in Appendix Figures C and F.

Next, although it was not our primary outcome of interest, we estimated the effect of abortion restrictions on births. We report estimates of the effect employing Poisson regression and 2-stage difference-in-differences in Appendix Table B and a visual depiction of the 2-stage difference-in-differences over time in Appendix Figure B. Finally, we report estimates of the effect of abortion restrictions on infant deaths, incorporating an adjustment for births (Appendix Table C).

We conducted the statistical analyses using R version 4.4.3 (RStudio, Boston, MA). All data and code used in these analyses are publicly available at CodeOcean (http://bit.ly/46oj9Ve).

RESULTS

Average marginal effect estimates based on our Poisson regressions and the 2-stage difference-in-differences results are shown in Table 1. Consistent findings emerged. Specifically, we observed a significant increase in total deaths per state-year that occurred in the first year of life. The Poisson estimation indicated an average 7.2% increase ($P<.001$) in infant deaths or 29.8 additional infant deaths per state-year. The 2-stage difference-in-differences estimates were similar, indicating 30.6 additional infant deaths ($P<.05$) per state-year. These results persisted when we adjusted for the number of births via an exposure term in the Poisson regression (Appendix Table C), where we estimated a 3.6% increase in the rate of infant death ($P<.05$). Further, using state-month panels (Appendix Table D), we estimated a 6.2% increase in infant deaths or 2.1 additional infant deaths per state-month ($P<.001$). Results were largely consistent when we considered bans and gestational limits separately.

Turning to the effects on infant death by age range, the Poisson estimates indicated a significant 6.5% increase ($P<.05$) in deaths of infants younger than 1 day, or approximately 10

TABLE 1— Average Effect of Abortion Restrictions on Count of Infant Deaths by Age at Death: United States, 2018–2023

	Deaths, <1 y, No. of Deaths (SE)	Deaths, <1 d, No. of Deaths (SE)	Deaths, 1–7 d, No. of Deaths (SE)	Deaths, 8–28 d, No. of Deaths (SE)	Deaths, 29–365 d, No. of Deaths (SE)	Deaths, 1 y	Deaths, 2 y
Poisson MFX	29.75*** (8.58)	9.90* (4.99)	2.04 (2.19)	2.63 (2.34)	13.35*** (3.86)	−2.56 (1.43)	−0.41 (0.95)
DID-2S[a]	30.80* (13.22)	6.70 (5.12)	3.04 (2.61)	4.78 (3.47)	15.89* (6.38)	−1.33 (1.69)	0.71 (1.21)

Note. DID-2S = 2-stage difference-in-differences regression; MFX = Poisson average marginal effects. n = 306 state-years. SEs are clustered by state.
[a]For the 2-stage difference-in-differences estimates, we used the method of Gardner.[21]
*$P<.05$; **$P<.01$; ***$P<.001$.

additional deaths per state-year. This estimate was comparable to the 2-stage difference-in-differences estimate, although that estimate was statistically insignificant. Neither estimation approach indicated a significant increase in deaths of infants aged 1 day through 1 week or infants aged 1 week through 1 month. However, both estimations indicated the largest and most statistically significant effect for infants aged 1 month to 1 year (an estimated 9.3% increase; $P < .001$).

Robustness Checks

We considered the effect of new abortion restrictions on the deaths of children aged 1 or 2 years to be placebo outcomes (Table 1). If the effect was causal, we would not expect to see an effect on the deaths of these children because the newly enacted abortion restrictions would not have been in place at the time of the child's birth. As anticipated, we observed no statistically significant effects on either outcome.

Next, we estimated an event study specification to examine posttreatment dynamics. This also allowed us to assess the presence of any pretreatment differences across treatment and control states, which would undermine the validity of the parallel trends assumption. Results using the 2-stage estimator are in Figure 1 for all outcome measures and indicate that the differences generally did not manifest until after the institution of a new abortion restriction. Furthermore, we saw an increase in total infant deaths from the first year to the second year after introducing a new restriction.

Secondary Analysis

The fact that larger effects manifested for infants older than 28 days required additional scrutiny. Accordingly, we assessed the extent to which the increase in infant deaths was attributable to deaths from causes other than issues arising during the perinatal period or congenital abnormality. We separately estimated the effect of new abortion restrictions on the number of infant deaths that occurred because of

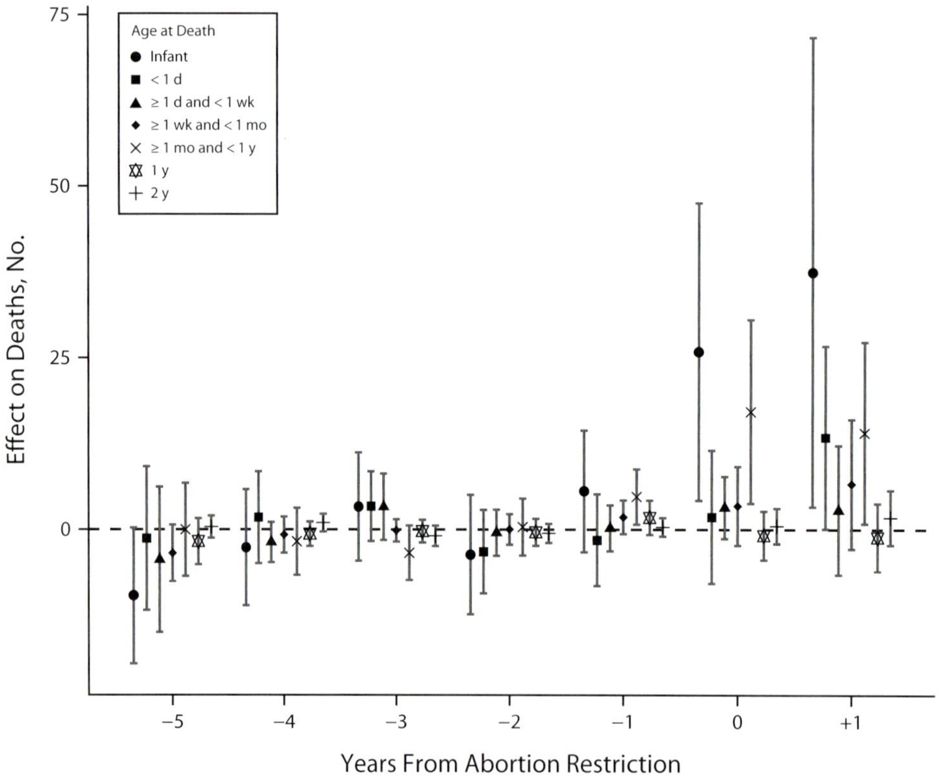

FIGURE 1— Difference-in-Differences Estimates of the Effect of State Abortion Restrictions on Infant and Early Childhood Deaths, by Age Group (0–2 Years), Relative to the Year of Restriction Enactment: United States, 2018–2023

Note. Error bars reflect 95% confidence intervals based on SEs clustered by state. "Infant" refers collectively to deaths among all infants aged < 1 year (the aggregation of all age categories < 1 year). Year 0 reflects a state's first calendar year in which a new abortion restriction was adopted, implying the first year is "partially" treated. Estimates used the 2-stage difference-in-differences estimator (Gardner[21]).

3 mutually exclusive and collectively exhaustive groups: (1) perinatal causes (i.e., deaths originating from issues in the fetal or perinatal period and up to 28 days from birth; *ICD-10* codes P00–P96), including conditions arising from maternal factors, birth trauma, and respiratory or cardiovascular diseases; (2) congenital causes (*ICD-10* codes Q00–Q99), including deaths from malformations, deformations, and chromosomal abnormalities (i.e., a subset of nonperinatal causes); and (3) other causes (all other *ICD-10* codes; Table 2). We estimated these relationships using Poisson regressions, and we report average marginal effects, reflecting effects in terms of the count of deaths of each type. Results using the 2-stage difference-in-differences estimator were generally consistent.

Results indicated that new abortion restrictions resulted in an increase of approximately 10.6 additional deaths owing to nonperinatal, noncongenital causes ($P < .01$), an 8.3% increase. This value was roughly equivalent to the estimated 11.6 additional deaths arising from perinatal causes ($P < .01$), an approximate 5.8% increase per state-year. Notably, the estimated increases in deaths among the 3 mutually exclusive groupings were not statistically distinguishable from one another (based on the pairwise z test, which yielded $P > .10$ in every case).

We also explored heterogeneity in the effect based on whether exceptions were allowed for fetal anomaly or the health of the mother. If such exceptions were meaningful, we should have seen a diminished effect in states that had such exceptions. Results are shown in Table 3 and continue to indicate a significant deleterious effect of new abortion restrictions on infant death. However, although we observed a negative point estimate for each exception dummy, neither was statistically significant.

Additional Robustness Checks

Beyond the earlier reported placebo and the event study estimations, we established the robustness of our findings in several ways. In Appendix Figure C, we demonstrate the robustness of our results to an additional estimator, reporting event study estimates associated with the extended form of Poisson 2-way fixed effect regression. We also repeated our analyses employing monthly panels. The monthly treatment schedule by state is depicted in Appendix Figure D. Results of an event study specification for the effect on total infant deaths are reported graphically in Appendix Figure E, based on the 2-stage difference-in-differences estimation, and in Appendix Figure F, based on the extended form of the Poisson estimation with 2-way fixed effects. In each case, we observed consistent results.

Finally, the impact of missingness in our sample is noteworthy. Recall that the CDC suppresses reports of death counts when the values fall between 1 and 9 for any given combination of observation characteristics (e.g., geography, time, cause). That is, the CDC reports a count only for values of 0 and values of 10 or more. This issue of value suppression has relatively little impact on the state-year panels. For example, we have just 1 suppressed value in the case of total infant deaths per state-year: Vermont in 2023. The issue became more pronounced when we began to split the death outcome by infant age range. From our panel of 306 state-year observations, we had 9 suppressed values for the count of deaths among infants aged 1 month through 365 days, 11 suppressed values for the count of deaths among infants younger than 1 day, 40 suppressed values for the count of deaths among infants aged 1 through 7 days, and 50 suppressed values for the count of deaths among infants aged 8 through 28 days. For these analyses, we imputed a random integer value between 1 and 9 to populate suppressed records and observed consistent results on repeated random imputation of the values. Furthermore, we observed consistent results omitting these observations and omitting the affected states from our

TABLE 2— Average Effect of Abortion Restrictions on Count of Infant Deaths by Cause of Death: United States, 2018–2023

Cause of Death	Poisson Average Marginal Effects, No. of Deaths (SE)
Perinatal[a]	11.64** (4.12)
Congenital[b]	7.44 (4.43)
Other[c]	10.57** (3.86)

Note. n = 306 state-years. SEs are clustered by state. Each row reflects a separate regression model (models were not estimated jointly).
[a]Perinatal causes include *International Classification of Diseases, 10th Revision* ([*ICD-10*] Geneva, Switzerland: World Health Organization; 1992) codes P00–P96.
[b]Congenital causes include *ICD-10* codes Q00–Q99.
[c]Other causes include all other *ICD-10* codes (mutually exclusive and collectively exhaustive).
*$P < .05$; **$P < .01$; ***$P < .001$.

TABLE 3— Average Effect of Abortion Restrictions on Count of Infant Deaths as Moderated by Legal Exception: United States, 2018–2023

	Fetal Exception,[a] Estimated Change in Infant Deaths (SE)	Health Exception,[b] Estimated Change in Infant Deaths (SE)
Abortion Ban	31.08* (12.10)	39.13** (15.12)
Abortion Ban × Fetal Exception[a]	−3.25 (12.19)	
Abortion Ban × Health Exception[b]		−13.54 (14.26)

Note. n = 306 state-years. SEs are clustered by state. Columns reflect a separate regression model (models were not estimated jointly). Rows referring to A × B indicate interaction terms between variables A and B. Estimates reflect Poisson marginal effects.
[a]Fetal exception refers to provisions in a state's abortion ban that allow exceptions for cases of fetal abnormality.
[b]Health exception refers to provisions in a state's abortion ban that allow exceptions for cases in which carrying a pregnancy to term would put the mother's health at risk.
*$P<.05$; **$P<.01$; ***$P<.001$.

analysis altogether. Results are available upon request.

DISCUSSION

In this work, we explored how the implementation of abortion restrictions enacted after *Dobbs* was decided influenced rates of infant mortality. Results indicated a statistically significant increase in infant deaths in abortion-restricting states, particularly among newborns (< 1 d) and older infants (1 mo to 1 y). Although deaths from perinatal, congenital, and other causes all increased, it is notable that we observed a significant and large increase in the latter. This result suggests that the increase in infant deaths was not exclusively attributable to deaths from complications during labor or congenital abnormalities. We also observed no evidence that these effects were significantly attenuated by the presence of legal exceptions for maternal health or fetal abnormality. Our findings are consistent with previous work establishing a relationship between Texas's SB-8 and infant deaths in Texas.[9] We expanded on that work by demonstrating that abortion restrictions lead to similar findings across a larger set of states with differing forms of restrictions and that these effects do not appear to be moderated by the presence of exceptions.

Our finding that the increase in deaths manifests among children older than 1 month, with a large and significant increase in nonperinatal, noncongenital causes, suggests that the effects do not exclusively reflect an increase in health complications at the time of birth.[23] Numerous possibilities might explain this finding. Greater economic costs associated with obtaining an abortion may shift the pool of mothers to those of lower socioeconomic means or other disadvantaged groups who are already at increased risk for experiencing an infant death.[24–26] Economic and social stress on families might also contribute to this finding, as noted in previous work demonstrating increased foster care placements in states with restricted abortion access.[8] Nonetheless, this result also differs slightly from findings in the Texas cohort, which suggested that the greatest increase in infant deaths was attributable to congenital abnormalities. This difference may be explained by the fact that we had a larger sample and, thus, additional statistical power. Alternatively, the different findings may reflect that the previous finding was specific to Texas.

The observation that including exceptions for maternal health or fetal abnormality did not lead to significant attenuation is, to our knowledge, a novel finding. Although this may be a function of limited statistical power, the increase in perinatal and congenital deaths in states with health exceptions suggests that such exceptions may not be regularly exercised by physicians or families in scenarios of congenital abnormalities or maternal health risk. This may stem from the statutory ambiguity in the conditions under which the exception applies, the limited guidance offered by restricting states in interpreting such exceptions, or the severity of penalties for incorrect use of exceptions.[27]

We also found that restriction-related increases in infant deaths are not exclusively attributable to perinatal causes or congenital abnormalities. Such deaths would presumably not be altered by the presence of legal exceptions to abortion restrictions. This suggests that improvements in outcomes might be possible with proper investment in support for child and maternal health after delivery. As discussed in previous work,[28] advocates in abortion-restricting states are increasingly focused on maternal and child health issues rather than abortion access to mitigate the downstream public health consequences of abortion restrictions. Our finding emphasizes the need for work that uncovers factors that contribute to the increase in mortality among older infants. If scholars can isolate these mechanisms, health care workers may be able to lessen the impact of bans in locations where legalizing abortion is politically infeasible.

Limitations

These findings are subject to limitations. First, although we used *ICD-10* codes to provide some insight into the causes of infant deaths, we could not observe the specific mechanism by which these effects manifested. Further work is required to understand how restrictions contribute to deaths in older infants. Second, we must emphasize that abortion restrictions are not assigned at random; they are more likely to be implemented in politically conservative states. We thus cannot claim that the effects would manifest if restrictions were implemented in more politically liberal states.

Third, although we explored birth-adjusted estimates (as seen in Appendix Table C), these analyses may be disconnected from infant deaths. As an example, the birth count we adjusted for in our estimations included children born in December, yet those children could not have contributed to deaths among infants older than 30 days in that year. Addressing this issue requires linked birth–death records, which are not available. Fourth, we were unable to evaluate whether excess infant deaths are experienced differentially by racial minorities and the lower socioeconomic class. Future work should investigate heterogeneity across demographic groups. Finally, the null effect for maternal and fetal health exceptions may have arisen because of a lack of statistical power. Accordingly, care must be taken not to overinterpret this null finding.

Public Health Implications

Numerous implications stem from these results. The loss of a child is traumatic for surviving parents and has long-term negative effects on parental mental health.[29–31] Loss of a sibling similarly has long-term negative effects on cognitive, socioemotional, and health outcomes for surviving children.[32] These negative effects of infant loss could worsen existing disparities for social groups who are differentially affected by abortion restrictions.[7,33] Additionally, as delivery carries significant risks for mothers, there is the obvious concern of compelling the delivery of infants with fatal congenital abnormalities.[29,34,35] Enacting such restrictions may impose a multifaceted penalty on women who are compelled to carry a relatively less viable pregnancy to term. Finally, these findings have implications for policymakers considering the implementation of abortion restrictions.[4–6,9] As noted in previous work, abortion restrictions increase mental distress in the general population. Excess infant deaths may further contribute to worsening mental health in states enacting abortion restrictions. AJPH

ABOUT THE AUTHORS

Michaela R. Anderson is with the Perelman School of Medicine, University of Pennsylvania, Philadelphia. Gordon Burtch is with the Questrom School of Business, Boston University, Boston, MA. Brad N. Greenwood is with the Costello College of Business, George Mason University, Fairfax, VA.

CORRESPONDENCE

Correspondence should be sent to Brad N Greenwood, PhD, George Mason University, 4400 University Dr, Fairfax, VA 22030 (e-mail: bgreenwo@gmu.edu). Reprints can be ordered at https://www.ajph.org by clicking the "Reprints" link.

PUBLICATION INFORMATION

Full Citation: Anderson MR, Burtch G, Greenwood BN. Abortion restrictions and infant mortality in the United States, 2018–2023. *Am J Public Health*. 2025;115(11):1895–1902.

Acceptance Date: June 18, 2025.

DOI: https://doi.org/10.2105/AJPH.2025.308228

ORCID iDs:
Gordon Burtch https://orcid.org/0000-0001-9798-1113

Brad N. Greenwood https://orcid.org/0000-0002-0772-7814

CONTRIBUTORS

M. R. Anderson and B. N. Greenwood interpreted the analysis. G. Burtch executed the analysis and interpreted the data. G. Burtch and B. N. Greenwood conceptualized and designed the analysis. B. N. Greenwood approved the final version of the article. All authors conceptualized, drafted, and revised the article.

CONFLICTS OF INTEREST

The authors declare no conflicts of interest.

HUMAN PARTICIPANT PROTECTION

This work is exempt from institutional review board review because no human participants were involved.

REFERENCES

1. *Dobbs v Jackson Women's Health Org.*, 142 S Ct 2228 (2022).
2. Center for Reproductive Rights. After *Roe* fell: abortion laws by state. 2023. Available at: https://reproductiverights.org/maps/abortion-laws-by-state. Accessed September 1, 2023.
3. Wilkinson TA, Bernard C. Abortion restrictions and the impact on families. *JAMA Pediatr.* 2024;178(1):15–16. https://doi.org/10.1001/jamapediatrics.2023.4735
4. Swanson K, Ravi A, Saleh S, Weia B, Pleasants E, Arvisais-Anhalt S. Effect of recent abortion legislation on Twitter user engagement, sentiment, and expressions of trust in clinicians and privacy of health information: content analysis. *J Med Internet Res.* 2023;25:e46655. https://doi.org/10.2196/46655
5. Anderson MR, Burtch G, Greenwood BN. The impact of abortion restrictions on American mental

health. *Sci Adv.* 2024;10(27):eadl5743. https://doi.org/10.1126/sciadv.adl5743

6. Thornburg B, Kennedy-Hendricks A, Rosen JD, Eisenberg MD. Anxiety and depression symptoms after the *Dobbs* abortion decision. *JAMA.* 2024;331(4):294–301. https://doi.org/10.1001/jama.2023.25599
7. Rader B, Upadhyay UD, Sehgal NK, Reis BY, Brownstein JS, Hswen Y. Estimated travel time and spatial access to abortion facilities in the US before and after the *Dobbs v Jackson Women's Health* decision. *JAMA.* 2022;328(20):2041–2047. https://doi.org/10.1001/jama.2022.20424
8. Adkins S, Talmor N, White MH, Dutton C, O'Donoghue AL. Association between restricted abortion access and child entries into the foster care system. *JAMA Pediatr.* 2024;178(1):37–44. https://doi.org/10.1001/jamapediatrics.2023.4738
9. Gemmill A, Margerison CE, Stuart EA, Bell SO. Infant deaths after Texas' 2021 ban on abortion in early pregnancy. *JAMA Pediatr.* 2024;178(8):784–791. https://doi.org/10.1001/jamapediatrics.2024.0885
10. Gemmill A, Franks AM, Anjur-Dietrich S, et al. US abortion bans and infant mortality. *JAMA.* 2025;333(15):1315–1323. https://doi.org/10.1001/jama.2024.28517
11. Lu MC, Johnson KA. Toward a national strategy on infant mortality. *Am J Public Health.* 2014;104(suppl 1):S13–S16. https://doi.org/10.2105/AJPH.2013.301855
12. Mannion E. Undue burdens: how the Texas abortion ban (SB 8) disproportionately affects low-income women. *Wash UJL & Pol'y.* 2023;72(1):259–282.
13. Maddow-Zimet I, Gibson C. Despite bans, number of abortions in the United States increased in 2023. March 2024. Available at: https://www.guttmacher.org/2024/03/despite-bans-number-abortions-united-states-increased-2023. Accessed July 25, 2025.
14. Aune D, Saugstad OD, Henriksen T, Tonstad S. Maternal body mass index and the risk of fetal death, stillbirth, and infant death: a systematic review and meta-analysis. *JAMA.* 2014;311(15):1536–1546. https://doi.org/10.1001/jama.2014.2269
15. *Roe v Wade*, 410 US 113 (1973).
16. Dimick JB, Ryan AM. Methods for evaluating changes in health care policy: the difference-in-differences approach. *JAMA.* 2014;312(22):2401–2402. https://doi.org/10.1001/jama.2014.16153
17. Abadie A, Athey S, Imbens GW, Wooldridge JM. When should you adjust standard errors for clustering? *Q J Econ.* 2022;138(1):1–35. https://doi.org/10.1093/qje/qjac038
18. Ciani E, Fisher P. Dif-in-dif estimators of multiplicative treatment effects. *J Econ Method.* 2019;8(1):20160011. https://doi.org/10.1515/jem-2016-0011
19. Chen J, Roth J. Logs with zeros? Some problems and solutions. *Q J Econ.* 2024;139(2):891–936. https://doi.org/10.1093/qje/qjad054
20. Baker AC, Larcker DF, Wang CC. How much should we trust staggered difference-in-differences estimates? *J Financ Econ.* 2022;144(2):370–395. https://doi.org/10.1016/j.jfineco.2022.01.004
21. Gardner J. Two-stage differences in differences. *arXiv preprint.* 2022;arXiv:2207.05943. https://doi.org/10.48550/arXiv.2207.05943
22. Wooldridge JM. Two-way fixed effects, the two-way Mundlak regression, and difference-in-differences estimators. *SSRN.* 2021. August 16, 2021. Available at: https://papers.ssrn.com/sol3/papers.cfm?abstract_id=3906345. Accessed July 25, 2025.
23. Ancel P-Y, Goffinet F, Kuhn P, EPIPAGE-2 Writing Group, et al. Survival and morbidity of preterm children born at 22 through 34 weeks' gestation in France in 2011: results of the EPIPAGE-2 cohort study. *JAMA Pediatr.* 2015;169(3):230–238. https://doi.org/10.1001/jamapediatrics.2014.3351
24. Vilda D, Hardeman R, Dyer L, Theall KP, Wallace M. Structural racism, racial inequities and urban–rural differences in infant mortality in the US. *J Epidemiol Community Health.* 2021;75(8):788–793. https://doi.org/10.1136/jech-2020-214260
25. Ratnasiri AW, Lakshminrusimha S, Dieckmann RA, et al. Maternal and infant predictors of infant mortality in California, 2007–2015. *PLoS One.* 2020;15(8):e0236877. https://doi.org/10.1371/journal.pone.0236877
26. Kim D, Saada A. The social determinants of infant mortality and birth outcomes in Western developed nations: a cross-country systematic review. *Int J Environ Res Public Health.* 2013;10(6):2296–2335. https://doi.org/10.3390/ijerph10062296
27. Sepper E, White K, Beasley A. The Texas Medical Board and the futility of medical exceptions to abortion bans. *JAMA.* 2024;331(24):2073–2074. https://doi.org/10.1001/jama.2024.9027
28. Daniel C, Mahoney A, Riley G. The politics of problem definition: abortion policy in Republican-controlled Louisiana. *Soc Sci.* 2024;13(8):387. https://doi.org/10.3390/socsci13080387
29. Rogers CH, Floyd FJ, Seltzer MM, Greenberg J, Hong J. Long-term effects of the death of a child on parents' adjustment in midlife. *J Fam Psychol.* 2008;22(2):203–211. https://doi.org/10.1037/0893-3200.22.2.203
30. Gold KJ, Leon I, Boggs ME, Sen A. Depression and posttraumatic stress symptoms after perinatal loss in a population-based sample. *J Womens Health (Larchmt).* 2016;25(3):263–269. https://doi.org/10.1089/jwh.2015.5284
31. Christiansen DM, Elklit A, Olff M. Parents bereaved by infant death: PTSD symptoms up to 18 years after the loss. *Gen Hosp Psychiatry.* 2013;35(6):605–611. https://doi.org/10.1016/j.genhosppsych.2013.06.006
32. Fletcher J, Vidal-Fernandez M, Wolfe B. Dynamic and heterogeneous effects of sibling death on children's outcomes. *Proc Natl Acad Sci U S A.* 2018;115(1):115–120. https://doi.org/10.1073/pnas.1709092115
33. Jones RK, Jerman J. Population group abortion rates and lifetime incidence of abortion: United States, 2008–2014. *Am J Public Health.* 2022;112(9):1284–1296. https://doi.org/10.2105/AJPH.2017.304042
34. Raymond EG, Grimes DA. The comparative safety of legal induced abortion and childbirth in the United States. *Obstet Gynecol.* 2012;119(2 pt 1):215–219. https://doi.org/10.1097/AOG.0b013e31823fe923
35. Stevenson A, Raymond E, Grossman D. Comparing mortality risk of induced abortion with mortality risk of staying pregnant. *Contraception.* 2023;127:110150. https://doi.org/10.1016/j.contraception.2023.110150

Social-Ecological Correlates of Involvement in Firearm-Related Violence in a Nationally Representative Survey of Adults

Krista R. Mehari, PhD, Jasmine N. Coleman, PhD, L. Taylor Stevens, MS, Albert D. Farrell, PhD, and Phillip N. Smith, PhD

Objectives. To examine social-ecological correlates of firearm-related violence involvement among adults.

Methods. Cross-sectional surveys were collected in the United States between August 2023 and September 2023 through an AmeriSpeak Panel (n = 1681), weighted to be nationally representative. Measures included self-reported involvement in firearm-related violence victimization and perpetration and hypothesized social-ecological risk factors.

Results. About 5.9% reported ever perpetrating firearm-related violence; 6.9% reported experiencing firearm-related victimization. In a fully adjusted model, factors associated with perpetration were greater traumatic stress symptoms, beliefs about gun use to enforce respect, positive attitudes about firearms, and firearm-related victimization. Factors associated with victimization were adverse childhood experiences, family and friends' histories of violence and suicide, traumatic stress symptoms, witnessing community violence, firearm-related perpetration, male sex, and lower income.

Conclusions. A range of factors across social-ecological domains were associated with firearm-related violence, emphasizing the need for a contextualized approach to understand firearm-related injuries and deaths. Posttraumatic stress and exposure to violence may be particularly important to understanding the cycle of firearm violence. Intervention strategies should be expanded to include individuals vicariously exposed to violence, not just those directly victimized. (*Am J Public Health*. 2025;115(11):1903–1912. https://doi.org/10.2105/AJPH.2025.308213)

AJPH November 2025, Vol. 115, No. 11

Homicide is a leading cause of death in the United States, representing a major health disparity. It accounts for 2.5% of deaths of Black Americans aged 15 years and older, but only 0.2% of White Americans in the same age range.[1] The vast majority (77%) of homicides in the United States are completed using firearms.[2] There is an urgent need to build a more comprehensive understanding of social-ecological factors that are associated with firearm-related violence involvement.

Social-ecological theory emphasizes the need to consider individual factors within the context of social and built environments (e.g., family, peers, neighborhoods).[3] However, existing research on predictors of firearm-related victimization in community or representative samples has had a heavy focus on demographic factors and policy.[4,5] Demographic factors associated with firearm-related violence involvement include living in metro areas, living in the South, having a lower income, being male, and being Black.[6,7] Individual-level factors include witnessing community violence.[8] Family-level factors include family violence.[8] Community-level factors include racial segregation, income inequality, disorder, concentrated disadvantage, and crime rates.[9,10]

This study used a social-ecological framework to examine the extent to which a range of hypothesized risk factors across multiple social-ecological domains were associated with firearm-related violence victimization and perpetration within a nationally representative sample of US adults. Its focus was on key social-ecological factors believed to be important by members of communities affected by violence who participated in participatory action research (Figure 1).[11]

METHODS

We recruited participants through an AmeriSpeak panel. AmeriSpeak is operated by NORC at University of Chicago and has a probability-based US sample of over 41 000 participants. Sampling through the NORC National Frame involved selecting addresses by combining information from the US Postal Service Delivery Sequence File with in-person listings that added rural households. We stratified the panel using US Census tracts or blocks based on race/ethnicity composition and concentrations of young adults; hard-to-reach populations were oversampled. After the first nonresponse, we sampled housing units for nonresponse follow-up using phone calls and in-person field visits. This sampling approach resulted in a panel within 1 to 2 percentage points of US Census data in terms of race/ethnicity, age, region, and rurality or urbanicity.[12] AmeriSpeak has the highest response rate of all commercially available US household panels.[13] Recruitment information was e-mailed to AmeriSpeak panel members or delivered over the telephone, depending on their preferences. Participants who opted into the study could complete the survey in English or Spanish, over the Internet or telephone, and received AmeriSpeak (cash-equivalent) points. The median survey completion time was 22 minutes.

Measures

Cultural factors. For this study, we developed a measure assessing norms about protection and defense based on participatory action research.[11] Participants responded to 6 items with the prompt, "How much do the people around you agree with the following statements?" on a 5-point rating scale from 1 (strongly disagree) to 5 (strongly agree). Factor analyses of these items supported 2 factors: prescriptive norms for protection and defense

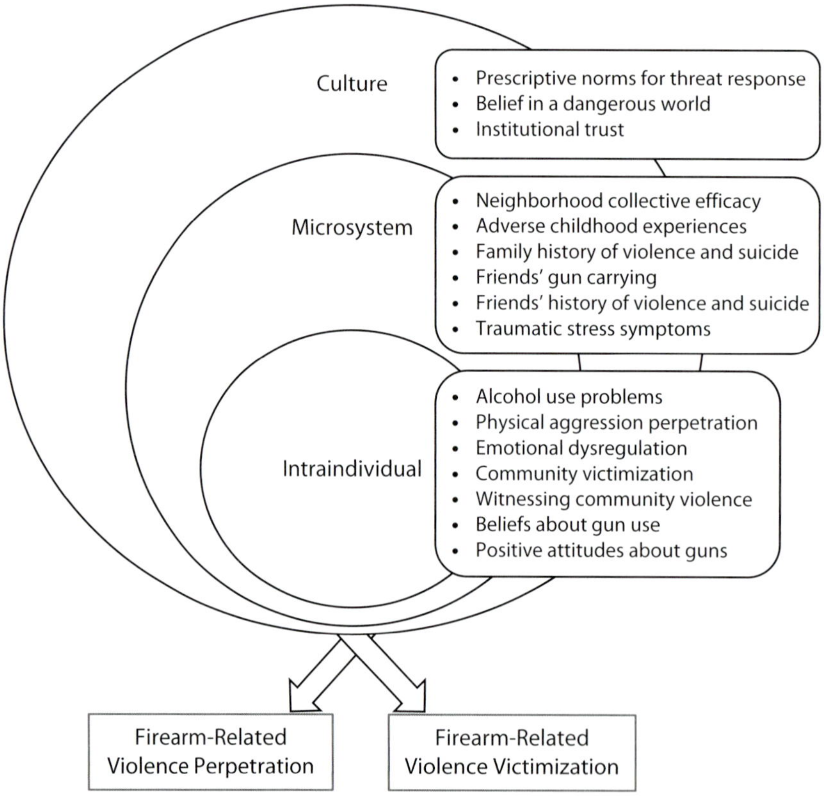

FIGURE 1— Proposed Model for Predicting Firearm-Related Violence Involvement With Hypothesized Predictors Categorized by Social-Ecological Domain

(e.g., "People should be prepared to defend their homes"; Cronbach's $\alpha = 0.82$) and prescriptive norms for reputation and respect (e.g., "When people get disrespected, they need to do something about it"; $\alpha = 0.77$). An adapted 5-item version of the Belief in a Dangerous World Scale[14] assessed participants' beliefs that the world is a dangerous place in which individuals are at risk from people who are inherently dangerous (e.g., "Many people are dangerous and will hurt others for no reason"; $\alpha = 0.65$). An adapted version of the World Values Survey of Institutional Trust[15] assessed how much participants trusted a list of institutions on a 4-point rating scale from 1 (not at all) to 4 (completely). Factor analyses identified 3 subscales: political (e.g., the government, politicians; $\alpha = 0.79$), law-and-order (e.g., the police, the justice system; $\alpha = 0.74$), and scientific (e.g., public health agencies like the Centers for Disease Control and Prevention; $\alpha = 0.80$).

Microsystemic factors. Microsystemic factors included community, family, and peers. An adapted version of the collective efficacy scale[16] assessed neighborhood informal control and social cohesion ($\alpha = 0.87$; e.g., "Can you count on your neighbors to intervene if a fight broke out in their home?"; 5-point scale from 1 [very unlikely] to 5 [very likely]). The Expanded Family ACEs scale[17] assessed childhood exposure to family adversity (e.g., "Did a parent or other adult in the household often or very often swear, insult, put you down, or humiliate you?"). For this study, we created 2 parallel measures to assess (1) family history of violence and suicide and (2) friends' history of violence and suicide based on participatory action research. Participants responded yes or no to 8 questions that assessed whether any close family members or friends had been injured or killed through violence or completed or attempted suicide. We assessed peer gun carrying by a single item asking how many of their friends carried guns, ranging from 1 (none of them) to 4 (all of them).[18]

Intraindividual factors. We assessed physical aggression by 5 items from the Problem Behavior Frequency Scale,[19] which asked participants to report their past 30-day frequency (1 [never] to 5 [10–19 times]) of specific aggressive behaviors (e.g., "hit or slapped someone"; $\alpha = 0.84$). The 3-item Alcohol Use Disorders Identification Test—Adapted assessed alcohol use problems (e.g., "How often did you have 6 or more drinks on one occasion in the past year?"; $\alpha = 0.82$).[20] The Primary Care posttraumatic stress disorder (PTSD) Screen for DSM-5[21] comprises 5 items that are asked if a participant endorses any lifetime exposure to a traumatic event (e.g., "Have you had nightmares about the event(s) or thought about the event(s) when you did not want to?"; $\alpha = 0.89$). We assessed emotion regulation by an adapted version of the Difficulties in Emotion Regulation—Short Form[22] (6 items; 1 [almost never] to 5 [almost always]). Subscales include Lack of Emotional Clarity (e.g., "I have no idea how I am feeling"; $\alpha = 0.88$) and Impulse Control Difficulties (e.g., "When I am upset, I become out of control"; $\alpha = 0.93$).

We assessed exposure to violence by 8 items from the Survey of Children's Exposure to Community Violence adapted for adults.[23] Participants indicated how often (1 [never] to 6 [≥ 20 times]) they were directly victimized by or witnessed 4 parallel events in the past 6 months: community victimization (e.g., "Been beaten up or mugged"; $\alpha = 0.77$) and witnessing community violence (e.g., "Seen someone else being attacked with a knife"; $\alpha = 0.80$). Beliefs About Gun Use is a 6-item measure developed for this study based on participatory action research.[11] Participants indicated how much they agreed with the acceptable use of firearms in a range of situations on a 5-point scale, from 1 (strongly disagree) to 5 (strongly agree). A factor analysis identified 2 factors: beliefs supporting gun use to enforce respect (e.g., "If you find out your partner is cheating on you, it's okay to go get a gun"; $\alpha = 0.87$) and beliefs supporting defensive gun use (e.g., "If someone breaks into your house, it's okay to go get a gun"; $\alpha = 0.80$). We assessed positive attitudes about guns by a measure developed for this study based on participatory action research. Participants identified their agreement with specific attitudes about firearms on a 5-point scale, from 1 (strongly disagree) to 5 (strongly agree); for example, "Guns are the best way to protect yourself" ($\alpha = 0.92$).

Demographic factors. Demographic factors were provided by AmeriSpeak and included age, sex, race or ethnicity, living in a metro area, education, and income. We assessed household firearm access by a single item, "Do you currently have a gun or guns?" with the response options of "No" (coded as no access), "Yes" (coded as personal ownership), or "There's a gun where I live, but it's not mine" (coded as household ownership).

Indicators of firearm-related violence involvement. Lifetime firearm-related victimization was assessed by 6 items. Three items were from the Survey of

Children's Exposure to Violence[23] (e.g., ever been shot at or ever been threatened with a gun), and 1 item was revised from the National Health Interview Survey[24]: "Have you ever had an accident or an injury from a firearm where any part of your body was hurt?" followed by a question confirming that they were injured by someone else. Two items were developed through a participatory action research study to assess lifetime firearm-related victimization by a current or former intimate partner; participants indicated whether a partner had ever "held or messed with a gun when they were angry at you" or "pointed a gun at you or held you at gunpoint."[11] We assessed lifetime firearm-related perpetration by 4 items developed for this study based on qualitative data and through participatory action research.[11] Two items were general: "Have you ever used a gun to defend yourself or someone else against a person or group of people?" and "Other than to defend yourself, have you ever used a gun against someone?" Two items examined lifetime firearm-related perpetration against a current or former intimate partner and were parallel to the victimization items.[11] These variables were treated as binary, with 1 = any lifetime involvement and 2 = no lifetime involvement.

Data Analysis Plan

We conducted demographics, correlations, and baseline differences in victimization and perpetration in SPSS version 29.0.2 (SPSS, Inc., Chicago, IL). We completed all subsequent analyses in MPlus version 8.11 (Los Angeles, CA: Muthén & Muthén). An a priori power analysis identified a full sample size goal of 1700, assuming the smallest subsample of 731 adults with firearm access. Power was estimated at 0.91 or higher to detect indirect effects as low as 0.023 using latent variables. Data were not clustered by location or household. We applied sampling weights in Mplus, such that parameters were estimated by maximizing a weighted loglikelihood function, and standard error computations used a sandwich estimator. Applying the sampling weights adjusted for both sample selection probabilities across 48 strata (including the intersections of race/ethnicity, age, education, and sex) as well as panel member nonresponses to the current survey (including age, sex, education, and race/ethnicity).[25] We used robust maximum likelihood estimation to address nonnormal data. We used full information maximum likelihood, which computes parameter estimates using all available data, to address missing data. All models had missing data for less than 4% of the overall sample, which is considered negligible.[26]

We used a model-building approach, in which only factors that were significantly correlated with firearm violence perpetration or victimization were included in the logistic regressions. First, we examined bivariate correlations between each variable and victimization and perpetration. Variables that were associated with either outcome were advanced to binary logistic regression models that paired hypothesized predictors within 1 domain of the social ecology (e.g., culture) with perpetration or victimization as the outcome. Next, variables that explained unique variance in the separate models were retained in the full, cross-domain models predicting perpetration or victimization. This approach enabled iterative testing while reducing model complexity and increasing interpretability of the results. We conducted multiple group models to determine whether firearm access moderated the relations between the hypothesized predictors and victimization or perpetration. An unconstrained model in which all coefficient paths were allowed to vary across firearm access subgroups was compared with a constrained model in which all coefficient paths were set to be equivalent across firearm access subgroups.

RESULTS

Demographic characteristics are reported in Table 1. Correlations among variables are reported in Table A (available as a supplement to the online version of this article at http://www.ajph.org). About 5.9% reported any firearm-related perpetration and 6.9% reported any firearm-related victimization. Participants with firearm access had higher firearm-related perpetration (9.51%) than participants with no firearm access (3.43%; $\chi^2_1 = 26.83$; $P < .001$), but there was no difference in firearm-related victimization across groups ($\chi^2_1 = 2.77$; $P = .10$). Separate analyses for each social-ecological domain investigated the extent to which variables within each domain uniquely predicted involvement in firearm-related violence (Table 2). Results of a full model that included all significant variables in all social-ecological domains are reported in Table 3. For both perpetration ($\chi^2_{12} = 18.01$; $P = .11$) and victimization ($\chi^2_9 = 12.16$; $P = .20$), the multiple group models indicated that patterns of relations did not vary by firearm access.

Firearm-Related Perpetration

Among cultural factors, higher trust in law-and-order (odds ratio [OR] = 0.51; 95% confidence interval [CI] = 0.31,

TABLE 1— Demographic Characteristics of Sample: United States, August–September 2023

	No. (%)
Sex at birth	
Male	793 (47.5)
Female	879 (52.5)
Race/ethnicity	
Non-Hispanic White	1032 (61.4)
Hispanic/Latinx	290 (17.3)
Non-Hispanic African American/Black	205 (12.2)
Non-Hispanic Asian	111 (6.6)
Non-Hispanic multiracial	31 (1.8)
Non-Hispanic other	11 (0.7)
Age, y	
18–24	193 (11.5)
25–34	286 (17.0)
35–44	287 (17.1)
45–54	244 (14.5)
55–64	289 (17.2)
65–74	293 (17.4)
≥ 75	90 (5.3)
Income, $	
< 30 000	352 (20.9)
30 000 to < 60 000	435 (25.9)
60 000 to < 100 000	415 (24.7)
≥ 100 000	480 (28.6)
Education	
Less than high school	142 (8.4)
High school graduate or equivalent	488 (29.0)
Vocational/tech school/some college/associates	448 (26.6)
Bachelor's degree	330 (19.6)
Postgraduate/professional degree	274 (16.3)
Metro	
Non-metro area	236 (14.1)
Metro area	1445 (85.9)

Note. n = 1681 based on a weighted sample.

0.84) and in scientific (OR = 0.64; 95% CI = 0.44, 0.93) institutions were associated with lower odds of perpetration. Among microsystemic predictors, more adverse childhood experiences (OR = 1.16; 95% CI = 1.08, 1.26), friends' history of injury or death from violence (OR = 2.39; 95% CI = 1.27, 4.48), and friends' gun carrying (OR = 1.91; 95% CI = 1.44, 2.55) were associated with higher odds of perpetration. Among intraindividual predictors, higher levels of traumatic stress symptoms (OR = 1.22; 95% CI = 1.03, 1.44), higher rates of witnessing community violence (OR = 1.82; 95% CI = 1.02, 3.23), higher levels of beliefs supporting gun use to enforce respect (OR = 1.74; 95% CI = 1.18, 2.58), more positive attitudes about guns (OR = 2.42; 95% CI = 1.63, 3.59), and ever experiencing firearm-related violence (OR = 6.54; 95% CI = 3.36, 12.72) were associated with higher odds of perpetration. Among demographic factors, being male was associated with higher odds (OR = 2.83; 95% CI = 1.56, 5.14), whereas having an income of $30 000 or more was associated with lower odds (OR = 0.40; 95% CI = 0.22, 0.71) of perpetration.

When all significant variables were entered simultaneously into the full model, only intraindividual and demographic factors were uniquely associated with firearm violence perpetration. Higher levels of traumatic stress symptoms (OR = 1.22; 95% CI = 1.01, 1.47), higher levels of beliefs supporting gun use to enforce respect (OR = 1.68; 95% CI = 1.13, 2.49), more positive attitudes about guns (OR = 2.16; 95% CI = 1.42, 3.28) and firearm-related victimization (OR = 6.30; 95% CI = 3.22, 12.32) were each uniquely associated with higher odds of perpetration.

Firearm-Related Victimization

Among cultural factors, higher trust in law-and-order institutions (OR = 0.59; 95% CI = 0.45, 0.78) was associated with lower odds of victimization. Among microsystemic factors, more adverse childhood experiences (OR = 1.19; 95% CI = 1.12, 1.26), family history of injury or death from violence (OR = 1.79; 95% CI = 1.26, 2.54), friends' gun carrying (OR = 1.26; 95% CI = 1.02, 1.56), and friends' histories of injury or death from violence (OR = 2.13; 95% CI = 1.49, 3.05) were associated with higher odds of victimization. Among intraindividual predictors, higher levels of traumatic

TABLE 2— **Odds of Perpetration and Victimization Predicted by Cultural, Microsystemic, Intraindividual, and Demographic Factors: United States, August–September 2023**

	Firearm Perpetration, OR (95% CI)	Firearm Victimization, OR (95% CI)
Model 1: cultural factors		
Prescriptive norms for defense and protection	1.39 (0.89, 2.17)	1.21 (0.97, 1.52)
Belief in a dangerous world	. . .	1.27 (0.99, 1.64)
Trust in political institutions	1.09 (0.60, 1.99)	. . .
Trust in law-and-order institutions	0.51 (0.31, 0.84)	0.59 (0.45, 0.78)
Trust in scientific institutions	0.64 (0.44, 0.93)	1.07 (0.84, 1.35)
Model 2: microsystemic factors		
Neighborhood collective efficacy	0.81 (0.57, 1.15)	0.88 (0.72, 1.08)
Adverse childhood experiences	1.16 (1.08, 1.26)	1.19 (1.12, 1.26)
Family history of violence and suicide	1.43 (0.81, 2.53)	1.79 (1.26, 2.54)
Friends' gun carrying	1.91 (1.44, 2.55)	1.26 (1.02, 1.56)
Friends' histories of violence and suicide	2.39 (1.27, 4.48)	2.13 (1.49, 3.05)
Model 3: intraindividual factors		
Physical aggression perpetration	2.10 (0.66, 6.70)	0.95 (0.29, 3.06)
Traumatic stress symptoms	1.22 (1.03, 1.44)	1.38 (1.25, 1.52)
Lack of emotional clarity	. . .	0.99 (0.91, 1.06)
Impulse control difficulties	0.99 (0.89, 1.11)	0.99 (0.88, 1.11)
Community victimization	0.79 (0.34, 1.82)	1.31 (0.55, 3.15)
Witnessing community violence	1.82 (1.02, 3.23)	2.84 (1.58, 5.11)
Beliefs supporting defensive gun use	1.02 (0.66, 1.59)	1.05 (0.87, 1.26)
Beliefs supporting gun use to enforce respect	1.74 (1.18, 2.58)	1.11 (0.81, 1.51)
Positive attitudes about firearms	2.42 (1.63, 3.59)	1.11 (0.91, 1.36)
Lifetime firearm victimization	6.54 (3.36, 12.72)	. . .
Lifetime firearm perpetration	. . .	5.67 (2.86, 11.26)
Model 4: demographic factors		
Metro area vs non-metro area	. . .	0.66 (0.43, 1.02)
Male adults vs female adults	2.83 (1.56, 5.14)	1.75 (1.25, 2.44)
Income of ≥ $30 000 vs < $30 000	0.40 (0.22, 0.71)	0.43 (0.30, 0.62)
Black vs White adults	. . .	1.38 (0.85, 2.24)

Note. CI = confidence interval; OR = odds ratio. n = 1681 based on a weighted sample. The table reports the results of binary logistic regression analyses in which odds ratios are adjusted for other factors in the same domain of the social ecology but not other domains. Cells with ellipses indicate that these values were not calculated because those variables did not explain a significant proportion of the variance in the bivariate models.

stress symptoms (OR = 1.38; 95% CI: = 1.25, 1.52), higher rates of witnessing community violence (OR = 2.84; 95% CI = 1.58, 5.11), and firearm-related violence perpetration (OR = 5.67; 95% CI = 2.86, 11.26) were associated with higher odds of victimization. Among demographic predictors, being male was associated with higher odds (OR = 1.75; 95% CI = 1.25, 2.44), whereas having an income of $30 000 or more was associated with lower odds (OR = 0.43; 95% CI = 0.30, 0.62) of victimization.

When all significant variables were entered simultaneously in the full model, microsystemic, intraindividual, and demographic factors explained unique variance in victimization. Specifically, adverse childhood experiences (OR = 1.12; 95% CI = 1.04, 1.19), family history of violence and suicide (OR = 1.54; 95% CI = 1.06, 2.25), friends' history of violence and suicide (OR = 1.59; 95% CI = 1.09, 2.31), higher levels of traumatic stress symptoms (OR = 1.23; 95% CI = 1.10, 1.38), greater rates of witnessing community violence (OR = 2.18; 95% CI = 1.45, 3.29), firearm-related violence perpetration (OR = 5.50; 95% CI = 2.59, 11.69), and

TABLE 3— Odds of Perpetration and Victimization Based on Cultural, Microsystemic, Intraindividual, and Demographic Factors (Fully Adjusted Model): United States, August–September 2023

	Firearm Perpetration, OR (95% CI)	Firearm Victimization, OR (95% CI)
Cultural factors		
Trust in law-and-order institutions	0.66 (0.39, 1.12)	1.12 (0.83, 1.51)
Trust in scientific institutions	0.94 (0.61, 1.46)	. . .
Microsystemic factors		
Neighborhood collective efficacy	. . .	. . .
Adverse childhood experiences	1.02 (0.92, 1.14)	1.12 (1.04, 1.19)
Family history of violence and suicide	. . .	1.54 (1.06, 2.25)
Friends' gun carrying	1.21 (0.83, 1.78)	1.07 (0.84, 1.35)
Friends' histories of violence and suicide	1.50 (0.75, 3.01)	1.59 (1.09, 2.31)
Intraindividual factors		
Traumatic stress symptoms	1.22 (1.01, 1.47)	1.23 (1.10, 1.38)
Witnessing community violence	1.30 (0.85, 1.99)	2.18 (1.45, 3.29)
Beliefs supporting gun use to enforce respect	1.68 (1.13, 2.49)	. . .
Positive attitudes about firearms	2.16 (1.42, 3.28)	. . .
Lifetime firearm victimization	6.30 (3.22, 12.32)	. . .
Lifetime firearm perpetration	. . .	5.50 (2.59, 11.69)
Demographic factors		
Male adults versus female adults	2.27 (1.08, 4.78)	1.66 (1.16, 2.38)
Income of ≥ $30 000 vs < $30 000	0.81 (0.37, 1.73)	0.57 (0.36, 0.89)

Note. CI = confidence interval; OR = odds ratio. n = 1681 based on a weighted sample. The table reports the results of binary logistic regression analyses that only included variables that explained unique variance in the domain-specific models (see Table 2); odds ratios are fully adjusted. Cells with ellipses indicate that these values were not calculated because those variables did not explain a significant proportion of the variance in the bivariate models.

being male (OR = 1.66; 95% CI = 1.16, 2.38) were each uniquely associated with higher odds of firearm-related victimization. In contrast, having an income of $30 000 or more was uniquely associated with lower odds of victimization (OR = 0.57; 95% CI = 0.36, 0.89).

DISCUSSION

This study represents an important step in developing a foundation of research to support the development and refinement of strategies to prevent and reduce firearm-related violence. Its primary aim was to use a social-ecological framework as a guide for exploring the breadth of factors that may be associated with firearm-related violence perpetration and victimization. As hypothesized, factors across multiple levels of the social ecology were associated with firearm violence victimization and perpetration.

Having engaged in firearm-related perpetration was associated with greater odds of firearm-related victimization and vice versa, underscoring that perpetration and victimization often co-occur within the same individual. Traumatic stress was uniquely associated with both types of involvement after we controlled for a range of other factors. The domain-specific models create a more complete picture of their shared correlates, indicating that lower trust in law-and-order institutions, adverse childhood experiences, friends' gun carrying, friends' histories of violence and suicide, and witnessing community violence are associated with firearm-related victimization and perpetration. A wealth of research has identified a relation between potentially traumatic events, such as childhood adversity (e.g., family violence) and witnessing community violence, and subsequent aggressive behaviors, and it has suggested that posttraumatic stress symptoms may at least partially explain those relations.[27–29] By definition, posttraumatic stress symptoms are preceded by a trauma, and interpersonal, violent assaults specifically predict PTSD.[30] However, posttraumatic stress also predicts increased risk and severity of subsequent aggression perpetration, as established by reviews and meta-analyses.[31,32] Similarly, having PTSD may also increase one's likelihood of further victimization; for example, 1 study showed that the female partners of male veterans were about 3 times more likely to perpetrate intimate partner violence when the veterans had PTSD.[33] In the case of firearm violence, symptom clusters associated with PTSD—such as the cognitive (e.g., distrust of others and the world) and mood (e.g., anger, fear) alterations as well as disruptions in arousal (e.g., hypervigilance)—are likely to motivate a person to engage in aggressive or provocative behavior, or to react strongly to perceived threats. Those behaviors may subsequently increase the likelihood that another person will respond to them with violence.

Another possible explanation for the relation between vicarious violent experiences and one's own firearm-related violence involvement is contagion. Prior research has found that every additional exposure to a person who has sustained a gunshot wound predicts an increased likelihood of being shot.[34] The specific mechanisms are unknown, although the findings may be caused by living in a high-violence area, having friends who carry firearms, or being involved in a cycle of victimization and violent retaliation that is marked by injury and death. Supporting this idea, friends' firearm carrying was associated with both firearm-related victimization and perpetration in the microsystemic-only model. This is a novel finding; no study identified in this literature review examined friends' firearm carrying as a predictor of firearm-related victimization or perpetration, although it does predict increases in one's own firearm carrying among youths and is likely associated with friends' general level of illegal activity, particularly in urban settings among youths.[35]

Two attitudes—positive attitudes toward guns and beliefs supporting gun use to enforce respect—predicted perpetration in the full model. The measure of beliefs supporting gun use to enforce respect taps heavily into themes related to retaliation for or prevention of violation of relationships. These items may shed important light on value systems that may provide justifications for firearm use when one's relationships are violated.

Importantly, race was not related to firearm-related perpetration even in bivariate correlations, and it was not related to firearm-related victimization after we controlled for other demographic factors. This finding underscores the need to move beyond an overreliance on a single demographic factor to explore why there is a higher prevalence of firearm-related injury and death among Black Americans—such as poverty, segregation, or other factors. Identifying malleable factors that explain the relation will make it possible to engage in effective public health prevention approaches.

Limitations

This study had some important limitations. The cross-sectional design made it impossible to point toward causality: the hypothesized predictors may be outcomes of firearm violence involvement, or the relations may be spurious. Longitudinal research is needed to understand how these variables are related to each other over time. In addition, although our results point to possible multilevel effects, we only had data from individuals, making it impossible for us to estimate group-level effects. Monomethod bias and recall error, especially related to traumatic events, may have inflated the results. Future research should examine possible within-domain and cross-domain interactions of possible predictors to determine factors that may mitigate or exacerbate the relations with firearm violence involvement, which can inform effective prevention.

Public Health Implications

Overall, this study represents an important step in disentangling preventable social-ecological correlates of involvement in firearm violence from static demographic factors. This study suggests that important targets of intervention include posttraumatic stress and the prevention of early adversity and witnessing violence. Of note, hospitals and law enforcement agencies often provide victim services for individuals who have sustained a firearm injury, which do not typically extend to close friends, family members, or witnesses; however, the results of this study suggest that those vicarious exposures may place individuals at risk for involvement in violence as perpetrators or victims. Interventions should be developed for individuals with vicarious experiences of firearm-related violence to interrupt the cycle of violence. AJPH

ABOUT THE AUTHORS

At the time of the study, Krista R. Mehari and L. Taylor Stevens were with the Department of Psychology and Human Development, Vanderbilt University, Nashville, TN, and the Department of Psychology, University of South Alabama, Mobile. Jasmine N. Coleman was with the Department of Psychology, University of Tennessee, Knoxville, and the Department of Psychology, University of South Alabama, Mobile. Albert D. Farrell was with the Department of Psychology, Virginia Commonwealth University, Richmond. Phillip N. Smith was with the Department of Psychology, University of South Alabama, Mobile.

CORRESPONDENCE

Correspondence should be sent to Krista R. Mehari, Psychology and Human Development, Peabody College of Education and Human Development, Vanderbilt University, 230 Appleton Pl #552, Nashville, TN 37203 (e-mail: krista.mehari@vanderbilt.edu).

Reprints can be ordered at https://www.ajph.org by clicking the "Reprints" link.

PUBLICATION INFORMATION

Full Citation: Mehari KR, Coleman JN, Stevens LT, Farrell AD, Smith PN. Social-ecological correlates of involvement in firearm-related violence in a nationally representative survey of adults. *Am J Public Health*. 2025;115(11):1903–1912.

Acceptance Date: June 8, 2025.

DOI: https://doi.org/10.2105/AJPH.2025.308213

ORCID iDs:
Krista R. Mehari https://orcid.org/0000-0002-7448-9393

Jasmine N. Coleman https://orcid.org/0000-0002-1034-1277

L. Taylor Stevens https://orcid.org/0000-0002-4543-2558

Phillip N. Smith https://orcid.org/0000-0002-9364-3907

CONTRIBUTORS

K. R. Mehari conceptualized and designed the work, oversaw the acquisition of data, interpreted data, drafted the work and critically revised it, and provided final approval of the version to be published. J. N. Coleman and L. T. Stevens participated in the acquisition of data, conducted data analysis, and drafted the work and critically revised it. A. D. Farrell participated in the conceptualization and design of the work, supervised data analysis, participated in the interpretation of data, and provided final approval of the version to be published. P. N. Smith conceptualized and designed the work, participated in the acquisition of data, revised the work critically for important intellectual content, and provided final approval of the version to be published.

ACKNOWLEDGMENTS

This study was funded by a grant from the Centers for Disease Control and Prevention (CDC; grant R01CE003298; principal investigators: K. R. Mehari and P. N. Smith). During the completion of this work, L. T. Stevens was supported by a training grant from the Eunice Kennedy Shriver National Institute of Child Health and Human Development (F31HD116419).

The results of this manuscript were presented at the 2024 National Research Conference on the Prevention of Firearm-Related Harms in Seattle, WA.

We thank the advisory board members, community research assistants, and qualitative interview participants, whose efforts and investment made this work possible.

Note. The contents are those of the authors and do not necessarily represent the official views of, nor an endorsement by, the CDC or the US Government. The CDC had no role in the study design, data collection procedures, data analysis or interpretation, or writing of the report.

CONFLICTS OF INTEREST

The authors declare that they have no conflicts of interest to report.

HUMAN PARTICIPANT PROTECTION

All procedures were approved by the University of South Alabama's institutional review board. The National Institutes of Health issued a Certificate of Confidentiality for this study.

REFERENCES

1. Centers for Disease Control and Prevention. Underlying cause of death, 2018–2022, single race results. CDC Wonder. Available at: https://wonder.cdc.gov/controller/datarequest/D158;jsessionid=83C550A0FD18FCB879951B0CF6E6. Accessed July 19, 2024.
2. Federal Bureau of Investigation. Expanded homicides reported in the United States. FBI Crime Data Explorer. Available at: https://cde.ucr.cjis.gov/LATEST/webapp/#/pages/explorer/crime/shr. Accessed May 21, 2025.
3. Bronfenbrenner U. Toward an experimental ecology of human development. *Am Psychol.* 1977;32(7):513–531. https://doi.org/10.1037/0003-066X.32.7.513
4. Schmidt CJ, Rupp L, Pizarro JM, Lee DB, Branas CC, Zimmerman MA. Risk and protective factors related to youth firearm violence: a scoping review and directions for future research. *J Behav Med.* 2019;42(4):706–723. https://doi.org/10.1007/s10865-019-00076-7
5. Morral AR, Schell TL, Jacobs T, Smart R. Visualizing firearm mortality and law effects: an interactive web-based tool, second edition. RAND Corporation. 2024. Available at: https://www.rand.org/pubs/tools/TLA243-6-v2.html. Accessed August 2, 2024.
6. Planty MG, Truman JL. Firearm violence, 1993–2011. US Department of Justice, Bureau of Justice Statistics. 2013. Available at: https://bjs.ojp.gov/library/publications/firearm-violence-1993-2011. Accessed November 10, 2023.
7. Lu Y, Baumler E, DeMello AS, Wood L, McGuire H, Temple JR. Firearm access, carriage and use in an ethnically diverse sample of young adults in Texas, USA. *Inj Prev.* 2024;30(6):521–525. https://doi.org/10.1136/ip-2023-044989
8. Osborne MC, Reidy DE, Temple JR, DeMello A, Lu Y. Examining the relation between early violence exposure and firearm-related experiences in emerging adulthood: a longitudinal cohort study. *Psychol Rep.* 2024;128(1):78–99. https://doi.org/10.1177/00332941241254313
9. Goin DE, Rudolph KE, Ahern J. Predictors of firearm violence in urban communities: a machine-learning approach. *Health Place.* 2018;51:61–67. https://doi.org/10.1016/j.healthplace.2018.02.013
10. Johnson BT, Sisti A, Bernstein M, et al. Community-level factors and incidence of gun violence in the United States, 2014–2017. *Soc Sci Med.* 2021;280:113969. https://doi.org/10.1016/j.socscimed.2021.113969
11. Smith PN, Cordell C, Stevens LT, et al. Project GRIP: an illustration of participatory action research with communities of people who own and use firearms. *Psychol Rep.* 2024;128(1):211–239. https://doi.org/10.1177/00332941241246467
12. NORC at the University of Chicago. Panel design. Available at: https://amerispeak.norc.org/us/en/amerispeak/about-amerispeak/panel-design.html. Accessed May 13, 2025.
13. American Association for Public Opinion Research. 2023 standard definitions: final dispositions of case codes and outcome rates for surveys. 2022. Available at: https://aapor.org/standards-and-ethics/standard-definitions. Accessed May 13, 2025.
14. Altemeyer B. The other "authoritarian personality." In: Zanna MP, ed. *Advances in Experimental Social Psychology.* Vol. 30. Cambridge, MA: Academic Press; 1998:47–92. https://doi.org/10.1016/S0065-2601(08)60382-2
15. González S, Smith C. *The Accuracy of Measures of Institutional Trust in Household Surveys: Evidence From the OECD Trust Database.* Paris, France: Organisation for Economic Co-operation and Development; 2017. https://doi.org/10.1787/d839bd50-en
16. Sampson RJ, Raudenbush SW, Earls F. Neighborhoods and violent crime: a multilevel study of collective efficacy. *Science.* 1997;277(5328):918–924. https://doi.org/10.1126/science.277.5328.918
17. Data Resource Center for Child and Adolescent Health. NSCH survey instruments. Available at: https://www.childhealthdata.org/learn-about-the-nsch/survey-instruments. Accessed August 28, 2024.
18. Keil S, Beardslee J, Schubert C, Mulvey E, Pardini D. Perceived gun access and gun carrying among male adolescent offenders. *Youth Violence Juv Justice.* 2020;18(2):179–195. https://doi.org/10.1177/1541204019865312
19. Farrell AD, Sullivan TN, Goncy EA, Le ATH. Assessment of adolescents' victimization, aggression, and problem behaviors: evaluation of the Problem Behavior Frequency Scale. *Psychol Assess.* 2016;28(6):702–714. https://doi.org/10.1037/pas0000225
20. Bush K, Kivlahan DR, McDonell MB, Fihn SD, Bradley KA, for the Ambulatory Care Quality Improvement Project (ACQUIP). The AUDIT alcohol consumption questions (AUDIT-C): an effective brief screening test for problem drinking. *Arch Intern Med.* 1998;158(16):1789–1795. https://doi.org/10.1001/archinte.158.16.1789
21. Prins A, Bovin MJ, Smolenski DJ, et al. The primary care PTSD screen for DSM-5 (PC-PTSD-5): development and evaluation within a veteran primary care sample. *J Gen Intern Med.* 2016;31(10):1206–1211. https://doi.org/10.1007/s11606-016-3703-5
22. Kaufman EA, Xia M, Fosco G, Yaptangco M, Skidmore CR, Crowell SE. The Difficulties in Emotion Regulation Scale Short Form (DERS-SF): validation and replication in adolescent and adult samples. *J Psychopathol Behav Assess.* 2016;38(3):443–455. https://doi.org/10.1007/s10862-015-9529-3
23. Martinez P, Richters JE. The Nimh Community Violence Project: II. Children's distress symptoms associated with violence exposure. *Psychiatry.* 1993;56(1):22–35. https://doi.org/10.1080/00332747.1993.11024618
24. National Center for Health Statistics. 2021 National Health Interview Survey. April 10, 2024. Available at: https://www.cdc.gov/nchs/nhis/2021nhis.htm. Accessed August 2, 2024.

25. NORC at the University of Chicago. AmeriSpeak panel technical overview. 2024. Available at: https://amerispeak.norc.org/content/dam/amerispeak/about-amerispeak/pdf/amerispeak-technical-overview.pdf. Accessed May 13, 2025.
26. Schafer JL. Multiple imputation: a primer. *Stat Methods Med Res.* 1999;8(1):3–15. https://doi.org/10.1177/096228029900800102
27. Litrownik AJ, Newton R, Hunter WM, English D, Everson MD. Exposure to family violence in young at-risk children: a longitudinal look at the effects of victimization and witnessed physical and psychological aggression. *J Fam Violence.* 2003;18(1):59–73. https://doi.org/10.1023/A:1021405515323
28. Farrell AD, Mehari KR, Kramer-Kuhn A, Goncy EA. The impact of victimization and witnessing violence on physical aggression among high-risk adolescents. *Child Dev.* 2014;85(4):1694–1710. https://doi.org/10.1111/cdev.12215
29. Overstreet S. Exposure to community violence: defining the problem and understanding the consequences. *J Child Fam Stud.* 2000;9(1):7–25. https://doi.org/10.1023/A:1009403530517
30. Creamer M. Posttraumatic stress disorder following violence and aggression. *Aggress Violent Behav.* 2000;5(5):431–449. https://doi.org/10.1016/S1359-1789(98)00017-2
31. Augsburger M, Maercker A. Associations between trauma exposure, posttraumatic stress disorder, and aggression perpetrated by women. A meta-analysis. *Clin Psychol Sci Pract.* 2020;27(1):e12322. https://doi.org/10.1037/h0101759
32. Bell KM, Orcutt HK. Posttraumatic stress disorder and male-perpetrated intimate partner violence. *JAMA.* 2009;302(5):562–564. https://doi.org/10.1001/jama.2009.1126
33. Jordan BK, Marmar CR, Fairbank JA, et al. Problems in families of male Vietnam veterans with posttraumatic stress disorder. *J Consult Clin Psychol.* 1992;60(6):916–926. https://doi.org/10.1037/0022-006X.60.6.916
34. Papachristos AV, Wildeman C, Roberto E. Tragic, but not random: the social contagion of nonfatal gunshot injuries. *Soc Sci Med.* 2015;125:139–150. https://doi.org/10.1016/j.socscimed.2014.01.056
35. Ross KM, Walsh CS, O'Connor KE, Sullivan TN. Ecological promotive and protective factors deterring gun carriage for young adults living in communities with high rates of community violence. *J Community Psychol.* 2023;51(3):1164–1180. https://doi.org/10.1002/jcop.23008

Silicosis Surveillance in California, 2019–2024: Tracking an Epidemic

Jennifer Flattery, MPH, Chelsea Woolsey, BS, Jane C. Fazio, MD, Sheiphali A. Gandhi, MD, MPH, Amy Heinzerling, MD, MPH, Robert J. Harrison, MD, MPH, and Kristin J. Cummings, MD, MPH

Objectives. To characterize the nature, burden, and trends of silicosis among California workers, including workers with engineered stone exposures.

Methods. We conducted multisource public health surveillance and generated descriptive statistics, compared engineered stone cases to cases with other silica exposures, and examined the utility of various data sources for silicosis surveillance.

Results. We received 1817 reports of possible silicosis for 648 individuals from 2019 to 2024 and confirmed 296 (46%) cases, including 243 (82%) associated with engineered stone exposures. Engineered stone cases were more likely to be younger, men, Latino, and from Los Angeles County than were non–engineered stone cases. Of engineered stone cases, at least 15 (6%) were known to have died, and 60 (25%) were referred for lung transplant, including 30 (12%) who received transplants. There was limited overlap between reporting mechanisms.

Conclusions. Multisource surveillance was effective for identifying a large number of individuals with silicosis, including people exposed to engineered stone. Outcomes were severe, and many patients had advanced disease. Results illustrate that worker screening and silica exposure mitigation are essential to prevent morbidity and mortality in the engineered stone countertop fabrication industry. (*Am J Public Health*. 2025;115(11):1913–1921. https://doi.org/10.2105/AJPH.2025.308225)

AJPH November 2025, Vol. 115, No. 11

Silicosis is a progressive, irreversible, fibrotic lung disease that results from the inhalation of respirable crystalline silica particles in the workplace. Silicosis is often disabling and can lead to respiratory failure and death, and there is no cure for severe disease other than lung transplantation. Silicosis is not a new disease, having been recognized by Hippocrates more than 2000 years ago, but the work and exposure contexts where it occurs have evolved along with industrial processes.[1] Silica occurs naturally in the earth's crust and is present in varying concentrations in nearly all rock. Silicosis has historically been recognized in a typically chronic form in older workers with decades of low to moderate exposure to dusty work environments involving natural stone, such as mining, foundries, sandblasting, tunneling, and construction.[2] More recently, silicosis has been recognized in the United States and around the world as associated with the fabrication of engineered stone (quartz) countertops. These cases typically involve considerably shorter periods of exposure among much younger workers with an accelerated form of disease.[2–7]

Engineered stone is manufactured by mixing crushed high-silica-content quartz with resins to create a composite material that can contain more than 90% silica, or more than 3 times the silica content of most natural stone.[8] Engineered stone has increased in popularity in the United States because of its cost, durability, and wide range of available colors and designs and is now the most commonly used material for countertops nationwide.[9]

Studies have shown that when engineered stone countertop material is cut, ground, or polished during fabrication, high levels of crystalline silica dust are generated that exceed regulatory limits set by the US Department of Labor Occupational Safety and Health Administration.[10–12] Efforts to prevent dust exposure, including engineering controls such as wet cutting methods for dust suppression and personal protective equipment, are complex and often not adequately protective.[11–13] Because of the difficulty in reducing dust to a level that would protect workers, Australia banned engineered stone containing more than 1% silica as of July 2024.[13] In response to the heightened silica exposure risk posed by engineered stone fabrication, the California Division of Occupational Safety and Health, California's workplace regulatory agency, has modified the existing silica standard to require specific exposure controls and medical monitoring for workers exposed to respirable crystalline silica while fabricating or finishing engineered stone.[14]

The first person in the United States known to have developed silicosis from engineered stone exposure was identified in Texas in 2014.[15] We began conducting case-based public health surveillance of silicosis in California in 2019 after a review of hospital discharge data identified a man aged 37 years who died from silicosis associated with engineered stone silica exposure.[4,5,16] In 2023, we reported the demographics, occupational history, and clinical features of the first 52 cases of engineered stone silicosis identified in California.[5,17] Surveillance efforts have since been significantly expanded. We update public health surveillance findings to further characterize the nature and extent of silicosis statewide, including a comparison of engineered stone worker characteristics with those of workers with other silica exposures.

METHODS

We identified silicosis cases through a combination of mechanisms:

1. Annual review of statewide hospital data (patient discharge and emergency department);
2. Voluntary direct health care provider reporting (physicians, tuberculosis [TB] controllers, and other local health department staff, pulmonary function laboratory technicians, and a transplant center);
3. Electronic case reporting (ECR) through the Reportable Conditions Knowledge Management System;
4. Worker screening as a result of case follow-up at a worksite; and
5. Voluntary direct reporting from other sources, including legal service providers.

After discovery of the index case in 2019, we examined hospital discharge data going back to 2006 to identify more silicosis cases and conducted screening at worksites associated with the index case. We have added additional data sources over time, including ECR and health care and legal service provider reporting in 2022.[18] We identified cases in hospital and ECR data using the *ICD-10* (*International Statistical Classification of Diseases and Related Health Problems, Tenth Revision* [Geneva, Switzerland: World Health Organization; 1992]) code for silicosis (J62.X). Some individuals were reported multiple times through multiple mechanisms or by only a single mechanism, which we considered "uniquely reported."

We recorded all reports in a relational database, with individual patients deduplicated.

Once we identified a report of silicosis, we obtained, reviewed, and abstracted medical records to ascertain additional case information and attempt to confirm the case. We confirmed cases using the National Institute for Occupational Safety and Health case definition for silicosis: history of occupational exposure to airborne silica dust and either imaging or pathology results interpreted as consistent with silicosis, as documented in medical records.[19] Those with engineered stone–associated silicosis met the confirmed case definition and additionally had a history of occupational exposure to engineered stone.

We recorded demographic data, occupational history, clinical information, and outcome data for all potential cases from initial reports and medical records. We calculated the ages at diagnosis, transplant, and death by subtracting date of birth from year of diagnosis, transplant date, and date of death, respectively. We calculated the interval from diagnosis to death by subtracting year of diagnosis from date of death. We defined outcome as the last patient disposition known to us based on reporting sources and medical records. Transplant status similarly reflects our most recent information, with mutually exclusive categories of transplanted, awaiting transplant, and denied transplant. We performed χ^2 analysis and generated descriptive statistics using SAS version 9.4 (SAS Institute, Cary, NC).

RESULTS

From January 2019 through December 2024, we received 1817 reports of silicosis for 648 individuals, including 313 (48%) with engineered stone exposures. Among the 648 reported individuals, we were able to confirm that 296 (46%) had silicosis. We determined an additional 73 (11%) not to be silicosis; 279 (43%) were missing essential information required for case confirmation. Among the 296 confirmed cases, 243 (82%) were associated with engineered stone exposure during countertop fabrication.

Table 1 shows that patients confirmed with silicosis were more likely to be men (99% vs 90%), to be Latino

TABLE 1— Demographic Characteristics of All Silicosis Cases Reported: California, 2019–2024

	All Potential Silicosis	Confirmed Silicosis	Confirmed Silicosis, Engineered Stone	Confirmed Silicosis, Non-Engineered Stone
Total, no. (%)	648	296 (46)	243 (38)	53 (8)
Male, no. (%)	584 (90)	292 (99)	242 (99.6)	50 (94)
Age, y, median (IQR)	50 (41–66)	47 (41–55)	46 (40–51)	65 (54–80)
Latino, no. (%)	435 (71)	262 (89)	237 (98)	25 (47)
Los Angeles County, no. (%)	247 (38)	150 (51)	138 (57)	12 (23)

Note. IQR = interquartile range.

(89% vs 71%), and to be from Los Angeles County (51% vs 38%) compared with all patients reported. Non–engineered stone workers with confirmed silicosis were older (median = 65 years; interquartile range [IQR] = 54–80) than were engineered stone workers with confirmed silicosis (median = 46 years; IQR = 40–51). Workers with confirmed engineered stone–associated silicosis were significantly more likely to be men (99.6% vs 94.0%; $P < .01$), to be Latino (98% vs 47%; $P < .001$), and to be from Los Angeles County (57% vs 23%; $P < .001$) than were workers with confirmed non–engineered stone–associated silicosis. The most commonly reported sources of silica exposure among workers with non–engineered stone silicosis were sandblasting, mining, cement work, glass manufacturing, brick manufacturing, and stone and tile cutting. Other occupations reported included dental technician, foundry worker, sculptor, and diatomaceous earth worker.

Engineered Stone Cases

Table 2 summarizes characteristics of confirmed engineered stone cases. Of the 105 workers with confirmed engineered stone silicosis in which country of origin was known, 69 (66%) were from Mexico, 20 (19%) from El Salvador, 7 (7%) from Guatemala, 4 (4%) from elsewhere in Latin America, 3 (3%) from countries outside Latin America, and 2 (2%) from the United States. Of the 114 confirmed engineered stone patients in which insurance status was known, 73 (64%) were covered under Medi-Cal, California's Medicaid program, 17 (15%) were uninsured or self-pay, 16 (14%) had private coverage, and 8 (7%) were covered by workers' compensation. The number of years of silica exposure was available for 166 (64%) workers with engineered stone silicosis, with a median of 19 years (IQR = 15–23), and

TABLE 2— Characteristics and Outcomes of Confirmed Engineered Stone–Associated Silicosis Cases: California, 2019–2024

Characteristic/Outcome (No. With Data Available)	No. (%) or Median (IQR)
Country of birth (105)	
Mexico	69 (66)
El Salvador	20 (19)
Guatemala	7 (7)
Other Latin America	4 (4)
Other	5 (5)
Years exposed (166)	19 (15–23)
Health insurance (114)	
Medi-Cal	73 (64)
Uninsured or self-pay	17 (15)
Private insurance	16 (14)
Workers' compensation	8 (7)
Outcomes (243)	
Death from silicosis	15 (6)
Age at death, y	46 (41–52)
Median interval from diagnosis to death in years	2
Referred for lung transplant	60 (25)
Transplanted (3 deceased)	30 (12)
Awaiting transplant (2 deceased)	24 (10)
Denied transplant (5 deceased)	6 (2)
Age at transplant, y	46 (38–51)

Note. IQR = interquartile range. Study population size was n = 243.

24 patients reporting 10 years of exposure or less. Among the 44 confirmed engineered stone patients with any information about TB, recognition of silicosis was delayed for 19 because of an initial diagnosis of TB, including 9 patients who received TB treatment before infection was ruled out and a silicosis diagnosis was made. We identified 5 confirmed engineered stone patients with silicotuberculosis.

We found that 60 (25%) of the 243 confirmed engineered stone patients were referred for lung transplant and 15 (6%) died as a result of their silicosis. Of the 60 transplant referrals, 30 (50%) received a transplant, 24 (40%) were waiting or being evaluated for transplant, and 6 (10%) were denied transplant. Ten (17%) of the 60 patients referred for transplant died (3 post-transplant, 2 while waiting, and 5 after denial). Patients who received transplants had a median age of 46 years at the time of transplant (IQR = 38–51) and 8 were younger than 40 years. Patients who died had a median age of 46 years at death (IQR = 41–52), including 3 who died before 40 years. The median interval from diagnosis to death was 2 years.

Reporting

Figure 1 illustrates the trend in silicosis case identification in California over time among those with confirmed engineered stone–associated silicosis and all other reported cases. Comparing the total number of cases from 2019 to 2021 before ECR and direct reporting by health care and legal services providers were added as data sources to the total number of cases in 2022 to 2024 shows that reporting of engineered stone cases increased 9-fold, whereas reporting of all other cases increased nearly 2.5-fold. Year of diagnosis was missing for 91 (37%) of 243 confirmed engineered stone cases, but among the 152 with data, 22 (15%) were diagnosed before 2019, when reporting began, and as early as 2006.

Among all individuals reported, 511 (79%) of 648 were uniquely reported through a single mechanism, whereas 145 (60%) of 243 confirmed engineered stone cases were uniquely reported through a single mechanism. Health care and legal service providers uniquely reported 106 (73%) of the 145 uniquely reported engineered stone cases, whereas hospital data and ECR were the largest sources for all other uniquely reported individuals (310/511 [61%]). Confirmed engineered stone cases were more likely to be reported by multiple reporting mechanisms compared with all cases (40% vs 21%).

Although the median was 1 report received per individual, the mean was 2.8, because some individuals were reported multiple times by multiple reporting sources, for multiple medical encounters, or both. Some individuals were reported by up to 4 different mechanisms. Reporting sources varied in volume and the ability to identify confirmed, engineered stone, and

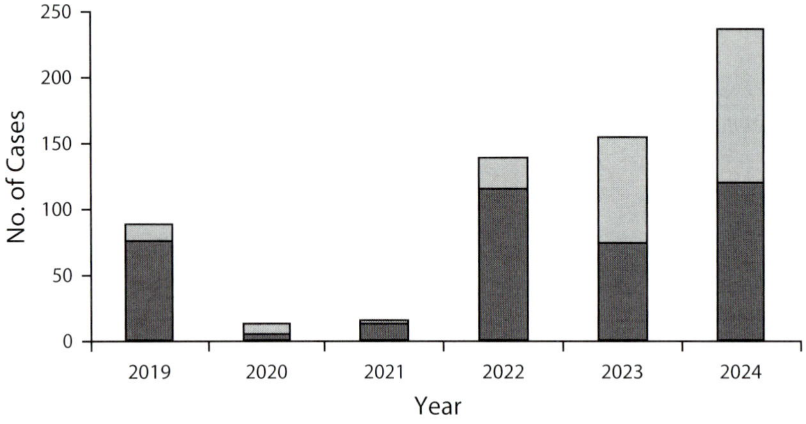

	2019	2020	2021	2022	2023	2024
Confirmed ES cases	13	7	2	24	80	117
All other reported cases	76	5	12	116	75	121

FIGURE 1— Silicosis Cases by Year Identified by California Department of Public Health: 2019–2024

Note. ES = engineered stone.

uniquely reported cases. Table 3 illustrates that across all 1817 reports received, 917 (50%) were received through ECR, 532 (29%) from hospital data, 161 (9%) from provider reports, 160 (9%) from legal services, and 46 (3%) from employee screening. We received 947 reports for confirmed engineered stone cases, with reports more likely to come from ECR, health care providers, and legal services than all other cases reported. Nearly 60% of all reports received for confirmed engineered stone cases were through ECR.

DISCUSSION

Since 2019, the California multisource silicosis surveillance system has processed 1817 reports for 648 individuals, of whom 243 were confirmed with engineered stone–associated silicosis. This is 1 of the largest case series of engineered stone silicosis reported worldwide and is especially noteworthy because nearly all cases were found through ongoing passive data collection, as opposed to active screening of engineered stone workers. Although the addition of case-finding mechanisms in the past 3 years has nearly tripled the number of all reported silicosis cases regardless of exposure, the number of confirmed engineered stone cases has increased 9-fold. This result illustrates the value of multisource surveillance and that without it, many cases may be unidentified; the burden of disease is likely underestimated because of reliance on physician reporting and can be better estimated by enhancing surveillance methods.

Historically, silicosis has been documented primarily in male-dominated industries. All but 4 of the 296 individuals with confirmed silicosis in our data set were men. Many of the reported cases that were determined not to have silicosis were women (23%), most commonly because of misdiagnosis or incorrect diagnosis codes in medical records. However, our surveillance data did identify 3 women with confirmed non–engineered stone–associated silicosis and 1 woman with confirmed engineered stone–associated silicosis. We have identified 2 additional women with potential engineered stone–associated silicosis but have not yet been able to confirm their diagnoses. To our knowledge, these are among the few women with engineered stone–associated silicosis reported worldwide.

Workers with confirmed non–engineered stone silicosis were significantly older and less likely to be Latino, compared with workers with confirmed engineered stone silicosis. Non–engineered stone patients worked in a variety of industries and occupations, including sandblasting, mining, glass product manufacturing, cement mixing and cutting, foundry work, and sand, rock, and brick work. Silica exposures are well documented in these work contexts, and historically workers in these environments develop chronic silicosis after decades of exposure.[2,20] We identified non–engineered stone patients across the state proportionate to state population distribution. This differs from engineered stone patients, 57% of whom resided in Los Angeles County, where 27% of the state population lives[21] but where there are high concentrations of engineered stone fabrication shops, and where several health care providers care for many silicosis patients and regularly report cases to the surveillance system.

Consistent with other publications on engineered stone silicosis, engineered stone silicosis patients in our data were primarily immigrants with a relatively short duration of exposure.[22–25] Although the median duration of exposure was 19 years, the range was from 1 to 39 years, with 24 patients (14% of those with data) reporting 10 years of exposure or less. Studies have demonstrated the relationship between exposure and disease[26,27] as well as the high levels of silica dust generated during engineered stone countertop fabrication,[10–12] illustrating the critical need

TABLE 3— Reports by Reporting Source for All Silicosis Cases Compared With Confirmed Engineered Stone–Associated Silicosis Cases: California, 2019–2024

Reporting Mechanism	All Reports, No. (%)	Reports for Confirmed Engineered Stone–Associated Cases, No. (%)
Total	1817 (100)	947 (52)[a]
Electronic case reporting	917 (50)	562 (59)
Hospital data	532 (29)	112 (12)
Health care provider	161 (9)	138 (15)
Legal	160 (9)	125 (13)
Active employee screening	46 (3)	10 (1)
Other	1 (0)	0 (0)

Note. The table represents reports, not individuals.
[a]This is a row percentage; the other percentages shown are column percentages.

to reduce exposures in the engineered stone fabrication industry. Although outcome reporting may not be timely given that it is captured in a surveillance system focused on reports at diagnosis, our surveillance data captured 15 deaths and 30 transplants, demonstrating the severe consequences of advanced disease in this young worker population. Transplant referral was made for a quarter of all confirmed engineered stone silicosis patients, and the youngest patient to receive a transplant was younger than 30 years. The median age at death was 46 years, with a median interval from diagnosis to death of 2 years, suggesting rapid disease progression and late diagnosis of disease.

These findings emphasize the importance of screening workers for disease and controlling workplace hazards. The California Division of Occupational Safety and Health's revised respirable crystalline silica standard contains new requirements, including that employers must conduct regular air monitoring, provide new protections for workers engaged in high-risk tasks, provide employee training, and test all high-risk workers for silicosis using more sensitive low-dose chest computed tomography scans as opposed to radiographs.[14] Employers also must report any confirmed silicosis cases to our surveillance system and the California Division of Occupational Safety and Health within 24 hours. These approaches may have an important impact on prevention, although enforcement of workplace standards can be challenging because the enforcing agency has limited resources and capacity.

Although silicosis is an occupational disease, only 7% of confirmed engineered stone cases with insurance information had medical care paid through workers' compensation. Instead, 79% of individuals with engineered stone–associated silicosis received publicly funded care or were uninsured. There is anecdotal information that many California engineered stone workers, although functioning as employees, are instead working as independent contractors,[5] which could affect their eligibility for workers' compensation. This results in cost shifting from employers' workers compensation insurance carriers to primarily publicly funded care and may dissuade workers from seeking care if they are not adequately covered by insurance. In general, the largely immigrant population of workers who are affected by engineered stone silicosis faces many barriers to health care and safe work environments.[28]

Early diagnosis is critical. The primary treatment of silicosis is limiting exposure in the workplace. Reducing exposures not only protects workers who have already been identified with silicosis from further exposure and may slow disease progression[29] but also decreases disease risk for other workers in the same work environment. Past studies in California have shown that worker medical screening and implementation of exposure controls in countertop fabrication shops are lacking.[10,30] Clinicians should routinely ask about work exposures and report any suspected cases of silicosis to their local or state health jurisdiction. Previous studies have demonstrated that delays in identification can result in more severe disease and poorer outcomes.[17]

It is well established that silicosis increases the risk of TB[31,32] and that TB and silicosis can be difficult to distinguish, both clinically and radiologically.[33] Because the patients we describe with engineered stone silicosis are young immigrant men from countries where TB is endemic, TB may be high in the differential diagnosis. We have previously documented delays in silicosis diagnosis because of initial diagnoses of TB.[5] Our current data include 5 confirmed engineered stone cases of silicotuberculosis as well as 19 engineered stone cases with silicosis diagnoses that were delayed because of first being diagnosed with TB, which was subsequently ruled out. Of those 19 cases, 9 cases were treated for TB before the silicosis diagnosis was recognized. Workers with silica exposures should be screened for both silicosis and TB, and clinicians should monitor those with silicosis for TB because of the increased risk posed by silicosis.

Strengths and Limitations

The data in this report are subject to several limitations. The data likely underrepresent total case counts in the state because it is well documented that silicosis, particularly in young engineered stone workers, is underrecognized and underdiagnosed.[34] Voluntary provider reporting was routinely done by 8 clinicians who had awareness and interest in the disease and was focused in 1 geographic area of the state. Low-wage immigrant workers may not have access to care or may not seek care because of fear of retaliation from employers or concerns about immigration status, all of which contribute to underdiagnosis and underrecognition. The medical records we reviewed were usually associated with only the medical encounter that was reported, limiting our knowledge of other care a patient may have received, and we relied primarily on patient self-report regarding their exposure to silica.

It is important to note that for the period we studied, silicosis reporting was not mandatory in California. Therefore, reporting was not done consistently for all cases, as voluntary health care provider and legal services reporting focused specifically on engineered stone cases and contained details about exposures, clinical status, and outcomes. Although hospital data and ECR identified individuals with silicosis statewide without regard to exposure source by using *ICD-10* codes indicating silicosis, medical records were generally more complete and detailed for younger patients with accelerated disease associated with engineered stone exposures, compared with older patients, whose exposures and silicosis diagnosis were many years earlier. As a result of the additional detail and more current histories, engineered stone case records were much more likely to provide the information necessary to meet the case definition for confirmation than were non–engineered stone records. We often identified non–engineered stone patients through diagnosis codes of silicosis in a historical problem list, but their encounters with the health care system were for other, non–silicosis-related medical conditions. More than 40% of all silicosis cases reported were missing essential information required for case confirmation or were still in the process of being confirmed. The age, ethnicity, and geographic distribution of individuals with unconfirmed cases more closely resembled those with confirmed non–engineered stone–associated silicosis than those with engineered stone–associated silicosis.

Our data demonstrate that multisource surveillance generates increased case finding. Case-finding mechanisms varied in timeliness and efficacy and had limited overlap. Nearly 80% of all silicosis cases and 60% of confirmed engineered stone cases were uniquely reported through only 1 reporting mechanism. Voluntary reporting by health care and legal service providers included detail and provided cases that were more easily confirmed, but the scope was limited to their practices and not geographically representative of the entire state. ECR provides real-time reporting of any health care encounter at a participating facility statewide with silicosis in the problem list. Currently, there are 3120 California facilities participating, and we have documented the value of using this mechanism to identify individuals with silicosis.[18] ECR has also been effective for providing updated information on case status and outcome and uniquely reported 20% of all reported silicosis cases.

The utility of ECR for surveillance should expand even more, as several large health care organizations do not yet participate. Hospital data are accessed annually and are therefore not timely, but they are effective for identifying cases with the most severe disease. The reporting mechanisms used for our surveillance system can be adopted by other public health jurisdictions for silicosis surveillance. In addition to accessing hospital and ECR data, media attention and outreach have been effective for raising health care provider awareness and enlisting voluntary provider reporting. Silicosis became a reportable disease in California in July 2025, which is anticipated to increase case finding significantly.

Public Health Implications

Using multisource surveillance in California, we identified an increasing number of accelerated engineered stone–associated cases among mostly young, Latino, immigrant men, as well as many cases of chronic silicosis from more traditional silica exposures. Given the lag time between exposure and diagnosis and extensive ongoing exposures, we expect many more engineered stone cases to be identified in the future. The outcomes for these young workers can be severe and illustrate the importance of identifying disease early and controlling workplace exposures. The addition of surveillance mechanisms, including ECR and voluntary reporting by informed health care and legal service providers, increased case finding significantly and are approaches that can be adapted by jurisdictions nationwide. AJPH

ABOUT THE AUTHORS

Jennifer Flattery, Chelsea Woolsey, Amy Heinzerling, Robert J. Harrison, and Kristin J. Cummings are with the Occupational Health Branch, California Department of Public Health, Richmond. Jane C. Fazio is with the David Geffen School of Medicine and Olive View Medical Center, University of California, Los Angeles. Sheiphali A. Gandhi is with the Division of Occupational, Environmental, and Climate Medicine, University of California, San Francisco.

CORRESPONDENCE

Correspondence should be sent to Jennifer Flattery, Occupational Health Branch, 850 Marina Bay Pkwy, Building P, 3rd Floor, Richmond, CA, 94804 (e-mail: Jennifer.flattery@cdph.ca.gov). Reprints can be ordered at http://www.ajph.org by clicking the "Reprints" link.

PUBLICATION INFORMATION

Full Citation: Flattery J, Woolsey C, Fazio JC, et al. Silicosis surveillance in California, 2019–2024:

tracking an epidemic. *Am J Public Health*. 2025;
115(11):1913–1921.
Acceptance Date: June 18, 2025.
DOI: https://doi.org/10.2105/AJPH.2025.308225
ORCID iDs:
Jennifer Flattery https://orcid.org/0000-0002-3158-4649

Chelsea Woolsey https://orcid.org/0009-0002-0223-7397

Jane C. Fazio https://orcid.org/0000-0002-3406-4542

Sheiphali A. Gandhi https://orcid.org/0000-0003-3156-7619

Amy Heinzerling https://orcid.org/0000-0001-8808-3004

Kristin J. Cummings https://orcid.org/0000-0002-5422-9199

CONTRIBUTORS

J. Flattery led the data acquisition, analysis, and interpretation and drafted the article. C. Woolsey contributed to the data acquisition, analysis, and interpretation. C. Woolsey, J. C. Fazio, S. A. Gandhi, A. Heinzerling, R. J. Harrison, and K. J. Cummings revised the article. J. C. Fazio, S. A. Gandhi, and A. Heinzerling contributed case reports. All authors made substantial contributions to the conceptualization and design of the work and approved the article.

ACKNOWLEDGMENTS

This study was supported in part by the National Institute for Occupational Safety and Health (NIOSH; grants 2U60OH008468, U19OH012293, 75D30122P14131, 75D30124P19702).

The authors thank the many reporters who identified silicosis cases and contributed information to the surveillance system.

Note. The findings and conclusions in this article are those of the authors and do not necessarily represent the views or opinions of the California Department of Public Health, the California Health and Human Services Agency, or NIOSH.

CONFLICTS OF INTEREST

The authors have no conflicts of interest to disclose.

HUMAN PARTICIPANT PROTECTION

The California Committee for the Protection of Human Subjects approved this project.

REFERENCES

1. Sherson D. Silicosis in the twenty-first century. *Occup Environ Med*. 2002;59(11):721–722. https://doi.org/10.1136/oem.59.11.721
2. Barnes H, Goh NSL, Leong TL, Hoy R. Silica-associated lung disease: an old-world exposure in modern industries. *Respirology*. 2019;24(12):1165–1175. https://doi.org/10.1111/resp.13695
3. Hoy RF, Dimitriadis C, Abramson M, et al. Prevalence and risk factors for silicosis among a large cohort of stone benchtop industry workers. *Occup Environ Med*. 2023;80(8):439–446. https://doi.org/10.1136/oemed-2023-108892
4. Centers for Disease Control and Prevention. Severe silicosis in engineered stone fabrication workers—California, Colorado, Texas, and Washington, 2017–2019. *MMWR Morb Mortal Wkly Rep*. 2019;68(38):813–818. https://doi.org/10.15585/mmwr.mm6838a1
5. Fazio JC, Gandhi SA, Flattery J, et al. Silicosis among immigrant engineered stone (quartz) countertop fabrication workers in California. *JAMA Intern Med*. 2023;183(9):991–998. https://doi.org/10.1001/jamainternmed.2023.3295
6. Pérez-Alonso A, Córdoba-Doña JA, Millares-Lorenzo JL, Figueroa-Murillo E, García-Vadillo C, Romero-Morillos J. Outbreak of silicosis in Spanish quartz conglomerate workers. *Int J Occup Environ Health*. 2014;20(1):26–32. https://doi.org/10.1179/2049396713Y.0000000049
7. Wu N, Xue C, Yu S, Ye Q. Artificial stone-associated silicosis in China: a prospective comparison with natural stone-associated silicosis. *Respirology*. 2020;25(5):518–524. https://doi.org/10.1111/resp.13744
8. National Institute for Occupational Safety and Health. Worker exposure to silica during countertop manufacturing, finishing and installation. DHHS (NIOSH) Publication No. 2015-106. Available at: https://www.osha.gov/sites/default/files/publications/OSHA3768.pdf. Accessed December 9, 2024.
9. Freedonia Group. US engineered stone countertops. Available at: https://www.freedoniagroup.com/industry-study/engineered-stone-countertops-4395.htm Accessed December 9, 2024.
10. Surasi K, Ballen B, Weinberg JL, et al. Elevated exposures to respirable crystalline silica among engineered stone fabrication workers in California, January 2019–February 2020. *Am J Ind Med*. 2022;65(9):701–707. https://doi.org/10.1002/ajim.23416
11. Qi C, Echt A. Engineering control of silica dust from stone countertop fabrication and installation. Available at: https://www.cdc.gov/niosh/surveyreports/pdfs/375-11a.pdf. Accessed December 9, 2024.
12. Occupational Safety and Health Administration. Lessons learned and initial findings from OSHA's emphasis program on silica in engineered stone. Available at: https://www.osha.gov/sites/default/files/publications/silica-hazard-alert.pdf. Accessed December 9, 2024.
13. Australian Department of Employment and Workplace Relations. Prohibition on the use of engineered stone. Available at: https://www.dewr.gov.au/engineeredstone Accessed December 9, 2024.
14. State of California. Standard for respirable crystalline silica for general industry. Available at: https://www.dir.ca.gov/oshsb/documents/Respirable-Crystalline-Silica-Non-Emergency-2nd-15-day.pdf. Accessed February 20, 2025.
15. Centers for Disease Control and Prevention. Notes from the field: silicosis in a countertop fabricator—Texas, 2014. *MMWR Morb Mortal Wkly Rep*. 2015;64(5):129–130. Available at: https://www.cdc.gov/mmwr/preview/mmwrhtml/mm6405a5.htm. Accessed August 26, 2025.
16. Heinzerling A, Cummings KJ, Flattery J, Weinberg JW, Materna B, Harrison R. Radiographic screening reveals high burden of silicosis among workers at an engineered stone countertop fabrication facility in California. *Am J Respir Crit Care Med*. 2021;203(6):764–766. https://doi.org/10.1164/rccm.202008-3297LE
17. Gandhi SA, Heinzerling A, Flattery J, et al. Active surveillance of engineered stone workers facilitates early identification of silicosis: a discussion of surveillance of occupational lung diseases. *New Solut*. 2023;33(2-3):119–129. https://doi.org/10.1177/10482911231189503
18. Centers for Disease Control and Prevention. Notes from the field: surveillance of silicosis using electronic case reporting—California, December 2022–July 2023. *MMWR Morb Mortal Wkly Rep*. 2023;72(46):1275–1276. https://doi.org/10.15585/mmwr.mm7246a4
19. National Institute for Occupational Safety and Health. Silicosis reporting guidelines. Available at: https://www.cdc.gov/niosh/surveillance/respiratorydisease/silicosis-reporting.html. Accessed December 9, 2024.
20. Bang KM, Attfield MD, Wood JM, Syamlal G. National trends in silicosis mortality in the United States, 1981–2004. *Am J Ind Med*. 2008;51(9):633–639. https://doi.org/10.1002/ajim.20607
21. US Census Bureau. California population change between census decades. Available at: https://www.census.gov/library/stories/state-by-state/california-population-change-between-census-decade.html. Accessed December 10, 2024.
22. Feary J, Devaraj A, Burton M, et al. Artificial stone silicosis: a UK case series. *Thorax*. 2024;79(10):979–981. https://doi.org/10.1136/thorax-2024-221715
23. Martínez González C, Prieto González A, García Alfonso L, et al. Silicosis in artificial quartz conglomerate workers. *Arch Bronconeumol (Engl Ed)*. 2019;55(9):459–464. https://doi.org/10.1016/j.arbres.2019.01.017
24. Kramer MR, Blanc PD, Fireman E, et al. Artificial stone silicosis: disease resurgence among artificial stone workers. *Chest*. 2012;142(2):419–424. [Erratum in: *Chest*. 2012;142(4):1080]. https://doi.org/10.1378/chest.11-1321
25. Hoy RF, Baird T, Hammerschlag G, et al. Artificial stone-associated silicosis: a rapidly emerging occupational lung disease. *Occup Environ Med*. 2018;75(1):3–5. https://doi.org/10.1136/oemed-2017-104428
26. National Institute for Occupational Safety and Health. Health effects of occupational exposure to respirable crystalline silica. 2002. Available at: https://www.cdc.gov/niosh/docs/2002-129/pdfs/2002-129.pdf?id=10.26616/NIOSHPUB2002129. Accessed December 10, 2024.
27. 't Mannetje A, Steenland K, Attfield M, et al. Exposure-response analysis and risk assessment for silica and silicosis mortality in a pooled analysis of six cohorts. *Occup Environ Med*. 2002;59(11):723–728. https://doi.org/10.1136/oem.59.11.723
28. Gandhi SA, Heinzerling A, Flattery J, Cummings KJ. Occupational contributions to respiratory health disparities. *Clin Chest Med*. 2023;44(3):635–649. https://doi.org/10.1016/j.ccm.2023.03.016
29. Carneiro APS, Barreto SM, Siqueira AL, Cavariani F, Forastiere F. Continued exposure to silica after diagnosis of silicosis in Brazilian gold miners. *Am J Ind Med*. 2006;49(10):811–818. https://doi.org/10.1002/ajim.20379
30. Spiegel A, Cummings KJ, Flattery J, Harrison R, Heinzerling A. Self-reported silica exposures and

workplace protections among engineered stone fabrication workers in California. *Am J Ind Med.* 2022;65(12):1022–1024. https://doi.org/10.1002/ajim.23432

31. Ehrlich R, Akugizibwe P, Siegfried N, Rees D. The association between silica exposure, silicosis and tuberculosis: a systematic review and meta-analysis. *BMC Public Health.* 2021;21(1):953. https://doi.org/10.1186/s12889-021-10711-1
32. Jamshidi P, Danaei B, Arbabi M, et al. Silicosis and tuberculosis: a systematic review and meta-analysis. *Pulmonology.* 2025;31(1):2416791. https://doi.org/10.1016/j.pulmoe.2023.05.001
33. Maboso B, Te Water Naude J, Rees D, Goodman H, Ehrlich R. Difficulties in distinguishing silicosis and pulmonary tuberculosis in silica-exposed gold miners: a report of four cases. *Am J Ind Med.* 2023;66(4):339–348. https://doi.org/10.1002/ajim.23460
34. Hoy RF, Sim MR. Correspondence on "Demographic, exposure and clinical characteristics in a multinational registry of engineered stone workers with silicosis" by Hua et al. *Occup Environ Med.* 2022;79(9):647–648. https://doi.org/10.1136/oemed-2022-108496

Multiple Social Demographics and Disparities in Smoking Cessation During Pregnancy in the United States, 2016–2022: An Intersectional Analytic Framework

Yangyang Cheng, MSc, Carmen C. W. Lim, PhD, Rodrigo Martin Carrillo-Larco, PhD, and Xiaolin Xu, PhD

AJPH November 2025, Vol. 115, No. 11

Objectives. To examine how multiple social demographics shape disparities in smoking cessation during pregnancy in an intersectional analytic framework.

Methods. We analyzed US National Vital Statistics System (2016–2022) data on 588 435 primiparous women with prepregnancy smoking. We constructed 192 intersectional strata to represent contexts defined by race/ethnicity, education, marital status, insurance status, and immigration status. We conducted a multilevel analysis of individual heterogeneity and discriminatory accuracy to estimate intersectional inequities in smoking cessation during pregnancy, predict cessation prevalence across strata, and assess the extent to which disparities were attributable to additive or interaction effects.

Results. Smoking cessation during pregnancy prevalence ranged from 27.2% to 89.4% across strata. Differences between intersectional strata explained 11.9% of the variation in smoking cessation, with educational level contributing most. Of the between-strata variation, 93.9% was explained by additive effects, whereas 6.1% was attributable to interaction effects.

Conclusions. Significant disparities in pregnancy smoking cessation are linked to multiple social demographics, highlighting the need for universal interventions paired with tailored support for disadvantaged groups to advance maternal health equity. (*Am J Public Health*. 2025;115(11):1922–1932. https://doi.org/10.2105/AJPH.2025.308237)

Maternal smoking during pregnancy is a preventable risk factor for adverse birth outcomes, such as preterm birth and infant death,[1] as well as long-term health effects, including lung disease and neurologic morbidity in offspring.[2] Over the past 30 years, the prevalence of smoking during pregnancy in the United States has declined substantially, largely because of tobacco control efforts.[3] However, a substantial number of pregnant women continue to smoke,[4] despite evidence demonstrating that quitting smoking during pregnancy can mitigate the risk of adverse outcomes.[5] A 2018 global review found that 53% of women continue to smoke daily during pregnancy.[3] Research indicates that historically marginalized populations have higher smoking rates and face greater challenges in quitting than do less marginalized groups.[6] Therefore, understanding how structural manifestations of social inequality, such as discrimination and marginalization, affect smoking cessation during pregnancy is crucial for developing tailored interventions.

Smoking cessation rates vary across sociodemographic groups, with observed disparities largely driven by structural discrimination and systemic disadvantage associated with historically marginalized positions, such as being among a racial/ethnic minority and having low socioeconomic status.[7]

Existing evidence indicates that a wide range of social demographics, including race/ethnicity, educational level, marital status, insurance status, and immigrant status, are associated with smoking cessation during pregnancy.[8] Most studies on smoking cessation inequities have examined social demographics primarily in isolation or focused on only a subset, thereby concealing heterogeneity in populations and failing to account for the intersections of multiple social demographics categories.[9,10]

However, a core tenet of intersectionality is that social categories are not independent and unidimensional but are intersecting and constructed through overlapping systems of power and oppression.[11] Rooted in Black feminist scholarship,[12] the concept of intersectionality also emphasizes how multiple social categories at the individual level interact with interlocking systems of privilege and oppression at the societal level to shape health patterns.[11] Scholars have increasingly called for a broader application of this framework, as conventional research has often neglected the structural roots of health inequities by failing to account for these intersecting systems.[13] Although there have been advancements in applying intersectionality to quantitative research, a significant gap remains. Adopting this approach can provide more robust insights into how overlapping social demographics contribute to health disparities among pregnant women.

More recently, a novel approach known as intersectional multilevel analysis of individual heterogeneity and discriminatory accuracy (I-MAIHDA), an application of the broader MAIHDA approach, has been developed to quantify the disparities in socioeconomic, psychosocial, and health conditions in an intersectional analytical framework.[14–16] In comparison with traditional regression analysis and other quantitative methods, I-MAIHDA offers superior practical, methodological, and theory-oriented advantages for assessing both between-group and within-group heterogeneity.[17] However, there has been limited research on the use of an I-MAIHDA approach to map the distribution of, and address, the intersection of social demographics in maternal smoking cessation.

We applied intersectionality as an analytical framework to examine how the intersectional strata constructed by race/ethnicity, education level, marital status, insurance status, and immigration status shape the disparities in smoking cessation prevalence during pregnancy by using the I-MAIHDA method. This approach can inform the development of tailored, resource-efficient interventions to improve smoking cessation outcomes during pregnancy.

METHODS

We obtained data from the US National Vital Statistics System, which was collected by the National Center for Health Statistics at the Centers for Disease Control and Prevention. The data include individual-level information on births, fetal deaths, and maternal status. The National Center for Health Statistics used standard documents, such as maternal and facility worksheets, to gather information on maternal and fetal health, including demographics, pregnancy complications, admission history, physical examinations, and delivery records for all live births in all 50 states and the District of Columbia. More details about National Vital Statistics System data collection and methodology can be found at https://www.cdc.gov/nchs/nvss/births.htm.

We retrieved 26 345 765 records from 2016 through 2022 from the National Vital Statistics System birth database. To avoid potential within-subject clustering owing to possible multiple pregnancies, we included only primiparous women who reported smoking before pregnancy in the study (n = 619 477). We excluded pregnant women with incomplete data on relevant demographics (n = 31 042). The detailed flowchart of participant inclusion and exclusion is presented in Figure A (available as a supplement to the online version of this article at http://www.ajph.org).

Smoking Cessation

Participants reported the average daily number of cigarettes smoked in the 3 months before pregnancy and during the first, second, and third trimesters of pregnancy. We categorized participants who smoked 1 or more cigarettes before pregnancy but not during the entire pregnancy (i.e., no smoking in any trimester, no smoking during the second and third trimesters, or no smoking during the third trimester) as having quit smoking.

Intersectional Social Contexts

We included 5 social demographics: race/ethnicity, educational level, marital status, insurance status, and immigrant status. We combined race/ethnicity into a single variable with 7 categories: non-Hispanic White, non-Hispanic Black, non-Hispanic American Indian or Alaska Native, non-Hispanic Asian, non-Hispanic Native Hawaiian or other Pacific Islander, non-Hispanic multiracial, and Hispanic. To ensure adequate sample sizes for analysis, we further divided race/ethnicity into non-Hispanic White, non-Hispanic Black, Hispanic, and other. We classified educational level as low (no high school diploma or equivalent), medium low (high school graduate or equivalent), medium high (some college or associate degree), high (bachelor's or more advanced degree). We classified women as married if they were married at any point between conception and childbirth and otherwise as unmarried. We classified insurance status as government (Medicaid, Indian Health Service, or other government insurance), private, or self-pay. We classified women as immigrants if they were born outside the United States but currently residing in the United States; otherwise, we defined them as nonimmigrants, meaning they were born and currently living in the United States.

Statistical Analysis

We described the characteristics of participants as counts (percentages) by smoking cessation status, and we tested differences among groups using the χ^2 test. We constructed 192 intersectional strata to represent intersectional contexts, defined by mutually exclusive combinations of race/ethnicity, educational level, marital status, insurance status, and immigrant status. To implement I-MAIHDA,[18] we employed a 2-level (multilevel) logistic regression model. We nested individuals (level 1) in intersectional strata (level 2). First, we estimated a null model (simple intersectional model) with random intercepts for intersectional strata, summarizing overall inequity. This model generated strata-specific predictions and quantified the degree of outcome heterogeneity both within and between strata. Based on this model, we estimated the variance partition coefficient (VPC), also known as the intraclass correlation coefficient, to measure the proportion of total variance in the outcome attributed to differences between strata by using the latent response approach:

$$(1) \qquad \text{VPC} = \frac{\sigma_u^2}{\sigma_u^2 + \frac{\pi^2}{3}} \times 100,$$

where σ_u^2 denotes the between-stratum variance and $\frac{\pi^2}{3}$ denotes the within-stratum variance equal to the variance of the standard logistic distribution. The VPC indicates the contextual influence of intersectional strata on individual inequalities, commonly referred to as the "general contextual effect" (GCE).[19] A higher VPC or GCE suggests a larger difference in prevalence between intersectional strata. Another measurement of GCE is the area under the receiver operating characteristic curve (AUC), which serves as a direct measure of a model's discriminatory accuracy. Higher AUC values indicate better differentiation between women who achieved smoking cessation and those who did not.

The GCE provides crucial insights into whether intervention strategies should be universal (low VPC/AUC) or tailored (high VPC/AUC). Proportionate universalism, which integrates universal interventions with additional tailored support for disadvantaged groups based on their unique contexts, serves as the guiding principle for intervention design.[20]

Then, we estimated 5 partial models to evaluate the contribution of each demographic to the between-stratum variance. These models extended the null model by adding 1 factor at a time as a fixed effect. We calculated the proportional change in variance (PCV) to measure the proportional reduction in between-stratum variance from the null model to the partial models:

$$\text{PCV} = \frac{\sigma^2_{u\ (null\ model)} - \sigma^2_{u\ (partial\ model)}}{\sigma^2_{u\ (null\ model)}} \times 100 \qquad (2)$$

where a high PCV indicates a substantial impact of the included demographic on observed disparities between strata.

Finally, we estimated a full model (intersectional interaction model) that expanded the null model by including all 5 variables used to construct the intersectional strata as fixed effects. This model estimated intersectional effects of strata and quantified the extent to which observed inequities between strata were explained by additive effects versus interaction effects. We used "intersectional effects" to denote the combined influence of multiple social demographics, encompassing both additive and interaction effects. By contrast, in qualitative frameworks, "intersectional effects" often emphasize concepts such as simultaneity, multiplicativity, or multiple jeopardy, highlighting how overlapping social positions reflect unique social experiences that are not reducible to statistical interaction effects as defined in quantitative research.[21] It is important to distinguish between these concepts to avoid conflating methodological techniques with theoretical foundations.

The VPC in the full model quantifies the proportion of the total variance remaining after adjusting for additive effects, attributable to interaction effects. Meanwhile, the PCV measures the proportion of between-stratum variance in the null model explained by additive effects, with the remaining variation (1 − PCV) attributable to interaction effects.

To assess potential confounding, we estimated 5 adjusted models based on the full model, each additionally including 1 of the following covariates: women's age at childbirth, delivery year, prepregnancy smoking frequency, receipt of Special Supplemental Nutrition Program for Women, Infants, and Children benefits, or husband's or partner's educational level. We selected these covariates based on their relevance to smoking behavior and cessation support.[8]

For each intersectional stratum, we applied maximum likelihood estimation to derive the total predicted prevalence (including additive effects and random intercept), the additive-only prevalence (additive effects only), and the interaction effects (the difference between the total and additive-only prevalence) with 95% confidence intervals (CIs).

We conducted all analyses using SAS version 9.4 (SAS Institute, Cary, NC) and R version 4.3.0 (RStudio, Boston, MA). We assessed statistical significance using the 2-sided test, with $P < .05$ considered significant.

RESULTS

We included 588 435 women who reported smoking before pregnancy in the final analysis (Figure A). Among them, 310 656 (52.8%) ceased smoking during pregnancy. Women who quit smoking were more likely to be of Hispanic ethnicity, have a higher educational level, be currently married, have private insurance, and be immigrants (Table 1). The stratum with the largest sample size was the unmarried, White nonimmigrant women with medium-low educational attainment and government insurance (n = 113 447), whereas the stratum with the smallest sample size was married Black immigrant women with low educational level and self-pay medical care (n = 1; Table A, available as a supplement to the online version of this article at http://www.ajph.org).

The intersectional multilevel models also showed the effects of intersectional strata and the variance attributable to between-strata differences (Table 2). The weighted predicted prevalence of smoking cessation was 66.4% (95% CI = 64.8, 67.9). The null model VPC revealed that 11.9% of the total variance in smoking cessation prevalence was attributable to between-stratum differences. The AUC value (AUC = 0.66) similarly indicated that intersectional strata had moderate discriminatory accuracy in classifying smoking cessation cases. Across the partial models, educational level contributed most to reducing the variation between strata (PCV = 41.2%), followed by race/ethnicity (PCV = 23.7%; Table B, available as a supplement to the online version of this article at http://www.ajph.org). The full model PCV indicated that 93.9% of the variation between strata was explained by the additive effects, which accounted for most of the differences in smoking cessation prevalence across intersectional strata, whereas the remaining 6.1% was attributable to interaction effects. After adjusting for the 5 covariates separately, the results generally remained consistent with the main analysis (Table C, available as a supplement to the online version of this article at http://www.ajph.org).

Predicted prevalence varied across intersectional strata, ranging from 27.2% to 89.4% (Figure 1; Table A). We observed the lowest predicted prevalence among White unmarried nonimmigrant women with a low educational level and self-pay medical care (27.2%). Conversely, we found the highest predicted prevalence among married Hispanic immigrant women with high educational level and private insurance (89.4%). As shown in Figure 2 (for 96 immigrant strata) and Figure B (available as a supplement to the online version of this article at http://www.ajph.org; for 96 nonimmigrant strata), regardless of combinations of the other 4 demographics, more highly educated women had a higher predicted prevalence of smoking cessation than did their less educated counterparts.

Despite the relatively small proportion of variance explained by interaction effects, a complex pattern of interactions emerged across certain strata. Among all strata, 21 showed a statistically significant positive interaction effect, for example, unmarried Hispanic immigrant women with low educational level and self-pay medical care had higher than expected prevalence, whereas 8 strata exhibited a negative effect, for example, unmarried White immigrant women with medium-low educational level and private insurance had lower than expected prevalence (Table A).

DISCUSSION

In this population-based study, we applied a novel I-MAIHDA approach to quantify the disparities in smoking cessation during pregnancy across intersectional social strata. To our knowledge, this is the first study to examine how intersections of multiple social demographics—such as race/ethnicity, education level, marital status, insurance status, and immigration status—shape smoking cessation

TABLE 1— **Participant Characteristics by Smoking Cessation: National Vital Statistics System, United States, 2016–2022**

Variable	All, No. (%)	Smoking Cessation, No. (%)		P
		No	Yes	
Total	588 435 (100.0)	277 779 (47.2)	310 656 (52.8)	
Race/ethnicity				<.001
Non-Hispanic White	461 508 (78.4)	229 918 (82.8)	231 590 (74.5)	
Non-Hispanic Black	47 429 (8.1)	19 367 (7.0)	28 062 (9.0)	
Hispanic	42 563 (7.2)	12 774 (4.6)	29 789 (9.6)	
Other	36 935 (6.3)	15 720 (5.7)	21 215 (6.8)	
Educational level				<.001
Low	108 126 (18.4)	66 377 (23.9)	41 749 (13.4)	
Medium low	247 094 (42.0)	127 152 (45.8)	119 942 (38.6)	
Medium high	185 082 (31.5)	73 258 (26.4)	111 824 (36.0)	
High	48 133 (8.2)	10 992 (4.0)	37 141 (12.0)	
Marital status				<.001
Unmarried	449 613 (76.4)	226 301 (81.5)	223 312 (71.9)	
Married	138 822 (23.6)	51 478 (18.5)	87 344 (28.1)	
Insurance status				<.001
Government	377 775 (64.2)	202 657 (73.0)	175 118 (56.4)	
Private	200 216 (34.0)	69 483 (25.0)	130 733 (42.1)	
Self-pay	10 444 (1.8)	5 639 (2.0)	4 805 (1.5)	
Immigrant status				<.001
Immigrant	18 982 (3.2)	4 956 (1.8)	14 026 (4.5)	
Nonimmigrant	569 453 (96.8)	272 823 (98.2)	296 630 (95.5)	
Delivery year				<.001
2016	121 005 (20.6)	55 652 (20.0)	65 353 (21.0)	
2017	107 135 (18.2)	50 294 (18.1)	56 841 (18.3)	
2018	96 509 (16.4)	45 622 (16.4)	50 887 (16.4)	
2019	84 983 (14.4)	40 111 (14.4)	44 872 (14.4)	
2020	74 690 (12.7)	35 915 (12.9)	38 775 (12.5)	
2021	59 844 (10.2)	28 517 (10.3)	31 327 (10.1)	
2022	44 269 (7.5)	21 668 (7.8)	22 601 (7.3)	
Age at delivery, y				<.001
<20	83 217 (14.1)	41 536 (15.0)	41 681 (13.4)	
20–24	233 613 (39.7)	112 257 (40.4)	121 356 (39.1)	
25–29	151 070 (25.7)	70 742 (25.5)	80 328 (25.9)	
30–34	82 367 (14.0)	36 090 (13.0)	46 277 (14.9)	
35–39	32 519 (5.5)	14 498 (5.2)	18 021 (5.8)	
≥40	5 649 (1.0)	2 656 (1.0)	2 993 (1.0)	
Smoking frequency before pregnancy, cigarettes per day				<.001
1-5	172 827 (29.4)	55 509 (20.0)	117 318 (37.8)	
6-10	188 396 (32.0)	87 480 (31.5)	100 916 (32.5)	
≥11	227 212 (38.6)	134 790 (48.5)	92 422 (29.8)	
WIC food during pregnancy				<.001
Yes	321 840 (54.7)	170 965 (61.5)	150 875 (48.6)	
No	260 964 (44.3)	103 925 (37.4)	157 039 (50.6)	
Unknown	5 631 (1.0)	2 889 (1.0)	2 742 (0.9)	

Continued

TABLE 1— Continued

Variable	All, No. (%)	Smoking Cessation, No. (%)		P
		No	Yes	
Husband/partner's educational level				<.001
Low	75 297 (12.8)	41 855 (15.1)	33 442 (10.8)	
Medium low	209 685 (35.6)	99 561 (35.8)	110 124 (35.4)	
Medium high	113 558 (19.3)	40 416 (14.5)	73 142 (23.5)	
High	29 396 (5.0)	6 120 (2.2)	23 276 (7.5)	
Unknown	160 499 (27.3)	89 827 (32.3)	70 672 (22.7)	

Note. WIC = Special Supplemental Nutrition Program for Women, Infants, and Children.

outcomes during pregnancy through an intersectionality framework.

By constructing intersectional strata defined by the aforementioned variables, we identified substantial disparities in cessation prevalence, which accounted for a relatively large proportion of the total variance. This suggests that the impact of intersectional social contexts on smoking cessation is significant and cannot be overlooked. Given the moderate GCE, health preventive and promotional interventions should adopt a framework of "proportionate universalism" to effectively reduce these disparities and increase smoking cessation rates. This approach balances universal access with tailored support for groups facing unique intersectional disadvantages, thereby promoting greater equity in smoking cessation outcomes.

Most of the differences across strata were explained by additive effects, with more than half of these attributable to variations in educational level and race/ethnicity differences. These underscore the utility of MAIHDA in identifying key contributors to observed disparities. The additive effects show that, on average, women who are non-White, have higher education, are married, have private insurance, and are immigrants were more likely to quit smoking during pregnancy. These findings were consistent with previous studies, as summarized in a meta-analysis.[8] Socioeconomically disadvantaged groups, such as women with lower educational level and self-pay medical care, face greater barriers to smoking cessation. These disparities are shaped by structural conditions such as smoking-promoting environments (e.g., greater density of tobacco retail outlets in low-income areas, high prevalence and acceptability of smoking in vulnerable communities), lack of access to cessation services, and intersectional discrimination-induced stressors.[22] Racial/ethnic and immigrant differences could partly be explained by differences in health care utilization and access to cessation treatments.[23,24] Disparities related to marital status can be attributed to support mechanisms (e.g., through marriage and employment) as well as social capital (e.g., trust and social participation).[25]

Only 6.1% of between-stratum variance was attributable to interaction effects. This likely reflects 2 primary factors: (1) sample fragmentation owing to the high number of strata, which reduced statistical power to detect interactions; and (2) the absence of key structural variables such as income and neighborhood environment, both of which are strongly linked to smoking behaviors and might have obscured a potential interaction effect.

Nevertheless, the limited interaction effects did not undermine the importance of mapping intersectional inequalities and provided evidence of heterogeneity of intersectional estimates around average main effects. For instance, we found that intersectional strata with White nonimmigrant women generally had lower cessation prevalence. Although White racial identity may be associated with relative privilege, the intersection of socioeconomic disadvantage contributed to a unique and often overlooked form of marginalization. These women frequently experience a sense of social marginalization linked to educational exclusion, economic precarity, and declining community infrastructures, factors associated with increased health-risk behaviors, including persistent tobacco use. By contrast, Hispanic immigrant women, even those with low education or self-pay medical care, exhibited relatively high cessation rates. This may reflect the buffering role of strong social networks and community-based protective factors.[26] This finding highlights the importance of an intersectional perspective, showing that protective social resources can counterbalance

TABLE 2— Intersectional Multilevel Models of Maternal Smoking Cessation: National Vital Statistics System, United States, 2016–2022

	Null Model	Full Model
Fixed effects, OR (95% CI)		
Race/ethnicity		
Non-Hispanic White (Ref)		1
Non-Hispanic Black		1.49 (1.37, 1.63)
Hispanic		2.42 (2.21, 2.64)
Other		1.42 (1.31, 1.54)
Educational level		
Low (Ref)		1
Medium low		1.44 (1.32, 1.58)
Medium high		2.09 (1.92, 2.27)
High		3.28 (2.99, 3.60)
Marital status		
Unmarried (Ref)		1
Married		1.20 (1.13, 1.28)
Insurance status		
Government (Ref)		1
Private		1.51 (1.41, 1.61)
Self-pay		0.86 (0.78, 0.94)
Immigrant status		
Nonimmigrant (Ref)		1
Immigrant		1.61 (1.50, 1.72)
Random effects		
Variance of random effects, stratum level	0.44	0.03
Summary results		
Weighted grand mean, % (95% CI)	66.4 (64.8, 67.9)	
Marginal R^2/conditional R^2	0.000/0.119	0.080/0.087
AIC/BIC	765 580.8/765 603.3	765 235.8/765 371.2
VPC,[a] %	11.9	0.8
PCV,[b] %		93.9
AUC	0.66	0.66

Note. AIC = Akaike information criterion; AUC = area under receiver operating characteristic curve; BIC = Bayesian information criterion; CI = confidence interval; OR = odds ratio; PCV = proportional change in variance; VPC = variance partition coefficient.
[a]Indicates the proportion of smoking cessation variance attributable to differences between intersectional strata.
[b]Measures the proportional reduction in between-stratum variance from the null model to the full model.

socioeconomic disadvantage but that inequities persist where such resources are lacking.

Furthermore, our research revealed substantial differences in smoking cessation prevalence across various intersectional strata, allowing us to identify vulnerable subgroups. For instance, married White nonimmigrant women with low education and government insurance (n = 7 293) had the second-lowest cessation rate, and their intersectional social contexts showed a negative interaction effect. Additionally, the largest stratum in our study—White unmarried nonimmigrant women with a medium-low educational level and government insurance (n = 113 447)—also had the relatively low cessation rate of 41%. Although it did not have among the lowest cessation rates, this stratum's substantial size may result in a considerable public health burden.

Strengths and Limitations

The strengths of this study include using whole-population data with a large sample size and a novel analytic approach. Our study also has limitations.

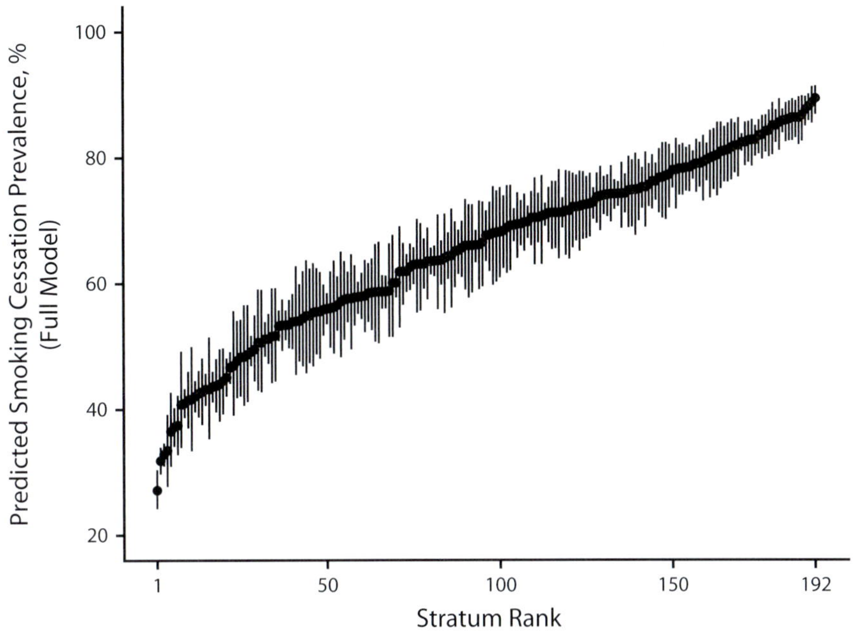

FIGURE 1— Predicted Smoking Cessation Prevalence by Stratum for All 192 Intersectional Strata: United States, 2016–2022

Note. Predictions used estimates from the full model based on total effects. Intersectional strata are ordered according to their rank from left to right, representing low to high. Markers indicate predicted value for each strata. Spikes indicate approximate 95% confidence intervals. For detailed information about the different intersectional strata, see Table A (available as a supplement to the online version of this article at http://www.ajph.org).

First, information on smoking frequency was self-reported, which may introduce recall bias. Second, sample sizes for certain strata were small, so comparisons among these strata should be interpreted with caution. Third, the model may not fully capture intersectional disadvantages because we did not include important variables (e.g., income, neighborhood environment, and stress exposure) owing to unavailable data, which may limit the comprehensiveness of the analysis. This limitation was further compounded by the purely quantitative approach we adopted. Our sole reliance on quantitative data means we may have missed out on the rich qualitative detail underlying the complex mechanisms of disadvantage. Future research could benefit from mixed-methods designs that integrate both qualitative and quantitative approaches to better capture these intricate processes. Fourth, our study population included only primiparous women who had live births, so the results cannot be applied to pregnancies that miscarried or ended for any other reason, restricting the generalizability of our findings.

Conclusions

Our study provides critical insights into the intersectional social disparities shaping smoking cessation during pregnancy. Our analysis reveals considerable variability in smoking cessation prevalence across different strata (particularly for educational level). Additive effects explained the majority of differences in cessation prevalence, whereas evidence of interaction effects emerged in strata with distinct intersectional contexts. These findings underscore the need for universal interventions, complemented by tailored support, to advance equity in maternal health outcomes.

Public Health Implications

Our findings suggest that interventions should adopt a proportionate universalism framework, combining universal measures with tailored approaches. In the current context of constrained public health funding and limited policy prioritization,[27] developing realistic and equitable measures is imperative. For universal measures, public health programs should ensure that all pregnant women have baseline access to smoking cessation interventions through integrated prenatal care. This includes routine screening for tobacco use during antenatal visits, intensive behavioral counseling with messages and self-help materials, and cognitive behavioral

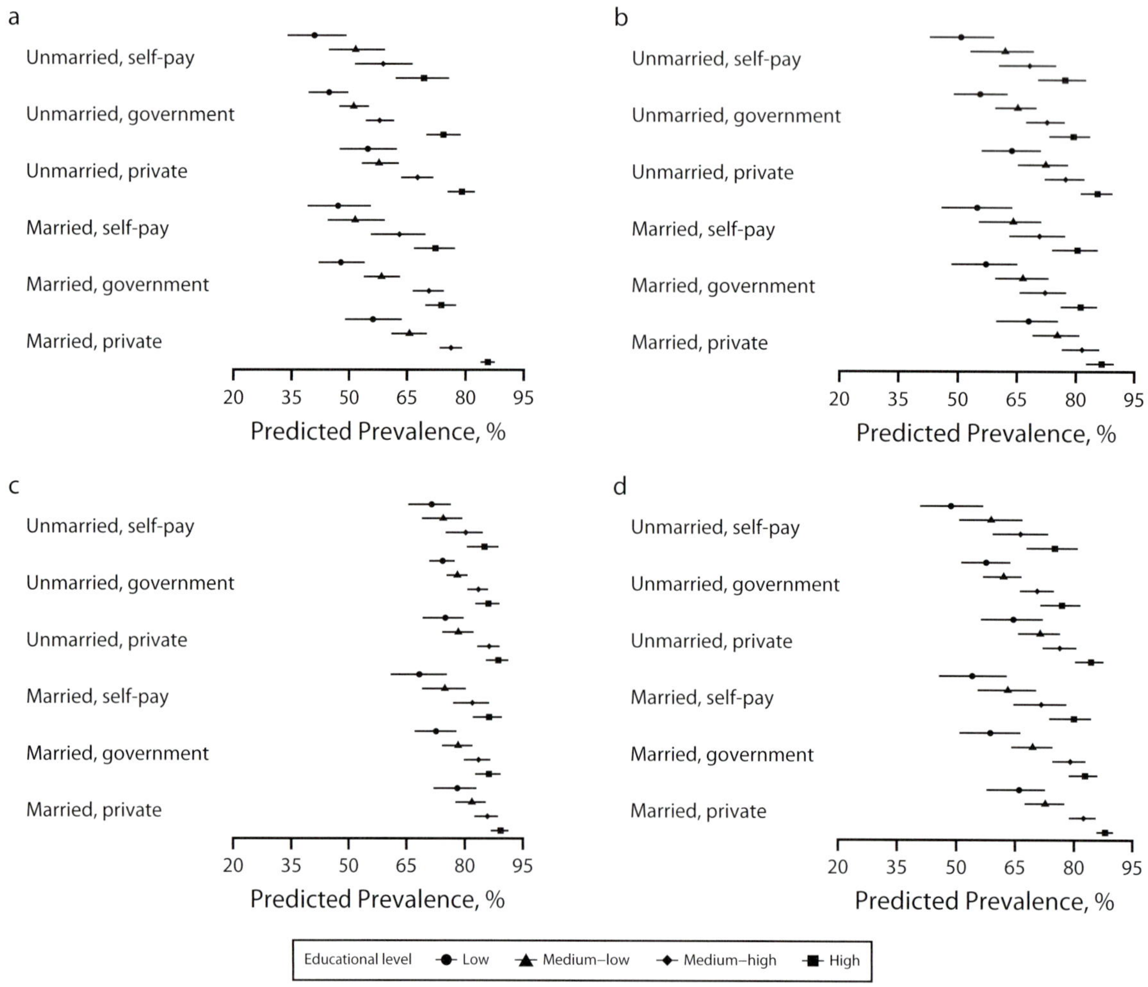

FIGURE 2— Predicted Smoking Cessation Prevalence by Stratum for 96 Strata in Immigrants Identifying as (a) White, (b) Black, (c) Hispanic, and (d) Other: United States, 2016–2022

Note. Predictions used estimates from the full model based on total effects. For detailed data on the smoking cessation prevalence, see Table A (available as a supplement to the online version of this article at http://www.ajph.org).

education from professional staff.[28] Universal digital interventions, such as online resources, telephone or SMS counseling, and smoking cessation apps, could spread awareness of prenatal smoking risks and cessation benefits, helping to shift population-level social norms.[29,30]

For tailored approaches, additional resources should be directed to those in intersectional strata experiencing both structural disadvantage and low cessation rates. For example, outreach programs embedded in community health centers or social service programs (e.g., the Special Supplemental Nutrition Program for Women, Infants, and Children) in socioeconomically deprived areas could include on-site cessation counseling, financial incentives for sustained abstinence, facilitated access to mobile health tools, and the distribution of culturally appropriate educational materials.[31–33] These services could address both structural barriers (e.g., health care access and economic precarity) and the absence of protective social contexts. Contextually and socially relevant interventions—such as peer support networks (both in-person and digital) and culturally competent educational initiatives along with language-concordant helplines and mailings—can strengthen social connectedness and enhance the availability and effectiveness of cessation interventions.[34,35] AJPH

ABOUT THE AUTHORS

Yangyang Cheng and Xiaolin Xu are with the School of Public Health, the Second Affiliated Hospital, Zhejiang University School of Medicine, Hangzhou, Zhejiang, China. Carmen C. W. Lim is with the National Centre for Youth Substance Use Research, School of Psychology, and the National Health and Medical Research Council Centre of Research Excellence in Achieving the Tobacco Endgame, School of Public Health, University of

Queensland, Brisbane, Australia. Rodrigo Martin Carrillo-Larco is with the Emory Global Diabetes Research Center, Hubert Department of Global Health, Rollins School of Public Health, Emory University, Atlanta, GA. Xiaolin Xu is also with the School of Public Health, Faculty of Medicine, University of Queensland, Brisbane, Australia.

CORRESPONDENCE

Correspondence should be sent to Xiaolin Xu, PhD, School of Public Health, Zhejiang University School of Medicine, Yuhangtang Rd 866, Hangzhou, Zhejiang 310058, China (e-mail: xiaolin.xu@zju.edu.cn). Reprints can be ordered at https://www.ajph.org by clicking the "Reprints" link.

PUBLICATION INFORMATION

Full Citation: Cheng Y, Lim CCW, Carrillo-Larco RM, Xu X. Multiple social demographics and disparities in smoking cessation during pregnancy in the United States, 2016–2022: an intersectional analytic framework. *Am J Public Health*. 2025;115(11):1922–1932.

Acceptance Date: June 22, 2025.

DOI: https://doi.org/10.2105/AJPH.2025.308237

ORCID iDs:

Yangyang Cheng https://orcid.org/0000-0001-6823-5015

Carmen C. W. Lim https://orcid.org/0000-0003-1595-6307

Rodrigo Martin Carrillo-Larco https://orcid.org/0000-0002-2090-1856

Xiaolin Xu https://orcid.org/0000-0002-8203-9878

CONTRIBUTORS

Y. Y. Cheng conducted the statistical analyses and data interpretation and drafted and revised the article. C. C. W. Lim and R. M. Carrillo-Larco revised the article critically for important intellectual content. X. L. Xu conceptualized the study design, revised the article, and supervised the project. All authors contributed to and approved the final version.

ACKNOWLEDGMENTS

Funding for this research was provided by the China Medical Board Open Competition Program (grant 21-416).

We appreciate the US National Center for Health Statistics for providing open access data.

CONFLICTS OF INTEREST

The authors have no conflicts of interest to disclose.

HUMAN PARTICIPANT PROTECTION

This study was considered exempt from institutional review board requirements because we used public de-identified data from the Centers for Disease Control and Prevention, National Center for Health Statistics, and the National Vital Statistics System.

REFERENCES

1. Pollack H, Lantz PM, Frohna JG. Maternal smoking and adverse birth outcomes among singletons and twins. *Am J Public Health*. 2000;90(3):395–400. https://doi.org/10.2105/ajph.90.3.395
2. Banderali G, Martelli A, Landi M, et al. Short and long term health effects of parental tobacco smoking during pregnancy and lactation: a descriptive review. *J Transl Med*. 2015;13:327. https://doi.org/10.1186/s12967-015-0690-y
3. Lange S, Probst C, Rehm J, Popova S. National, regional, and global prevalence of smoking during pregnancy in the general population: a systematic review and meta-analysis. *Lancet Glob Health*. 2018;6(7):e769–e776. https://doi.org/10.1016/S2214-109X(18)30223-7
4. Martin JA, Osterman MJK, Driscoll AK. Declines in cigarette smoking during pregnancy in the United States, 2016–2021. *NCHS Data Brief*. 2023(458):1–8.
5. Bérard A, Zhao JP, Sheehy O. Success of smoking cessation interventions during pregnancy. *Am J Obstet Gynecol*. 2016;215(5):611.e611–611.e618. https://doi.org/10.1016/j.ajog.2016.06.059
6. Lee J, Contrera Avila J, Ahluwalia JS. Differences in cessation attempts and cessation methods by race/ethnicity among US adult smokers, 2016–2018. *Addict Behav*. 2023;137:107523. https://doi.org/10.1016/j.addbeh.2022.107523
7. Nguyen-Grozavu FT, Pierce JP, Sakuma KK, et al. Widening disparities in cigarette smoking by race/ethnicity across education level in the United States. *Prev Med*. 2020;139:106220. https://doi.org/10.1016/j.ypmed.2020.106220
8. Riaz M, Lewis S, Naughton F, Ussher M. Predictors of smoking cessation during pregnancy: a systematic review and meta-analysis. *Addiction*. 2018;113(4):610–622. https://doi.org/10.1111/add.14135
9. Passey ME, Longman JM, Adams C, Johnston JJ, Simms J, Rolfe M. Factors associated with provision of smoking cessation support to pregnant women—a cross-sectional survey of midwives in New South Wales, Australia. *BMC Pregnancy Childbirth*. 2020;20(1):219. https://doi.org/10.1186/s12884-020-02912-0
10. Ezegbe C, Neil AL, Magnussen CG, et al. Maternal smoking during pregnancy: trends and determinants in the Conception to Community Study. *Birth*. 2021;48(1):76–85. https://doi.org/10.1111/birt.12515
11. Bowleg L. The problem with the phrase women and minorities: intersectionality—an important theoretical framework for public health. *Am J Public Health*. 2012;102(7):1267–1273. https://doi.org/10.2105/AJPH.2012.300750
12. Crenshaw K. Demarginalizing the intersection of race and sex: a Black feminist critique of antidiscrimination doctrine, feminist theory, and antiracist politics. *Univ Chic Legal Forum*. 1989:1989(1):138–167.
13. Samra R, Hankivsky O. Adopting an intersectionality framework to address power and equity in medicine. *Lancet*. 2021;397(10277):857–859. https://doi.org/10.1016/S0140-6736(20)32513-7
14. Forrest LN, Beccia AL, Exten C, Gehman S, Ansell EB. Intersectional prevalence of suicide ideation, plan, and attempt based on gender, sexual orientation, race and ethnicity, and rurality. *JAMA Psychiatry*. 2023;80(10):1037–1046. https://doi.org/10.1001/jamapsychiatry.2023.2295
15. Kobayashi LC, Peterson RL, Yu X, et al. Life course financial mobility and later-life memory function and decline by gender, and race and ethnicity: an intersectional analysis of the US KHANDLE and STAR cohort studies. *Lancet Healthy Longev*. 2024;5(9):100613. https://doi.org/10.1016/S2666-7568(24)00129-6
16. Erhart M, Müller D, Gellert P, O'Sullivan JL. Mapping intersectional sociodemographic inequalities in measurement and prevalence of depressive symptoms: an intersectional multilevel analysis of individual heterogeneity and discriminatory accuracy using data from a population-based nationwide survey in Germany. *J Clin Epidemiol*. 2024;173:111446. https://doi.org/10.1016/j.jclinepi.2024.111446
17. Evans CR. Overcoming combination fatigue: addressing high-dimensional effect measure modification and interaction in clinical, biomedical, and epidemiologic research using multilevel analysis of individual heterogeneity and discriminatory accuracy (MAIHDA). *Soc Sci Med*. 2024;340:116493. https://doi.org/10.1016/j.socscimed.2023.116493
18. Evans CR, Leckie G, Subramanian SV, Bell A, Merlo J. A tutorial for conducting intersectional multilevel analysis of individual heterogeneity and discriminatory accuracy (MAIHDA). *SSM Popul Health*. 2024;26:101664. https://doi.org/10.1016/j.ssmph.2024.101664
19. Merlo J, Wagner P, Austin PC, Subramanian SV, Leckie G. General and specific contextual effects in multilevel regression analyses and their paradoxical relationship: a conceptual tutorial. *SSM Popul Health*. 2018;5:33–37. https://doi.org/10.1016/j.ssmph.2018.05.006
20. Carey G, Crammond B, De Leeuw E. Towards health equity: a framework for the application of proportionate universalism. *Int J Equity Health*. 2015;14:81. https://doi.org/10.1186/s12939-015-0207-6
21. Guan A, Thomas M, Vittinghoff E, Bowleg L, Mangurian C, Wesson P. An investigation of quantitative methods for assessing intersectionality in health research: a systematic review. *SSM Popul Health*. 2021;16:100977. https://doi.org/10.1016/j.ssmph.2021.100977
22. Matthews KA, Gallo LC. Psychological perspectives on pathways linking socioeconomic status and physical health. *Annu Rev Psychol*. 2011;62:501–530. https://doi.org/10.1146/annurev.psych.031809.130711
23. Tong E, Saito N, Tancredi DJ, et al. A transnational study of migration and smoking behavior in the Mexican-origin population. *Am J Public Health*. 2012;102(11):2116–2122. https://doi.org/10.2105/AJPH.2012.300739
24. Williams RK, Levine MA. Vermont's comprehensive public health framework for tobacco control and prevention. *Prev Med*. 2020;140:106152. https://doi.org/10.1016/j.ypmed.2020.106152
25. Pennanen M, Broms U, Korhonen T, et al. Smoking, nicotine dependence and nicotine intake by socio-economic status and marital status. *Addict Behav*. 2014;39(7):1145–1151. https://doi.org/10.1016/j.addbeh.2014.03.005
26. Shaw RJ, Pickett KE, Wilkinson RG. Ethnic density effects on birth outcomes and maternal smoking

during pregnancy in the US linked birth and infant death data set. *Am J Public Health*. 2010;100(4):707–713. https://doi.org/10.2105/AJPH.2009.167114

27. Mallapaty S. 25 million deaths: what could happen if the US ends global health funding. *Nature*. 2025;641(8061):17–18. https://doi.org/10.1038/d41586-025-01191-z
28. Patnode CD, Henderson JT, Coppola EL, Melnikow J, Durbin S, Thomas RG. Interventions for tobacco cessation in adults, including pregnant persons: updated evidence report and systematic review for the US Preventive Services Task Force. *JAMA*. 2021;325(3):280–298. https://doi.org/10.1001/jama.2020.23541
29. Nian T, Guo K, Liu W, et al. Non-pharmacological interventions for smoking cessation: analysis of systematic reviews and meta-analyses. *BMC Med*. 2023;21(1):378. https://doi.org/10.1186/s12916-023-03087-z
30. Bricker JB, Watson NL, Mull KE, Sullivan BM, Heffner JL. Efficacy of smartphone applications for smoking cessation: a randomized clinical trial. *JAMA Intern Med*. 2020;180(11):1472–1480. https://doi.org/10.1001/jamainternmed.2020.4055
31. Berlin I, Berlin N, Malecot M, Breton M, Jusot F, Goldzahl L. Financial incentives for smoking cessation in pregnancy: multicentre randomised controlled trial. *BMJ*. 2021;375:e065217. https://doi.org/10.1136/bmj-2021-065217
32. Haas JS, Linder JA, Park ER, et al. Proactive tobacco cessation outreach to smokers of low socioeconomic status: a randomized clinical trial. *JAMA Intern Med*. 2015;175(2):218–226. https://doi.org/10.1001/jamainternmed.2014.6674
33. Olaiya O, Sharma AJ, Tong VT, et al. Impact of the 5As brief counseling on smoking cessation among pregnant clients of Special Supplemental Nutrition Program for Women, Infants, and Children (WIC) clinics in Ohio. *Prev Med*. 2015;81:438–443. https://doi.org/10.1016/j.ypmed.2015.10.011
34. Barnett MJ, Fealy S, Wilson A. Barriers and enablers for smoking cessation amongst pregnant women: an umbrella review. *Women Birth*. 2019;32(4):310–317. https://doi.org/10.1016/j.wombi.2018.10.007
35. Vijayaraghavan M, Dove MS, Stewart SL, et al. Racial/ethnic differences in the response to incentives for quitline engagement. *Am J Prev Med*. 2018;55(6 suppl 2):S186–S195. https://doi.org/10.1016/j.amepre.2018.07.018

Changes in E-Cigarette and Cigarette Sales in California and Neighboring States Following a Law Prohibiting Flavored Tobacco Product Sales

Fatma Romeh M. Ali, PhD, Adam M. Leventhal, PhD, Megan C. Diaz, PhD, Elisha W. Crane, MPH, and Kristy Marynak, PhD, MPP

Objectives. To assess changes in e-cigarette and cigarette sales, overall and by flavor type, following implementation of California's law prohibiting flavored tobacco product sales.

Methods. E-cigarette and cigarette retail sales data were licensed from Circana, categorized by flavor, and summed into quarters during 2019 to 2024. We used difference-in-differences regressions with 2-way fixed effects to compare quarterly sales per capita before and after implementation of the California law in California, California-adjacent states, and 32 control states.

Results. Prohibiting flavored tobacco product sales in California was associated with a 36.98% reduction in total milligrams of e-cigarette nicotine sold and a 10.55% reduction in cigarette pack sales, compared with control states. Declines in flavored product sales were partially offset by increased sales of products marketed as nontobacco flavored that contain synthetic cooling agents or other additives that deliver multisensory flavor experiences. California's law was not associated with statistically significant sales changes in neighboring states.

Conclusions. California's flavored tobacco law resulted in overall declines in e-cigarette and cigarette sales, without affecting neighboring states. Restrictions on the sale of all tobacco products that deliver multisensory flavor experiences may lead to further declines in sales. (*Am J Public Health*. 2025;115(11):1933–1937. https://doi.org/10.2105/AJPH.2025.308182)

AJPH November 2025, Vol. 115, No. 11

Strong evidence supports prohibiting sales of flavored tobacco products, which drive youth tobacco use and related disparities.[1] Characterizing flavors other than tobacco, except menthol, are prohibited at the federal level for cigarettes and prefilled e-cigarettes. California banned sales of flavored tobacco products, including menthol cigarettes, effective December 21, 2022.[2] Simultaneously, cigarette and e-cigarette manufacturers began marketing products that deliver multisensory flavor experiences without characterizing flavor descriptors, such as "clear" e-cigarettes with coolants and "nonmenthol" cigarettes containing tropical flavorants or coolants.[3–6]

This study assessed pre- and postpolicy changes in e-cigarette and cigarette sales, overall and by flavor, in California and neighboring states. A difference-in-differences (DID) analysis compared those sales changes against changes in control states to isolate the ban's effect.

METHODS

Sales data are based on custom research by the National Foundation for the Centers for Disease Control and Prevention, Inc. using Circana retail point of sale scanner data for multi-outlet and convenience stores (Circana LLC, Chicago, IL), including brick-and-mortar stores but excluding online and tobacco specialty stores. We excluded e-cigarettes sold without e-liquids. We summed sales into quarters from the second quarter of 2019 (2019 Q2) to the second quarter of 2024 (2024 Q2), for a total of 21 quarters.

We categorized e-cigarette flavors as tobacco, menthol, mint, clear or other cooling, other (fruit, sweets, combined fruit or sweet and cooling, such as banana ice), or unknown, based on data source flavor names and online searches for ambiguous flavors. "Clear or other cooling" included products marketed as "clear," "clear ice," or "unflavored," informed by lab testing of "clear" products[6] and online descriptions. "Unflavored" e-cigarettes lacking cooling sensations were classified as unknown. Cigarette flavors were categorized as menthol, nonmenthol cooling or tropical (e.g., Camel Crisp, Newport Green, Newport EXP, Camel Crush Oasis), tobacco, or unknown.[3–5]

E-cigarette sales were measured by total nicotine sold (mg), calculated as e-liquid volume (mL) × nicotine concentration (mg/mL) × units sold.[7] One 20-cigarette pack equaled 1 unit.

We used DID analysis with 2-way fixed-effects generalized linear model regressions with state-clustered standard errors to compare quarterly e-cigarette and cigarette sales per capita in California with sales in 3 neighboring states (Arizona, Nevada, Oregon) and 32 control states, before versus after policy implementation, overall and by flavor. The analysis adjusted for state- and time-fixed effects and state-level covariates (age–race distribution, population size, unemployment, tobacco control policies, and COVID-19 metrics). We calculated the effect on cooling or tropical products by subtracting the effect on tobacco and nontobacco flavored sales from the total sales effect. Visual checks and tests confirmed the DID parallel trends assumption (Figures A and B in Appendix, available as a supplement to the online version of this article at http://www.ajph.org). Statistical significance was set at $P < .05$ (further details in "Supplemental Information: Methods" in online Appendix).

RESULTS

In the first 6 quarters after California's law (2023 Q1 to 2024 Q2), e-cigarette nicotine sales decreased 18.0% in California but rose 52.8% in neighboring states and 29.9% in control states, compared with the 6-quarter prepolicy period (Figure 1 and Figure C). Menthol, mint, and other nontobacco flavored sales decreased 55.0% in California but increased 68.5% in neighboring states and 34.8% in control states. Tobacco-flavored sales increased 27.6% in California but declined 12.7% and 12.9% in neighboring and control states. Clear or other cooling e-cigarette sales increased across all groups: 6159.6% (19.7% of postpolicy sales) in California, 523.2% (0.2% of sales) in neighboring states, and 319.2% (0.1% of sales) in control states. Notably, 93.6% of California's remaining flavored e-cigarette sales after the law were disposable e-cigarettes.

Total cigarette sales decreased 21.1% in California and roughly 12% in neighboring (−12.4%) and control (−12.1%) states. Menthol cigarette sales dropped 95.4% in California, versus 14.3% and 13.1% in neighboring and control states. Tobacco-flavored sales declined 6.4% in California, versus 11.8% and 11.6% declines in neighboring and control states. Nonmenthol cooling or tropical flavored sales increased 40 535.9% (6.5% of sales) in California, while neighboring and control states sales approached zero. Despite the overall increase in nonmenthol cooling or tropical-flavored cigarette sales in California during 2023 Q1 to 2024 Q2, fluctuations occurred. In 2023 Q1, cooling and tropical-flavored sales increased 7356.4% and 7851.9%, respectively, compared with 2022 Q4 (Figure D). After a stable period, in early 2024, cooling cigarette sales increased 14.7% whereas tropical-flavored sales decreased 96.7%.

DID regression results show that California's flavored tobacco ban led to a 36.98% (−25.41 mg) drop in average quarterly e-cigarette sales per capita versus control states (Table A). Tobacco-flavored e-cigarette sales increased 53.52% (4.96 mg), whereas nontobacco flavor sales (excluding clear or other cooling) decreased 66.32% (−39.38 mg; $P < .001$) versus control states. Clear or other cooling flavored sales increased 9.01 mg per capita versus control states. The rise in tobacco and clear or other cooling e-cigarette sales in California partially offset the decline in nontobacco flavored e-cigarettes sold, by 12.6% and 22.9%, respectively. California-adjacent states showed no statistically significant changes in e-cigarette nicotine sales versus control states. For cigarettes, following California's ban, average quarterly cigarette sales per capita fell 10.55% (−0.87 packs), and menthol sales decreased 94.86% (−2.35 packs), whereas tobacco-flavored sales increased 12.90% (0.75 packs) versus control states (all $P < .001$). Nonmenthol cooling or tropical sales increased 0.73 packs per capita versus control states. The rise in tobacco and nonmenthol cooling or tropical cigarette sales partially offset California's menthol decline (31.9% and 31.1%, respectively). California-adjacent states showed no significant cigarette sales change versus controls.

DISCUSSION

California's flavored tobacco sales ban was associated with statistically significant

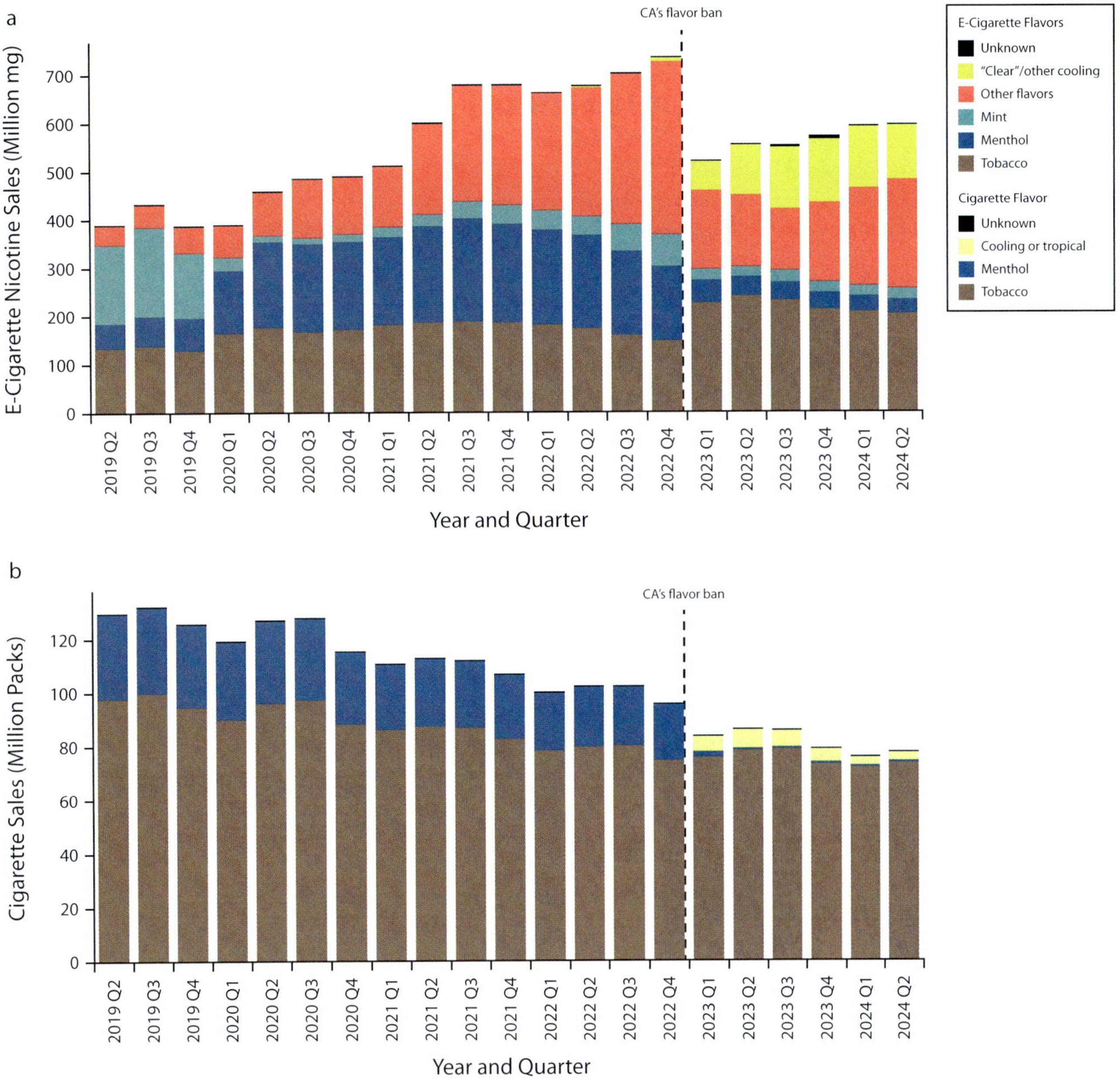

FIGURE 1— California's Quarterly E-Cigarette and Cigarette Sales by Flavor, 2019 Q2–2024 Q2

Note. Q = quarter. E-cigarette and cigarette point-of-sale data are licensed from Circana for convenience stores, gas stations, grocery stores, drug stores or pharmacies, mass merchandiser outlets, club stores, dollar stores, and military sales; Internet and vape shop sales were not recorded. E-cigarette accessories and devices sold without e-liquids were excluded. E-Cigarette nicotine sales (mg) were calculated as the product of e-liquid volume (mL), nicotine concentration (mg/mL), and unit sales. Cigarette units are measured in packs of 20 cigarettes each. E-cigarette Other Flavors category includes fruit, clove or spice, chocolate, alcoholic drink (such as wine, cognac, or other cocktails), candy or desserts/other sweets, some other flavor; e-cigarette Clear or Other Cooling includes products with flavor names such as clear, clear ice, or unflavored, which likely contain nonmenthol synthetic cooling agents (e.g., Flum Pebble Clear, EB Design BC5000 Clear). Cigarette flavors are tobacco, menthol (contains menthol), nonmenthol cooling or tropical (e.g., Camel Crisp, Newport Green, Newport EXP, Camel Crush Oasis). Figure C (available as a supplement to the online version of this article at http://www.ajph.org) presents the quarterly sales of e-cigarettes and cigarettes by flavor, for both neighboring states and control states.

declines in e-cigarette nicotine and cigarette packs sold during the first 1.5 years of implementation. These declines remained after we adjusted for control state trends, state-level demographic and economic factors, and tobacco control policies. In California-adjacent states, sales increases relative to controls did not persist after we adjusted for confounders. This finding—that flavored tobacco bans decrease state tobacco sales without affecting neighbors—aligns with prior Massachusetts ban evaluations.[8–9]

After the policy, sales of tobacco-flavored e-cigarettes and e-cigarettes without a characterizing flavor descriptor, but delivering multisensory experiences (e.g., Camel Crisp nonmenthol cigarettes; Flum Pebble "clear" e-cigarettes) increased in California but not control states. However, this increase was smaller than the decrease in nontobacco-flavored sales, resulting in an overall sales decline. Disposable e-cigarettes constituted 94% of California's remaining noncompliant flavored e-cigarette sales, with notable increases in sales of "clear" or "unflavored" products. Testing of 19 "clear" disposables found that all contained WS-3 coolant and 18 contained menthol.[6] Notwithstanding, these data demonstrate the impact of enforcement. In April 2023, the California attorney general sent letters to manufacturers of cigarettes with tropical or cooling flavorants, determining that the products were presumptively flavored under the state law.[10] By early 2024, R.J. Reynolds' tropical product sales in California were negligible.[11] California further strengthened its law, effective January 1, 2025, to prohibit products providing a "cooling sensation," including "clear" products with flavored statements or images.[12]

This study, the first to evaluate the impact of California's flavored tobacco sales law, has limitations. First, additional factors might affect California's tobacco sales, although DID regression with state and time fixed effects, covariates, and a control group aimed to minimize bias. Second, estimates rely on Circana data at the time of analysis, and newer data may vary. Finally, the study excluded tobacco specialty stores, online orders, and illicit sales, potentially underestimating the law's effect. Complementary surveys could further document behavioral changes after the ban.

PUBLIC HEALTH IMPLICATIONS

California's flavored tobacco ban successfully reduced in-state e-cigarette and cigarette sales without affecting sales in neighboring states. Decreases in flavored sales were partially offset by increased sales of products marketed as "nonmenthol" or "clear" containing synthetic cooling agents and other additives that deliver multisensory flavor experiences. Comprehensive policies that prohibit the sale of these alternatives could better curb youth-appealing products and protect public health. *AJPH*

ABOUT THE AUTHORS

Fatma Romeh M. Ali and Elisha W. Crane are with the National Foundation for the Centers for Disease Control and Prevention, Inc. (CDC Foundation), Atlanta, GA. Adam M. Leventhal is with the Institute for Addiction Science, University of Southern California, Los Angeles. Megan C. Diaz is with the Truth Initiative Schroeder Institute, Washington, DC. At the time of this study, Kristy Marynak was with the CDC Office on Smoking and Health, Atlanta, GA.

CORRESPONDENCE

Correspondence should be sent to Fatma Romeh M. Ali, CDC Foundation, 600 Peachtree St NE #1000, Atlanta, GA 30308 (e-mail: fali@cdcfoundation.org). Reprints can be ordered at http://www.ajph.org by clicking the "Reprints" link.

PUBLICATION INFORMATION

Full Citation: Ali FRM, Leventhal AM, Diaz MC, Crane EW, Marynak K. Changes in e-cigarette and cigarette sales in California and neighboring states following a law prohibiting flavored tobacco product sales. *Am J Public Health*. 2025;115(11): 1933–1937.

Acceptance Date: April 25, 2025.

DOI: https://doi.org/10.2105/AJPH.2025.308182

ORCID iDs:

Fatma Romeh M. Ali https://orcid.org/0000-0001-5017-1869

Adam M. Leventhal https://orcid.org/0000-0002-1217-525X

Megan C. Diaz https://orcid.org/0000-0001-6915-2529

Kristy Marynak https://orcid.org/0000-0002-3385-6468

CONTRIBUTORS

F. R. M. Ali led the study's conceptualization and design, conducted formal analysis and methodology, carried out the investigation, interpreted the data, and took the lead in drafting and revising the article. A. M. Leventhal and M. C. Diaz provided valuable insights into the study's conceptualization and methodology, contributed to data interpretation and investigation, and participated in drafting and revising the manuscript. E. W. Crane conducted data investigation, ensuring accurate curation and validation, and contributed to the manuscript revision. K. Marynak played a key role in the study's conceptualization and design, data investigation, and interpretation, as well as drafting and revising the manuscript. All authors have reviewed and approved the final version of this study.

ACKNOWLEDGMENTS

This work was funded by the Bloomberg Initiative to Reduce Tobacco Use through the CDC Foundation with a grant from Bloomberg Philanthropies.

Note. The funders had no role in the design and conduct of the study, data collection, management, analysis, interpretation of the data, preparation, review, approval of the manuscript, or decision to submit the manuscript for publication. The findings and conclusions in this report are those of the authors and do not necessarily represent the official position of the US Centers for Disease Control and Prevention or the CDC Foundation.

CONFLICTS OF INTEREST

The authors declare no conflicts of interest. M. C. Diaz has received tobacco-related consulting work from the World Health Organization and owns 4 shares of Philip Morris International for research purposes. No other authors have reported financial disclosures.

HUMAN PARTICIPANT PROTECTION

This research did not involve human participation; therefore, institutional review board oversight was not sought.

REFERENCES

1. Bold KW, Kong G, O'Malley SS. The scientific basis for the regulation of flavors in tobacco products. *Annu Rev Clin Psychol.* 2024;20(1):381–406. https://doi.org/10.1146/annurev-clinpsy-080921-075624
2. SB 793 - California Legislature. 2019–2020 Regular Session. Plural Policy. Available at: https://pluralpolicy.com/app/legislative-tracking/bill/details/state-ca-20192020-sb793/450654. Accessed July 14, 2025.
3. Page MK, Paul EE, Leigh NJ, et al. Still "Cool": tobacco industry responds to state-wide menthol ban with synthetic coolants. *Tob Control.* 2025; 34(2):254–258. https://doi.org/10.1136/tc-2023-058149
4. Meza LR, Galimov A, Sussman S, et al. Proliferation of "non-menthol" cigarettes amid a state-wide

flavour ban. *Tob Control.* 2025;34(1):135–137. https://doi.org/10.1136/tc-2023-058074

5. Jabba SV, Erythropel HC, Anastas PT, Zimmerman JB, Jordt SE. Synthetic cooling agent and other flavor additives in "non-menthol" cigarettes marketed in California and Massachusetts after menthol cigarette bans. *JAMA.* 2023;330(17):1689–1691. https://doi.org/10.1001/jama.2023.17134
6. Minetti ET, Erythropel HC, Keith R, et al. Cardiovascular health effects and synthetic cooling agents in e-cigarettes labeled as "clear" marketed in Massachusetts after the tobacco product flavoring ban. *medRxiv.* [Preprint] 2024.04.18.24305863. https://doi.org/10.1101/2024.04.18.24305863
7. Ali FRM, Diaz MC, Armour BS, Crane E, Tynan MA, Marynak KL. Trends in US e-cigarette sales measured in milligrams of nicotine, 2019–2024. *Am J Prev Med.* 2025;68(6):1173–1178. https://doi.org/10.1016/j.amepre.2025.02.007
8. Ali FRM, King BA, Seaman EL, Vallone D, Schillo B. Impact of Massachusetts law prohibiting flavored tobacco products sales on cross-border cigarette sales. *PLoS One.* 2022;17(9):e0274022. https://doi.org/10.1371/journal.pone.0274022
9. Kingsley M, McGinnes H, Song G, Doane J, Henley P. Impact of Massachusetts' statewide sales restriction on flavored and menthol tobacco products on tobacco sales in Massachusetts and surrounding states, June 2020. *Am J Public Health.* 2022;112(8):1147–1150. https://doi.org/10.2105/AJPH.2022.306879
10. Miller BM. Letter to Jonathan Reed re: California Flavor Ban Notice of Determination. Available at: https://oag.ca.gov/prop65/ag-letters. Accessed July 14, 2025.
11. R.J. Reynolds Tobacco Company. American Petroleum and Convenience Store Association v Rob Bonta. First Amended Complaint for Declaratory and Injunctive Relief and Verified Petition for Writ of Mandate. E-filed December 4, 2023. Available at: https://www.publichealthlawcenter.org/sites/default/files/case/RJR-Bonta-Complaint.pdf. Accessed July 14, 2025.
12. California Office of the Attorney General. Restrictions on flavored tobacco products. 2024. Available at: https://oag.ca.gov/system/files/media/2024-dle-18.pdf. Accessed July 14, 2025.

Differences in Breastfeeding Rates Among African Americans, Black Immigrants, and Hispanic Black Individuals Compared to Other Race/Ethnicity Groups for Infants Born Between 2011 and 2022, United States

Amira A. Roess, PhD, MPH, and Rebecca C. Robert, PhD, MS

AJPH November 2025, Vol. 115, No. 11

Objectives. To compare breastfeeding initiation (BFI), breastfeeding duration, and exclusive breastfeeding (EBF) of Black subgroups and other race groups in the United States.

Methods. We analyzed National Survey of Child Health data for infants born between 2011 and 2022 (n = 89 067). Multivariable generalized linear models identified determinants of BFI, duration, and EBF (6 months).

Results. African Americans (i.e., non-Hispanic Black Americans) had significantly lower breastfeeding rates compared with other race/ethnicity groups; Black immigrants had among the highest rates. BFI was significantly lower for African Americans (58.5%) and Hispanic Black (78.5%) individuals, and significantly higher for Black immigrants (88.8%) compared with non-Hispanic White persons (84.1%). Among those who initiated, African Americans and Hispanic Black individuals had lower duration rates.

Conclusions. African Americans were the only group with BFI rates below the Healthy People 2020 goal; Black immigrants were above the goal. That Hispanic Black individuals had lower rates compared with Hispanic persons who are not Black suggests the potential impact of structural and medical racism on health behaviors. The results underscore the importance of differentiating Black subgroups in public health practice and research. (*Am J Public Health*. 2025;115(11):1938–1941. https://doi.org/10.2105/AJPH.2025.308242)

Human (breast) milk provides protection from sudden infant death syndrome, infectious diseases, asthma, obesity, and type 2 diabetes in infants, and from breast and ovarian cancer in females, all of which disproportionately affect Black Americans.[1] Healthy People 2020's goal for breastfeeding initiation (BFI; 81.9%) was met by non-Hispanic White and Hispanic populations by 2014, but was unmet by Black Americans.[2,3]

Research on breastfeeding rates demonstrates that current federal race/ethnicity classifications are problematic because they mask differences in breastfeeding, and likely other health-related behaviors and outcomes among the Black American population.[4,5] For example, in a low-income Washington, DC, population, Black immigrants achieved significantly higher BFI rates compared with African Americans,[5] and the same was found in a national study.[6] A systematic review of breastfeeding practices among African immigrants living in high-income countries demonstrated high BFI (90%).[7] Other small studies report greater odds for BFI among Black immigrants compared with Black/African Americans (non-Hispanic, nonimmigrants) in the United States.[6,8,9]

We did not find literature estimating breastfeeding rates among the three main Black American subgroups (Hispanic Black, Black immigrant, African American) nationally over time. Our objective was to estimate rates of BFI, breastfeeding duration (any breastfeeding at 1, 3, 6, and 12 months), and exclusive breastfeeding at 6 months (EBF) among Black subgroups and compare them to other race/ethnicity groups nationally.

METHODS

We conducted a secondary analysis using National Survey of Children's Health (NSCH) deidentified data collected between January 1, 2016, and December 31, 2022. Data were included on children born between 2011 and 2022 and aged 5 years or younger at the time of the survey (n = 89 067).

Outcome

BFI (yes/no) information was collected on all children aged 5 years or younger ("Was this child ever breastfed or fed breastmilk?"). Any breastfeeding (yes/no) at 1, 3, 6, and 12 months was calculated for children who reached that age at the time of the survey using the question, "How old was this child when he or she completely stopped breastfeeding or being fed breast milk?" EBF (yes/no) was calculated by NSCH for all children aged 6 months to 5 years.

Determinants

Covariates were based on a literature review: maternal age at birth (continuous), caregiver education (categorical), married or living with partner (dichotomous), low birthweight status (dichotomous), year of birth (continuous), household federal poverty level (defined by NSCH; categorical), and infant's race/ethnicity (non-Hispanic White, non-Hispanic Asian, non-Hispanic American Indian/Alaska Native, non-Black Hispanic, and Black, which included three subgroups). Black immigrants reported Black race, not Hispanic, and born abroad or had 1 or more parents born abroad. Hispanic Black individuals reported Black race and Hispanic ethnicity (regardless of immigrant status). African Americans reported as Black race, not Hispanic, and not immigrant.

Statistical Analysis

We conducted correlation analyses to assess for multicollinearity among covariates (≥ 0.8 indicating collinearity) and bivariate analyses to estimate associations between each covariate and BFI. We employed multivariable generalized linear modeling with a logit link and robust standard errors to estimate adjusted odds ratios (AORs) and 95% confidence intervals (CIs) between BFI and covariates. We conducted 5 additional models (1 per remaining dichotomous outcome) using only the sample who had initiated breastfeeding to determine if race/ethnicity differences persisted once breastfeeding began (Table B, available as a supplement to the online version of this article at https://ajph.org). We applied weights to generate nationally representative results as recommended by NSCH.[10] We conducted analyses with Stata version 16 (StataCorp LP, College Station, TX).

RESULTS

Most infants were born to mothers aged 25 to 34 years (57.0%), had a caregiver with at least a high-school education (74.6%), and lived in a household that was 200% or more above the federal poverty level (59.6%). Most caregivers were married or living with a partner (81.7%). The three largest race/ethnicity groups were non-Hispanic White (54.5%), non-Black Hispanic (25.0%), and African Americans (9.7%; Table A, available as a supplement to the online version of this article at https://ajph.org).

BFI was highest among Black immigrants (88.8%) and lowest among African Americans (58.5%), and rates for Hispanic Black individuals were between the other two Black groups (Figure 1). These same patterns continued across all breastfeeding outcomes (any breastfeeding at 1, 3, 6, and 12 months and EBF; Figure 1). Overall, the BFI rate during the study period reached the Healthy People 2020 goal by 2020, but not for African Americans who had the lowest BFI rates of all other race/ethnicity groups each year—from 42.6% (2014) to 68.8% (2021; Figure A, available as a supplement to the online version of this article at https://ajph.org).

Caregivers who were married or living with a partner, compared with neither, demonstrated significantly higher BFI (83.8% vs 65.4%) as did caregivers who completed high school compared with less than high school (77.1% vs 65.9%; Tables A and B). In the adjusted model, compared with non-Hispanic White individuals, African Americans demonstrated significantly lower odds of BFI (AOR = 0.41; 95% CI = 0.36, 0.48), while Black immigrants showed significantly higher odds (AOR = 1.96; 95% CI = 1.38, 2.79). All other race/ethnicity

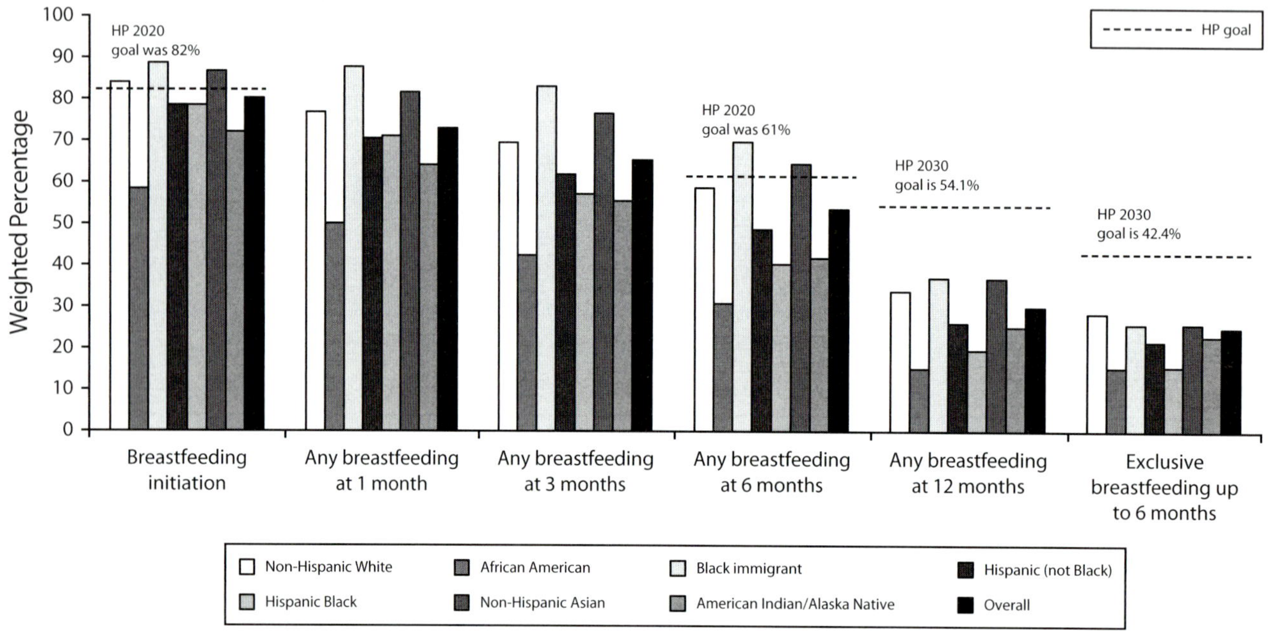

FIGURE 1— Weighted Mean Percentage of Breastfeeding Rates by Race/Ethnicity of Infants Born Between 2011 and 2022: United States

Note. HP = Healthy People. Breastfeeding initiation and any breastfeeding at 6 months were not included in 2030 goals; exact percentages for breastfeeding provided in Appendix Tables A and C (available as a supplement to the online version of this article at https://www.ajph.org).

AJPH November 2025, Vol. 115, No. 11

groups had BFI rates similar to non-Hispanic White individuals (Table B).

Among those who initiated breastfeeding, compared with non-Hispanic White individuals, African Americans and Hispanic Black individuals demonstrated significantly lower rates for all breastfeeding behaviors, while Black immigrants demonstrated significantly higher rates (Figure 1, Figures A and B [available as supplements to the online version of this article at https://ajph.org]).

DISCUSSION

We sought to disentangle differences in breastfeeding rates among Black Americans, a group with historically low rates. Using national data, we found significant differences in breastfeeding rates between Black subgroups, a finding supported by previous studies of higher BFI for Black immigrants compared with African Americans among low-income populations.[5,6,8] African American is the only racial/ethnic group that falls well below the Healthy People 2020 BFI goal of 82% and additionally demonstrated the lowest rates for any breastfeeding in the first year of life and for EBF. In contrast, rates for Black immigrants were among the highest compared with other groups.

Among those who initiated breastfeeding, African Americans and Hispanic Black individuals showed the lowest rates of EBF, and any breastfeeding at 3 months and after. Research is needed to understand why duration rates remain lower among these two subgroups, even after initiating. Other research has shown worse health outcomes for Hispanic Black populations compared with Hispanic individuals of other races, and the same mechanisms underpinning these findings may be at play here: historical and lasting structural racism directed at Black individuals throughout the Americas.[11,12] Black immigrants likely benefit from familial and cultural support to foster healthy behaviors like breastfeeding, and this may offer a protective mechanism against structural racism that is not available to the same degree for African Americans.[7] In addition, lower breastfeeding rates among Hispanic Black individuals compared with Hispanic individuals who are not Black highlight the potential impact of structural and medical racism on health behaviors.

Limitations of NSCH data include missing important determinants of breastfeeding, like delivering in a Baby-Friendly hospital and delivery mode. Since data were collected for children aged 5 years and younger, recall bias may affect results. Nevertheless, NSCH provides nationally representative detailed breastfeeding and race/ethnicity data that are largely unavailable elsewhere.

PUBLIC HEALTH IMPLICATIONS

This study marks the first, to our knowledge, to examine breastfeeding rates among three Black race subgroups (Black immigrant, Hispanic Black, African American) in a national sample over time. African Americans experienced the lowest initiation and duration rates, Hispanic Black individuals followed with the next lowest rates, while Black immigrants achieved among the highest rates. Combining African American, Black immigrant, and Hispanic Black subgroups masks important differences and overestimates rates among African Americans; likewise, combining Hispanic Black and non-Black Hispanic individuals under "Hispanic" ethnicity overestimates rates among Hispanic Black individuals. Granular racial/ethnic data can lead to culturally relevant interventions targeting structural and medical racism to address the complex causes of inequities in breastfeeding and other health behaviors. AJPH

ABOUT THE AUTHORS

Amira A. Roess is with the College of Public Health, George Mason University, Fairfax, VA. Rebecca C. Robert is with the Conway School of Nursing, The Catholic University of America, Washington, DC.

CORRESPONDENCE

Correspondence should be sent to Amira A. Roess, College of Public Health, George Mason University, 4400 University Dr, Fairfax, VA 22030 (e-mail: aroess@gmu.edu). Reprints can be ordered at https://ajph.org by clicking the "Reprints" link.

PUBLICATION INFORMATION

Full Citation: Roess AA, Robert RC. Differences in breastfeeding rates among African Americans, Black immigrants, and Hispanic Black individuals compared to other race/ethnicity groups for infants born between 2011 and 2022, United States. *Am J Public Health*. 2025;115(11): 1938–1941.

Acceptance Date: July 2, 2025.

DOI: https://doi.org/10.2105/AJPH.2025.308242

ORCID iDs:

Amira A. Roess https://orcid.org/0000-0003-2321-1575

Rebecca C. Robert https://orcid.org/0000-0003-1660-9681

CONTRIBUTORS

A. A. Roess led the data analysis. A. A. Roess and R. C. Robert conceptualized the study, wrote the brief, and approved the final version.

CONFLICTS OF INTEREST

The authors have no conflicts of interest to declare.

HUMAN PARTICIPANT PROTECTION

This study is a secondary analysis using National Survey of Children's Health deidentified data and is not considered human participant research; thus, no institutional review board approval was required.

REFERENCES

1. Meek JY, Noble L, Section on Breastfeeding. Policy Statement: Breastfeeding and the use of human milk. *Pediatrics*. 2022;150(1):e2022057988. https://doi.org/10.1542/peds.2022-057988
2. The Surgeon General's Call to Action to Support Breastfeeding. Washington, DC: US Department of Health and Human Services, Office of the Surgeon General; 2011.
3. Marks KJ, Nakayama JY, Chiang KV, et al. Disaggregation of breastfeeding initiation rates by race and ethnicity—United States, 2020–2021. *Prev Chronic Dis*. 2023;20:E114. https://doi.org/10.5888/pcd20.230199
4. Griffith DM, Johnson J, Zhang R, Neighbors HW, Jackson JS. Ethnicity, nativity and the health of American Blacks. *J Health Care Poor Underserved*. 2011;22(1):142–156. https://doi.org/10.1353/hpu.2011.0011
5. Roess AA, Robert RC, Kuehn D, et al. Disparities in breastfeeding initiation among African American and Black immigrant WIC recipients in the District of Columbia, 2007–2019. *Am J Public Health*. 2022; 112(4):671–674. https://doi.org/10.2105/AJPH.2021.306652
6. Campbell AG, Naz S, Peña A. Breastfeeding behaviors by race/ethnicity and foreign-born status in the United States: an analysis of the US National Survey of Children's Health. *Breastfeed Med*. 2024; 19(11):870–880. https://doi.org/10.1089/bfm.2024.0271
7. Odeniyi AO, Embleton N, Ngongalah L, Akor W, Rankin J. Breastfeeding beliefs and experiences of African immigrant mothers in high-income countries: a systematic review. *Matern Child Nutr*. 2020;16(3):142–156. https://doi.org/10.1111/mcn.12970
8. Griswold MK, Crawford SL, Perry DJ, et al. Experiences of racism and breastfeeding initiation and duration among first-time mothers of the Black Women's Health Study. *J Racial Ethn Health Disparities*. 2018;5(6):1180–1191. https://doi.org/10.1007/s40615-018-0465-2
9. Hawkins SS, Gillman MW, Shafer EF, Cohen BB. Acculturation and maternal health behaviors: findings from the Massachusetts birth certificate. *Am J Prev Med*. 2014;47(2):150–159. https://doi.org/10.1016/j.amepre.2014.02.015
10. Data Resource Center for Child and Adolescent Health. National Survey of Children's Health. Available at: https://www.childhealthdata.org/learn-about-the-nsch/NSCH. Accessed January 29, 2025.
11. Cuevas AG, Dawson BA, Williams DR. Race and skin color in Latino health: an analytic review. *Am J Public Health*. 2016;106(12):2131–2136. https://doi.org/10.2105/AJPH.2016.303452
12. Safon CB, Heeren T, Kerr S, et al. Racial and ethnic disparities in breastfeeding continuation among US Hispanic mothers: identification of mechanisms. *Breastfeed Med*. 2023;18(1):3–13. https://doi.org/10.1089/bfm.2022.0196

UNITED STATES POSTAL SERVICE® Statement of Ownership, Management, and Circulation (All Periodicals Publications Except Requester Publications)

1. Publication Title: American Journal of Public Health	2. Publication Number: 0090-0036	3. Filing Date: 09/30/2025
4. Issue Frequency: Monthly	5. Number of Issues Published Annually: 12	6. Annual Subscription Price: $993–$1445 Online + Print

7. Complete Mailing Address of Known Office of Publication *(Not printer) (Street, city, county, state, and ZIP+4®)*
American Public Health Association
800 I St., NW, Washington, DC 20001-3710

Contact Person: Brian Selzer
Telephone *(Include area code)*: 202-777-2464

8. Complete Mailing Address of Headquarters or General Business Office of Publisher *(Not printer)*
American Public Health Association
800 I St., NW, Washington, DC 20001-3710

9. Full Names and Complete Mailing Addresses of Publisher, Editor, and Managing Editor *(Do not leave blank)*

Publisher *(Name and complete mailing address)*
American Public Health Association
800 I St., NW, Washington, DC 20001-3710

Editor *(Name and complete mailing address)*
Denys Lau, PhD, American Public Health Association
800 I St., NW, Washington, DC 20001-3710

Managing Editor *(Name and complete mailing address)*
Brian Selzer, American Public Health Association
800 I St., NW, Washington, DC 20001-3710

10. Owner *(Do not leave blank. If the publication is owned by a corporation, give the name and address of the corporation immediately followed by the names and addresses of all stockholders owning or holding 1 percent or more of the total amount of stock. If not owned by a corporation, give the names and addresses of the individual owners. If owned by a partnership or other unincorporated firm, give its name and address as well as those of each individual owner. If the publication is published by a nonprofit organization, give its name and address.)*

Full Name	Complete Mailing Address
American Public Health Association	800 I St., NW, Washington, DC 20001-3710

11. Known Bondholders, Mortgagees, and Other Security Holders Owning or Holding 1 Percent or More of Total Amount of Bonds, Mortgages, or Other Securities. If none, check box → ☐ None

Full Name	Complete Mailing Address
District of Columbia	Washington, DC

12. Tax Status *(For completion by nonprofit organizations authorized to mail at nonprofit rates) (Check one)*
The purpose, function, and nonprofit status of this organization and the exempt status for federal income tax purposes:
☑ Has Not Changed During Preceding 12 Months
☐ Has Changed During Preceding 12 Months *(Publisher must submit explanation of change with this statement)*

13. Publication Title	14. Issue Date for Circulation Data Below	
American Journal of Public Health	09/30/2025	

15. Extent and Nature of Circulation	Average No. Copies Each Issue During Preceding 12 Months	No. Copies of Single Issue Published Nearest to Filing Date
a. Total Number of Copies *(Net press run)*	897	890
b. Paid Circulation *(By Mail and Outside the Mail)* (1) Mailed Outside-County Paid Subscriptions Stated on PS Form 3541 (Include paid distribution above nominal rate, advertiser's proof copies, and exchange copies)	577	615
(2) Mailed In-County Paid Subscriptions Stated on PS Form 3541 *(Include paid distribution above nominal rate, advertiser's proof copies, and exchange copies)*	0	0
(3) Paid Distribution Outside the Mails Including Sales Through Dealers and Carriers, Street Vendors, Counter Sales, and Other Paid Distribution Outside USPS®	29	30
(4) Paid Distribution by Other Classes of Mail Through the USPS (e.g., First-Class Mail®)	0	0
c. Total Paid Distribution *[Sum of 15b (1), (2), (3), and (4)]*	606	645
d. Free or Nominal Rate Distribution *(By Mail and Outside the Mail)* (1) Free or Nominal Rate Outside-County Copies included on PS Form 3541	0	0
(2) Free or Nominal Rate In-County Copies Included on PS Form 3541	0	0
(3) Free or Nominal Rate Copies Mailed at Other Classes Through the USPS (e.g., First-Class Mail)	0	0
(4) Free or Nominal Rate Distribution Outside the Mail *(Carriers or other means)*	0	0
e. Total Free or Nominal Rate Distribution *(Sum of 15d (1), (2), (3) and (4))*	0	0
f. Total Distribution *(Sum of 15c and 15e)*	606	645
g. Copies not Distributed *(See Instructions to Publishers #4 (page #3))*	291	245
h. Total *(Sum of 15f and g)*	897	890
i. Percent Paid *(15c divided by 15f times 100)*	100	100

* If you are claiming electronic copies, go to line 16 on page 3. If you are not claiming electronic copies, skip to line 17 on page 3.

UNITED STATES POSTAL SERVICE® Statement of Ownership, Management, and Circulation (All Periodicals Publications Except Requester Publications)

16. Electronic Copy Circulation	Average No. Copies Each Issue During Preceding 12 Months	No. Copies of Single Issue Published Nearest to Filing Date
a. Paid Electronic Copies	10,132	15,870
b. Total Paid Print Copies (Line 15c) + Paid Electronic Copies (Line 16a)	10,738	16,515
c. Total Print Distribution (Line 15f) + Paid Electronic Copies (Line 16a)	10,738	16,515
d. Percent Paid (Both Print & Electronic Copies) (16b divided by 16c × 100)	100	100

☑ **I certify that 50% of all my distributed copies (electronic and print) are paid above a nominal price.**

17. Publication of Statement of Ownership
☑ If the publication is a general publication, publication of this statement is required. Will be printed in the 11/01/2025 issue of this publication. ☐ Publication not required.

18. Signature and Title of Editor, Publisher, Business Manager, or Owner: [signature] Director of Publications — Date: 09/29/2025

I certify that all information furnished on this form is true and complete. I understand that anyone who furnishes false or misleading information on this form or who omits material or information requested on the form may be subject to criminal sanctions (including fines and imprisonment) and/or civil sanctions (including civil penalties).

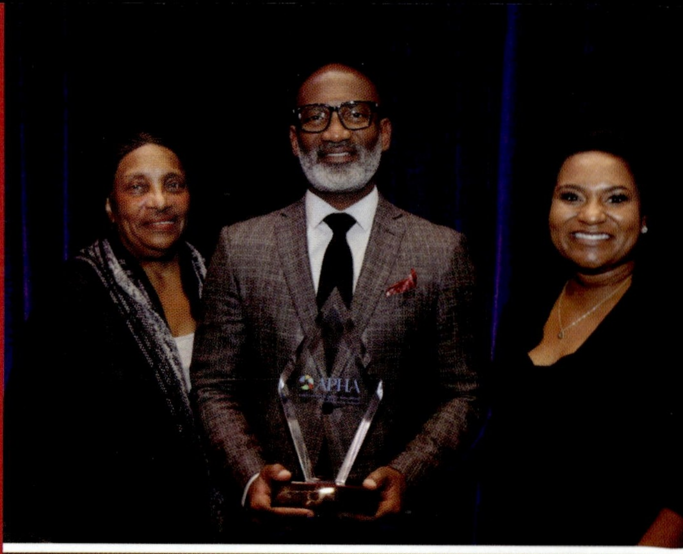

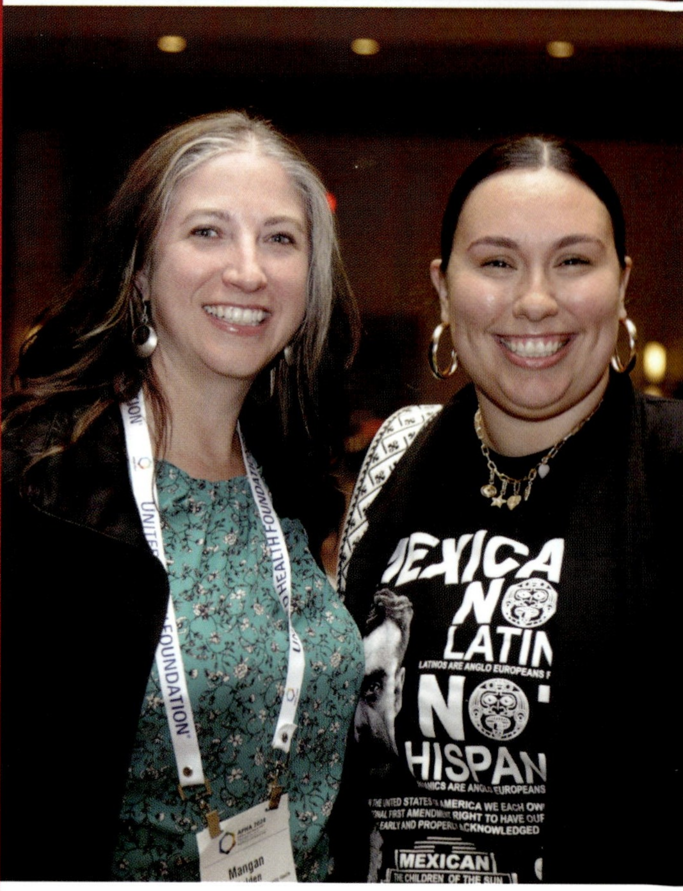